Pocket Guide
to
Low Sodium
Foods

Pocket Guide to Low Sodium Foods

Bobbie Mostyn

InData Group, Inc.

Pocket Guide to Low-Sodium Foods. Copyright @ 2003 by Bobbie Mostyn. All rights reserved. This book, or parts thereof, may not be reproduced in any form without permission from the publisher, exceptions are made for brief excerpts used in published reviews. Published by InData Group, Inc., P.O. Box 11908, Olympia, WA 98508-1908.

Printed in the United States of America

Cover design: Gray Ponytail Studios - www.grayponytail.com

Pocket Guide to Low-Sodium Foods Web site:

www.lowsaltfoods.com

Library of Congress Cataloging-in-Publication Data

Mostyn, Bobbie
  Pocket guide to low sodium foods / Bobbie Mostyn. -- 2003 ed.
    p.cm.
    Includes index.
    LCCN 2002117596
    ISBN 0-9673969-1-3

  1. Food--Sodium content--Tables.   I. Title.
TX553.S65M67 2003   613.2'85
                                                QBI03-200284

DEDICATED TO:

*My husband, Mike - without your continued support and help
this whole project would not be possible -
you are the light of my life!*

*All my friends and family - thanks for your understanding
and patience for all the calls and emails
that went unanswered.*

*Food manufacturers and restaurants who are
reducing the sodium in their product offerings -
thanks for your interest in our well-being -
we, in turn, will support your products.*

*Those who are watching their sodium intake -
hopefully this guide makes your food
choices a little bit easier.*

CONTENTS

INTRODUCTION ix
   Using Less Salt ix
   Become Sodium Conscious xi
   Note to the Hypertensive xii

DINING OUT xiv
   Fast Foods Quick Reference xv

FOOD LABELING GUIDELINES xvi
   What the Label Tells You xvi
   Nutritional Content Claims xvii
   Calories and Nutrients xviii
      Calories xviii
      Fats and Cholesterol xviii
      Carbohydrates, Sugar and Fiber xx
      Sodium xxii

USING THIS GUIDE xxiii
   Nutritive Criteria xxv

READING THE NUTRITIVE VALUES xxvii

ABBREVIATIONS AND SYMBOLS xxviii

FOOD MEASUREMENTS AND EQUIVALENTS xxix

CONTENTS

PART 1 – GROCERY PRODUCTS

Baking & Cooking Needs 3
Beverages 12
Breads, Rolls & Bread Products 21
Breakfast Products 31
Condiments & Sauces 38
Dairy Products & Alternatives 55
Desserts & Sweets 64
Diet & Nutritional Foods 88
Dinners, Entrees & Side Dishes 92
Ethnic Foods 107
Fish & Seafood 115
Fruits 120
Meat, Poultry & Alternatives 123
Pasta, Noodles, Rice & Grains 132
Snack Foods 134
Soups, Stews & Chili 143
Vegetables, Beans & Legumes 147

PART 2 – QUICK-SERVE RESTAURANT CHAINS 159

RESTAURANT QUICK REFERENCE 205

RESOURCES 215

INDEX 219

INTRODUCTION

Salt is contributing to a U.S. health crisis and the medical community is sounding the alarm. According to recent estimates, Americans consume 4,000-6,000 milligrams (mg) of sodium per day – two to three times more than the National Institutes of Health recommended level of 2,400mg (or about 1 teaspoon salt).

There is reason for concern. Excessive sodium has been linked to the development of high blood pressure (or hypertension). Once developed an individual's risk for heart attack, stroke, kidney and other problems increases significantly.

More than 50 million Americans (one in four adults) have high blood pressure and that number is expected to increase as our population ages. In fact, fifty percent of people over the age of 60 develop hypertension.

Nevertheless, there is good news. Studies show that a substantial decrease in the amount of sodium consumed can lower blood pressure and may even help prevent hypertension. Medical experts are now recommending sodium reduction for everyone, not just hypertensive patients.

USE LESS SALT

Reducing one's intake of salt is not easy. Nearly everything we eat contains some natural sodium. Additionally, we have become accustomed to salty foods, thanks in part to our busy lifestyles that have increased our use of convenience and fast foods. Unfortunately, the more salt we consume, the more we crave. It's a vicious cycle, but it can be modified.

Although lifestyle changes may be difficult, particularly when it comes to eating, you can retrain your tastebuds to enjoy less salt in about 6-8 weeks. If you start gradually, using a little less salt each day, not only will your use of sodium decrease, but also your craving. In fact, many foods that used to taste good will now taste salty.

The majority of sodium in your diet comes from three main sources:

- salt added at the table and to cooking
- processed and convenience products
- restaurant and fast food meals

Tips to Reducing Salt

Eliminate the saltshaker. Don't salt before you taste. Break the habit of automatically reaching for the saltshaker.

Choose lower sodium foods. Eat more fruits and vegetables and use less prepared foods (the less processing, the less sodium). Look for foods labeled *sodium free, low sodium, reduced sodium, unsalted* and *no salt added.* (See Nutritional Content Claims, page xvii, for more information.)

Read the label. Know how much sodium is in each serving. Be alert to "salty" terms, like *brine, cured, marinated, pickled* and *smoked.* Notice serving sizes. What is listed may be smaller than what you will actually eat.

Use less salt in cooking. In most recipes salt can be reduced or, in many cases, omitted without compromising the flavor. Use more herbs and spices, particularly onion and garlic powder. Also, low-sodium bouillon can add extra flavor, as can wine, vinegar, lemon or lime juice.

Prepare low-salt recipes. Get a good low-sodium cookbook. Many are available at your local bookstore. Also, search the Internet where there is an abundance of low-salt recipes.

Order low-sodium foods at restaurants. Ask how foods are prepared and whenever possible request that no salt be added to your entree. Find restaurants that feature "heart-healthy" meals or will accommodate your dietary restrictions. (NOTE: "Heart-healthy" usually indicates a menu item is low fat or low cholesterol and may not always be low sodium.)

NOTE: Although salt and sodium are used interchangeably, there is a difference. Sodium is a mineral that combines with chlorine to form salt. Salt contains 40% sodium and 60% chlorine.

BECOME SODIUM CONSCIOUS

Many people think they are not consuming a lot of salt because they do not use it at the table or in their cooking. Although the saltshaker contributes about 25% of the salt we consume, the majority of it comes off the grocery shelves.

As you become more sodium conscious, you will discover disparities among brands. For instance, some tomato pastes have as much as 440mg sodium, but others only have 100mg. They taste the same but when you add it up, it's 330mg less sodium.

Foods High in Sodium

Bakery items – bagels, breads, donuts and pastries

Canned foods – soups, meats, fish, sauerkraut, beans and vegetables

Convenience foods – frozen dinners, pizza, cereals and packaged mixes (such as pancakes, food "helpers," stuffing and rice dishes)

Dairy products – cheese and cottage cheese

Deli items – bacon, luncheon meats, corned beef, smoked meats or fish, sardines, anchovies and mayonnaise-based salads (like cole slaw and potato salad)

Snack foods – crackers, chips and dips

Condiments – mustard, ketchup, mayonnaise, salad dressings, pickles, olives, capers, salsas and packaged seasoning mixes

Sauces – gravy, steak or BBQ, pasta, teriyaki and soy sauces

Baking needs – self-rising flour, baking and biscuit mixes, bouillon cubes, batter and coating mixes, breadcrumbs, corn syrup, cooking wines, meat tenderizers, monosodium glutamate (MSG), baking powder and baking soda

Beverages – tomato and vegetable juices, Bloody Mary and chocolate drink mixes

---

Use the *Pocket Guide to Low-Sodium Foods* to find low-salt substitutes for the previous high-sodium products. For example, instead of using a teriyaki marinade (which may have as much as 3,050mg sodium per tablespoon), substitute one of the many grilling sauces with less than 140mg per tablespoon. You will find that nearly every type of food has a low-salt alternative.

HIDDEN SOURCES OF SODIUM

There are numerous sources of sodium that you may not be aware. Certain dentifrices, aspirin and medications that contain ibuprofen (such as Advil and Nuprin) contain sodium, as do antacids, like Rolaids, Alka-Seltzer and Bromo-Seltzer (some have as much as 761mg). Check labels for low-sodium alternatives or ask your pharmacist or healthcare provider for suggestions.

Also, many households have water-softening systems that contain sodium chloride. To remedy this, potassium chloride (potassium replaces the salt) may be used instead. Of course, if it is still a concern you can always drink bottled water.

NOTE TO THE HYPERTENSIVE

"High blood pressure is a time bomb in your blood vessels, just waiting to explode in a stroke or heart attack," says Pat Kendall, Ph.D., R.D., a nutrition specialist at Colorado State University Cooperative Extension. "It just keeps ticking away, speeding the artery-clogging process until the blood vessels finally burst."

Scary stuff, but there is new research that has determined diet can have a positive effect on blood pressure. Funded by the National Heart, Lung and Blood Institute (NHLBI), the Dietary Approaches to Stop Hypertension (DASH) clinical study shows that the DASH diet not only lowers blood pressure, but may help prevent and control hypertension. Based on 2,000 calories a day, the DASH diet is low in fats and cholesterol and plentiful in fruits, vegetables and low-fat dairy products.

Subsequent research (DASH-2) indicates the lower the sodium intake, the lower the drop in blood pressure and recommends eating 1500mg or less sodium per day. *(To order the DASH Diet, see Resources, pg 215.)*

SALT SUBSTITUTES

If you are taking certain diuretics and other prescription drugs for the treatment of hypertension, be cautious of salt substitutes. Many contain potassium which may adversely affect your medication. Additionally, many foods that are low in sodium also have added potassium. Check with your healthcare provider before using salt substitutes or consuming potassium-enhanced foods.

Other Culprits That Raise Blood Pressure

Caffeine (including coffee, tea, soft drinks, chocolate and some medications) – may temporarily increase blood pressure

Licorice – consumed in large amounts

Phenylalanine (used in sugar-free foods that contain aspartame, such as Nutra-Sweet and Equal) – may elevate blood pressure in sensitive individuals

Alcohol – more than 1 glass of wine or 24 oz of beer is considered excessive and may cause a rise in blood pressure

Cold and cough remedies - decongestants (such as, pseudoephedrine, phenylpropanolamine, dextromethorphan) found in many cough and cold medications may elevate blood pressure

Appetite suppressants - ingredients (like diethylpropion) found in many weight reducing agents may raise blood pressure

---

NOTE: Diet is only one part of the prevention and treatment of hypertension. Other factors include exercise, maintaining a healthy weight, quitting smoking and increasing your intake of calcium and magnesium. Before making any major changes in salt consumption or beginning an exercise program, be sure to talk with your healthcare provider.

DINING OUT

The most difficult time to control salt consumption is when dining out. Making good nutritional choices can often be difficult, particularly when we don't know what has been added to the foods we order. For example, a healthy garden salad with low-fat dressing oftentimes has more sodium than a hamburger and french fries. Hard to believe, but depending on how it is prepared, what we think is healthy may not be low sodium.

Another fast food misconception is chicken or fish sandwiches being a better choice than beef. There may be less fat, but not salt. In most instances added seasonings, coatings, deep frying and other preparations create a much higher sodium meal.

Perhaps one day, with enough public pressure, nutritional data will be available at all restaurants. In the meantime, follow the suggestions below in selecting healthier, low-sodium menu items.

Watch the Salt

- Order the smallest portion or eat half the meal (save the rest for the next day)
- Avoid fried foods (batter is usually salted)
- Skip the butter and condiments (better yet, bring your own low-salt versions)
- Stay away from soups and creamed sauces
- Ask for salad dressings and sauces on the side (so you can control the amount used)
- Choose oil and vinegar or vinaigrettes over creamy dressings
- Select steamed, broiled, grilled and roasted foods

PLAN AHEAD

If you know you will be dining out, eat a low-salt breakfast and lunch. If you have too much salt at one meal, keep your sodium intake low for the next couple of meals.

You can also place low-sodium condiments, like ketchup, mustard, mayonnaise and salad dressing, in small plastic containers and take them with you. The important thing is you do not have to deprive yourself. Just use moderation. Remember, low salt does not mean no salt.

FAST FOODS QUICK REFERENCE

Wondering where to get a hamburger and french fries with the lowest sodium? Which pizza won't put you over the top in your daily salt consumption? For your convenience a *Restaurant Quick Reference* has been included (see page 205-214). Use this to find the best places to get your favorite meals and stay within low-sodium guidelines.

FOOD LABELING GUIDELINES

The Food and Drug Administration (FDA) regulates food labeling to assure consumers that the information they receive is accurate and not misleading. Labels contain a lot of uesful information to help you make healthy food choices.

WHAT THE LABEL TELLS YOU

Serving Size - Identified in familiar units (such as cups or tablespoons) followed by the metric equivalent (i.e. grams) and is determined by the amount typically eaten.

Amount per Serving - Nutritional information is based on one serving. In this example, if you eat 2 cups you need to double the calories, nutrients and *% Daily Value*.

Nutrition Facts

Serving Size 1 cup (55g)
Servings Per Container about 8

Amount Per Serving

Calories 170	Calories from Fat 10

	% Daily Value*
Total Fat 1 g	**2** %
Saturated Fat 0g	**0** %
Cholesterol 0mg	**0** %
Sodium 85mg	**4** %
Total Carbohydrate 41g	**14** %
Dietary Fiber 7g	**28** %
Sugars 21g	
Protein 6g	

Vitamin A 0%	■	Vitamin C 0%
Calcium 0%	■	Iron 6%

*Percent Daily Values are based on a 2,000 calorie diet. Your daily values may be higher or lower depending on your calorie needs.

	Calories	2,000	2,500
Total Fat	Less than	65g	80g
Sat Fat	Less than	20g	25g
Cholesterol	Less than	300mg	300mg
Sodium	Less than	2,400mg	2,400mg
Total Carbohydrate		300m	375mg
Dietary Fiber		25g	30 g

Calories from Fat - This is the amount of fat multiplied by 9 (number of calories per gram of fat). Dietary guidelines suggest no more than 30% of daily calories come from fat. To calculate percentage, divide *Calories from Fat* by *Calories* (in this example, $10 \div 170 = 6\%$).

Nutrients - All values are listed in grams except for *Cholesterol* and *Sodium* which are in milligrams. Use these figures to compare fat, sodium, etc. between products. If a nutrient is not shown, there is no significant amount in the product.

% Daily Value - How much of the *Recommended Daily Values* (RDVs) each nutrient provides. Calculations are based on 2,000 calories. In this example, sodium is 4% (2,400g divided by 85g). This is another way to compare similar products.

Ingredients - Listed in order from most to least amount.

NUTRITIONAL CONTENT CLAIMS

The FDA has provided guidelines for claims and descriptions manufacturers may use on food labeling. Based on one serving, they include:

	FREE	LOW	REDUCED/ LESS	LIGHT/ LITE
Cal	< 5 calories	40 calories or less	25% less than normal	50% less than normal
Fat	< 0.5g fat	3g or less fat	25% less than normal	50% less than normal
Sat Fat	< 0.5g sat fat & < 0.5g trans fatty acids	1g or less saturated fat	25% less than normal	50% less than normal
Chol	< 2mg chol & 2g or less sat fat	< 20mg chol & 2g or less sat fat	25% less than normal	50% less than normal
Sug	< 0.5g sugar		25% less than normal	50% less than normal

	FREE	VERY LOW	LOW	UNSALTED/NSA
Sod	< 5mg sod	< 35mg sod	<140mg sod	No salt added to normally salted food

NOTE: *Low fat* and *non fat* do not mean low sodium or low sugar; manufacturers often replace the fat with added salt and sugar.

CALORIES AND NUTRIENTS

CALORIES

Calories measure the amount of energy contained in foods and are calculated based on the amount of carbohydrates, fat and protein within the food. (Alcohol also provides calories.)

Once consumed and digested, food is converted to glucose which fuels everything the body does (walk, talk, breathe, etc.). The more active an individual, the greater the caloric need. When the body takes in more calories than it requires, the extra energy is stored as body fat.

The amount of calories needed is different for every individual. For food labeling purposes, the *% Daily Values* are based on 2,000 calories a day. If your caloric needs are more or less than this, adjust accordingly when determining your daily requirements.

FATS AND CHOLESTEROL

Fats and cholesterol go hand-in-hand. Not only are fats found in foods containing cholesterol, but saturated fats raise LDL cholesterol levels (the bad stuff), contributing to clogged arteries and hypertension.

Types of Fat

Saturated - Usually solid at room temperature (comes mainly from animal products, but also present in some plant foods, i.e. cocoa butter, palm and coconut oils).

Monounsaturated - Liquid at room temperature, but solidify in the refrigerator (found in plant foods, such as olive oil, canola oil, avocados and nuts).

Polyunsaturated - Liquid at room temperature and in the refrigerator (examples are vegetable oils, including corn oil, safflower oil and sunflower oil).

Trans fatty acids - Result of hydrogenation and used for shelf stability or solidifying a fat product (found in margarine, packaged and baked goods, and fast foods).

Not all fats are harmful and have been classified as either good or bad. Saturated fat is considered bad, it raises cholesterol and is the leading cause of heart disease. Monounsaturated and polyunsaturated fats help lower cholesterol and are considered good. (Although too much of any fat raises blood cholesterol levels, all fats should be used in moderation.) Trans fatty acids, considered saturated and classified as bad, not only raise total blood cholesterol but also raise LDL (the bad) and lower HDL (the good).

Only total fat (a combination of all four fats) and saturated fat are listed on food labels. To determine if a product has trans fatty acids look for *hydrogenated* or *partially hydrogenated* in the ingredients. Be aware that many low-fat, low-cholesterol products may have trans fatty acids.

The American Heart Association (AHA) suggests total fat should comprise no more than 30% of the calories coming from fat and no more than 10% from saturated fat (7% if you have heart disease, diabetes, or high LDL cholesterol). Choose fats with 2g or less saturated fat per serving.

CHOLESTEROL

Cholesterol is a waxy, fat-like substance produced naturally in the body and is necessary for many bodily functions. The body manufactures all the cholesterol it needs and circulates it via the bloodstream, which separates it into "good" and "bad" lipoproteins.

The bad, or low-density lipoproteins (LDL), stick to the blood vessel walls. The good, or high-density lipoproteins (HDL), unstick LDLs and excrete it from the arteries. This is why the ratio of HDL to LDL is important. Over time these deposits (along with fat) build up, causing the arteries to clog. As the arteries narrow, the flow of blood decreases and blood pressure increases. This build-up of fatty deposits is also a major factor in coronary disease and strokes.

Cholesterol is found mainly in animal foods (meat, poultry, fish, egg yolks and dairy products), it is not found in plant foods. The daily recommendation for cholesterol is less than 300mg.

CARBOHYDRATES, FIBER AND SUGAR

Carbohydrates are the body's supplier of energy. Once consumed carbohydrates are converted into two basic forms: simple (found in sugars) and complex (comprised of starches and fibers). Except for fiber (which is not digestible), all carbohydrates turn directly into sugar (glucose) in the bloodstream and affect blood glucose in different ways.

Carbohydrates

Simple carbohydrates - generally have no nutritive value and produce a rapid rise in blood glucose followed by a rapid fall.
Complex carbohydrates - are more nutritious and produce a slower, more sustained blood glucose response.

Foods high in complex carbohydrates are usually low in calories, saturated fat and cholesterol. They are found primarily in plant foods, such as fruits, vegetables, whole grains, beans and legumes. They also are present in dairy products.

Daily caloric intake of carbohydrates should be between 55-60% (or 25-35 grams) with an emphasis on complex carbohydrates.

FIBER

Fiber is the part of food that is not digested and is found only in plants. There are two types of fiber – soluble and insoluble.

Soluble fiber – dissolves in fluids of the large intestine. It is found in oats, barley, rye, nuts, fruits, vegetables, psyllium seeds (used in fiber laxatives), beans and legumes. Consumed in large amounts, soluble fiber can decrease blood cholesterol, improve blood glucose levels and appears to reduce hypertension. It also may help with weight loss by increasing the feeling of fullness.

Insoluble fiber – does not dissolve in the intestinal fluids, but passes straight through and helps maintain regularity. It is found in whole grains, seeds, bran, fruit and vegetable skins. It also is associated with reduced risk of colon cancer.

The amount of fiber also affects blood glucose. The more fiber in a food, the slower the digestion and absorption of sugars. To help understand fiber's influence on blood glucose, the glycemic index (GI) was developed. Using glucose (the highest rated GI) as a standard, a food is ranked by how fast it is digested and how much it causes blood glucose to rise. We will not get into GI rankings in this book, but suffice to say, this new information is changing the way nutritionists and the medical society are looking at carbohydrates.

The recommended level of total insoluble and soluble fiber is 20-35 grams per day. Look for a minimum of 3 grams of fiber, but 5 grams or more is better.

SUGAR

Sugar consumption has been on the increase and experts believe diets high in sugar are contributing to many of today's health problems.

Current research indicates long-term consumption of a diet high in refined (simple) carbohydrates produces higher insulin levels, which plays a roll in hypertension. As insulin levels elevate, adrenaline production is stimulated, which can cause blood vessel constriction and increased sodium retention. Additionally, high carbohydrate intake has been linked to increased LDL and decreased HDL cholesterol.

The RDVs have no sugar guidelines, however, the US Department of Agriculture (USDA) advises limiting sugar to 10 teaspoons (47g) a day (based on a 2,000-calorie diet).

SODIUM

Sodium is essential to the body. About 500mg a day is needed to help regulate fluids and maintain normal functioning of nerves and muscles. If excess sodium is not used, fluid builds up (water retention) increasing the work of the heart and kidneys.

Select foods that contain less than 5 percent of the daily value for sodium. You can also make low sodium choices by looking at the milligrams of sodium. Most experts suggest limiting any food above 480mg sodium per serving.

USING THIS GUIDE

With our increasingly busy lifestyles, making healthy, low-sodium food choices at the supermarket and when dining out is challenging. Most of us do not have time to compare the labels of thousands of grocery items. We also have no idea of what's in the fast foods we are consuming.

This is where the *Pocket Guide to Low Sodium Foods* can help. It includes common products found in most grocery stores and menu items from 61 national restaurant chains. It's small enough to put in a purse or coat pocket and can be used as a quick reference when grocery shopping or eating out.

Only low-salt foods within acceptable Nutritive Criteria (see pg xxv) are listed. Calories, fat, saturated fat, cholesterol, carbohydrates, fiber, sugar and sodium are shown for each food product. These are the most important nutrients to consider for healthy eating.

The book is broken down into two parts: *Grocery Products* and *Quick-Serve Restaurant Chains*.

GROCERY PRODUCTS

All foods are listed alphabetically within the following 17 categories and approximates the aisles of your supermarket.

Baking & Cooking Needs
Beverages
Breads, Rolls & Bread Products
Breakfast Products
Condiments & Sauces
Dairy Products & Alternatives
Desserts & Sweets
Diet & Nutritional Foods

Dinners, Entrees & Side Dishes
Ethnic Foods
Fish & Seafood
Fruits
Meat, Poultry & Substitutes
Pasta, Noodles, Rice & Grains
Snack Foods
Soups, Stews & Chilis
Vegetables, Beans & Legumes

Generic nutrient analysis is shown for each food type (listed by amount of sodium in ascending order) and represents the average or typical values for that particular food. This is followed by brand named products in alphabetical order and, when applicable, are divided into subcategories, such as *Canned*, *Frozen* and *Ready-to-Eat*. Only low-salt foods within the Nutritive Criteria are listed. (NOTE: Products exceeding these guidelines may be shown if substantially less than the non-brand product.)

QUICK-SERVE RESTAURANT CHAINS

This section includes national fast-food and quick-serve restaurant chains listed in alphabetical order. Although fast foods are loaded with fat and sodium and are not necessarily the best choice for healthy, low-sodium diets, they are a fact of life. Use the *Pocket Guide to Low-Sodium Foods* to help you make the wisest selections.

Restaurant menu selections are broken down into categories, such as *Sandwiches, Salads, Side Dishes and Desserts*. Only low-salt foods within the Nutritive Criteria are listed. However, if all choices within a category exceed sodium guidelines, the menu item with the least amount of salt is listed as a reference. Additionally, some lower fat items (i.e. chicken and fish), may be shown even though salt content is higher than the nutritive guidelines.

Unfortunately, not all restaurant chains were willing or responsive to requests to reprint nutritional data. In order to give readers some idea of sodium content for these eateries, menu items with the least salt are listed. Foods are grouped as follows: 150mg sodium or less, 250mg sodium or less and increases in increments of 250mg up to 1000mg. If all items in a category are exceed 1000mg sodium, the lowest item(s) is listed. Although excessive in sodium, individuals who consume these foods may want to eat a smaller portion to keep within daily guidelines.

NUTRITIVE CRITERIA

The amount of sodium per serving determines which foods are listed in the guide. However, the criteria is different for fast foods. If we used the same criteria, there would be very few selections, consequently sodium amounts have been raised. No foods above these guidelines are listed except for those previously noted.

	Maximum Sodium	
	Grocery	Fast Food
Main dishes (i.e. frozen dinners, sandwiches)	> 500g	> 550g
Sides (i.e. baked goods, desserts, vegetable dishes)	> 200g	> 250g
Condiments and individual foods	> 150g	> 200g

All information contained in the *Pocket Guide to Low-Sodium Foods* is based on nutritional data provided by the US Department of Agriculture, food manufacturers, restaurant chains and author calculations.

Data is for informational purposes only and is subject to change. No endorsement is intended of companies and their products, nor is any adverse judgment implied for companies and products not mentioned.

Availability of products, menu items and variations in serving sizes or product ingredients may occur dependent upon geographical region, local suppliers, season of the year and production changes. Read manufacturer's product labels or contact individual restaurants for the most up-to-date analysis of food items. Data was collected during 2002-2003.

AUTHOR'S NOTE: Read labels and continue to re-read them. I have been fooled many times by favorite low-sodium foods that suddenly have more salt listed than the last time I used them.

ABBREVIATIONS AND SYMBOLS

all	all varieties/flavors		NSA	no salt added
approx	approximately		orig	original
avg	average		oz	ounce
cal	calories		pc	piece(s)
carb	carbohydrate		pkg	package
choc	chocolate		pkt	packet
chol	cholesterol		prep	prepared to product
envl	envelop			directions
FF	fat free		refrg	refrigerated
fl oz	fluid ounce		reg	regular
g	gram		sat	saturated fat
lb	pound		serv	serving
LF	low fat		sm	small
mayo	mayonnaise		sod	sodium
med	medium-sized		sq	square
mg	milligram(s)		tbsp	tablespoon
micro	microwave		tsp	teaspoon
misc	miscellaneous		veg	vegetable
most	most varieties		w/	with
NF	nonfat		w/o	without

-    nutritional data unavailable

<   less than

FOOD MEASUREMENTS AND EQUIVALENTS

1 1/2 tsp	=	1/2 tbsp	=	0.25 oz	=	7 grams
3 tsp	=	1 tbsp	=	0.5 oz	=	14 grams
2 tbsp	=	1/8 cup	=	1 oz	=	28 grams
4 tbsp	=	1/4 cup	=	2 oz	=	55 grams
8 tbsp	=	1/2 cup	=	4 oz	=	115 grams
16 tbsp	=	1 cup	=	8 oz	=	225 grams

LIQUID

1/2 fl oz	=	15 ml	=	1 tbsp
1 fl oz	=	30 ml	=	1/8 cup
2 fl oz	=	60 ml	=	1/4 cup
4 fl oz	=	120 mil	=	1/2 cup
8 fl oz	=	240 ml	=	1 cup
16 fl oz	=	480 ml	=	1 pint
2 cups	=	1 pint	=	1/2 quart
4 cups	=	2 pints	=	1 quart
4 pints	=	2 quarts	=	1/2 gallon
8 pints	=	4 quarts	=	1 gallon

READING THE NUTRITIVE VALUES

Food	Cal	Fat	Sat	Chol	Carb	Fib	Sug	Sod
FROSTING								
Vanilla, ready-to-spread, 2 tbsp	140	5	2	0	23	0	20	70
Cream cheese, ready-to-spread, 2 tbsp	140	5	2	0	23	0	20	80
Chocolate, ready-to-spread, 2 tbsp	130	5	2	0	21	0	18	90
BRANDS . . .								
MIX								
Calorie Control Lemon, Vanilla, Choc, or Cream Cheese (typ), 2 tbsp	93	3	1	0	8	0	1	27
Estee, all, prep, 2 tbsp	67	1	0	0	13	0	-	0
READY-TO-SPREAD								
Betty Crocker Soft Whipped								
Fluffy White, 2 tbsp	100	5	2	0	15	0	14	25
Vanilla, 2 tbsp	100	5	2	0	15	0	14	25

* An asterisk indicates product is available online, check *Resources*, pgs 215-218, for additional information.

Generic foods are listed first, followed by brand-name products. Values are an average for all foods of this type.

Nutritional information unavailable.

If the nutrient value on a food label is:		Low Sodium Guide uses:
<5	(less than 5mg or g)	5
<1	(less than 1mg or g)	1
tr	(trace amount present)	0
nutrient not listed	(no significant amount present)	0

NOTE: All nutrient values have been rounded off to the nearest whole number.

PART 1

GROCERY PRODUCTS

BAKING & COOKING NEEDS

ALMOND PASTE

(see Pastry Fillings, pg 8)

BAKING CHOCOLATE & CHIPS

Food	Cal	Fat	Sat	Chol	Carb	Fib	Sug	Sod
Baking chocolate:								
Semi-sweet, 1 oz	140	9	5	0	16	2	14	0
Sweet, 1 oz	120	7	4	0	16	2	16	0
Unsweetened, 1 oz	148	16	9	0	8	4	0	4
White, 1 oz	160	12	6	5	16	0	16	30
Chips:								
Choc, semi-sweet, 1 oz	140	8	5	0	18	2	14	0
Butterscotch, 1 oz	160	8	7	0	18	0	18	30
White, 1 oz	160	8	7	0	18	0	18	40
Peanut butter, 1 oz	160	8	8	0	14	0	12	70
Cocoa powder, unsweetened, 2 tbsp	25	1	1	0	6	3	0	2

BRANDS . . .
Most brands are within the generic range.

BAKING MIXES

(also see mixes for specific items, i.e. Biscuits, Brownies, Cakes, Cookies, etc.)

Food	Cal	Fat	Sat	Chol	Carb	Fib	Sug	Sod
All-purpose baking mix, 1/4 cup	129	5	1	0	19	1	1	383
BRANDS . . . *(1/4 CUP UNLESS NOTED)*								
Atkins Bake Mix	110	2	0	0	6	3	1	220
Ener-G Brown Rice Mix	148	4	0	0	25	3	2	35
Fran Gare's Decadent Desserts								
Choc Bake Mix	93	3	0	0	10	4	0	106
Almond Bake Mix	120	7	0	0	8	3	0	153

BAKING POWDER & SODA

(see Leavening Agents, pg 7)

BATTER, SEASONING & COATING MIXES

(also see Breadcrumbs, Cracker & Sweet Crumbs, pg 4)

Food	Cal	Fat	Sat	Chol	Carb	Fib	Sug	Sod
Tempura batter mix, 1/4 cup	100	0	0	0	23	0	0	175
Batter mix, 1/4 cup	100	0	0	0	22	1	0	690
Seasoning & coating mix, 1/4 pkg	80	4	0	0	10	0	1	800

BAKING & COOKING NEEDS
Breadcrumbs, Cracker & Sweet Crumbs

Food	Cal	Fat	Sat	Chol	Carb	Fib	Sug	Sod
BATTER, SEASONING AND COATING MIXES								
BRANDS . . . *(1/4 CUP UNLESS NOTED)*								
Golden Dipt Tempura, 1 oz	100	0	0	0	20	0	1	150
Ka-Me Tempura	200	0	0	0	44	0	0	10
Louisiana Fish Fry Fish Fry, 2 tsp	20	0	0	0	5	0	0	5
Seasoned Fish Fry, 2 tsp	20	0	0	0	5	0	0	135
Shake 'N Bake Chicken Herb & Garlic, 2 tsp	20	1	0	0	4	0	1	160
NOTE: This is Shake 'N Bake's lowest sodium coating mix.								
Sun Luck Tempura	100	0	0	0	23	1	1	50
Tony Chachere's Fish Fry Creole	120	0	0	0	26	1	2	35
Zatarain's Fish Fry, SF, 1 tbsp	45	0	0	0	0	0	0	0
Wonderful Fish Fry, 1 tbsp	45	0	0	0	0	0	0	0

BREADCRUMBS, CRACKER & SWEET CRUMBS

Food	Cal	Fat	Sat	Chol	Carb	Fib	Sug	Sod
Cracker meal, 1/4 cup	110	1	0	0	23	1	0	8
Cookie crumbs, 1/4 cup	140	6	2	10	26	0	14	110
Graham cracker crumbs, 1/4 cup	107	3	1	0	17	1	3	200
Breadcrumbs, plain, 1/4 cup	107	1	0	0	20	1	1	233
Breadcrumbs, seasoned, 1/4 cup	110	1	0	0	21	1	1	795
BRANDS . . .								
BREADCRUMBS *(1/4 CUP UNLESS NOTED)*								
*4C Plain, SF	200	4	0	0	40	1	1	0
Seasoned, SF	83	1	0	0	17	1	1	4
*Ener-G	175	6	0	0	28	0	1	36
*Hol-Grain Brown Rice, SF	40	0	0	0	9	0	0	0
*Nu-World Foods Amaranth	122	2	0	0	22	3	0	2
*Taam	187	0	0	0	44	0	0	26
CRACKER MEAL								
Most brands are within the generic range.								
MISC CRUMBS AND BREADING *(1/4 CUP UNLESS NOTED)*								
Kellogg's Corn Flake	80	0	0	0	18	0	2	160
*Streit's Matzo Meal, NSA	110	0	0	0	24	1	0	0
Sun Luck Panko Breading, 1 oz	110	1	0	0	21	1	1	85
SWEET CRUMBS								
Most brands are within the generic range.								

COCONUT

Food	Cal	Fat	Sat	Chol	Carb	Fib	Sug	Sod
Coconut milk, 1/4 cup	111	12	11	0	2	0	2	7
Shredded coconut, unsweetened, 1 oz	187	18	16	0	7	5	0	10
Sweetened, 1 oz	142	10	9	0	14	1	10	74

Food	Cal	Fat	Sat	Chol	Carb	Fib	Sug	Sod

COCONUT

BRANDS . . . *(1 OZ UNLESS NOTED)*

Baker's Angel Flake, Sweetened	140	12	10	0	12	2	10	0

CORNMEAL

Cornmeal, white or yellow:

Degermed, 1/4 cup	126	0	0	0	27	3	0	1
Whole-grain, 1/4 cup	111	1	0	0	24	2	0	11
Self-rising, 1/4 cup	123	1	0	0	26	3	0	465

BRANDS . . .
Most brands are within the generic range.

CORNSTARCH

Cornstarch, 1 tbsp	31	0	0	0	7	0	0	1

BRANDS . . .
Most brands are within the generic range.

EGGS - DRIED/POWDERED

Egg whites, powdered, 1 tbsp	53	0	0	0	1	0	0	173

BRANDS . . .

***Deb El** Just Whites, 2 tsp	12	0	0	0	0	0	0	51
Whole Eggs, 2 tsp	80	6	2	245	1	0	1	75
***Ener-G** Egg Replacer, 1 1/2 tsp	14	0	0	0	4	0	0	6
Egg White Replacer, 1 1/2 tsp	19	0	0	0	0	0	0	62

FATS, OILS & COOKING SPRAYS

Cooking spray, 1/3 sec spray	0	0	0	0	0	0	0	0
Lard or shortening, 1 tbsp	115	13	5	12	0	0	0	0
Oil, all varieties, 1 tbsp (avg)	119	14	2	0	0	0	0	0

BRANDS . . .
Most brands are within the generic range.

FAT SUBSTITUTES

BRANDS . . . *(1 TBSP UNLESS NOTED)*

Mrs. Bateman's ButterLike	36	1	0	5	8	0	0	20
***Rokeach** Neutral Nyafat	99	11	-	0	0	0	0	0

FLAVORINGS & EXTRACTS

Flavorings & extracts, 1 tsp (avg)	10	0	0	0	0	0	0	0

BRANDS . . .
Most brands are within the generic range.

BAKING & COOKING NEEDS
Flour

Food	Cal	Fat	Sat	Chol	Carb	Fib	Sug	Sod

FLOUR

Food	Cal	Fat	Sat	Chol	Carb	Fib	Sug	Sod
Rice flour, white, 1 cup	578	2	1	0	127	4	0	0
Brown, 1 cup	574	4	1	0	121	7	0	13
Cake flour, 1 cup	496	1	0	0	107	2	0	0
Rye flour, dark, 1 cup	415	3	0	0	88	29	4	1
Light, 1 cup	374	1	0	0	82	15	0	2
All-purpose flour, 1 cup	495	2	0	0	99	3	0	3
Wheat flour, whole-grain, 1 cup	407	2	0	0	87	15	3	6
Soy flour, 1 cup	366	17	3	0	30	8	0	11
Potato flour, 1 cup	571	1	0	0	133	9	0	88
Self-rising flour, 1 cup	443	1	0	0	93	3	0	1588

BRANDS . . .

Most brands are within the generic range.

FROSTING, ICING & DECORATIONS

FROSTING

Food	Cal	Fat	Sat	Chol	Carb	Fib	Sug	Sod
Vanilla frosting, ready-to-spread, 2 tbsp	140	5	2	0	23	0	20	70
Cream cheese frosting, ready-to-spread, 2 tbsp	140	5	2	0	23	0	20	80
Choc frosting, ready-to-spread, 2 tbsp	130	5	2	0	21	0	18	90

BRANDS . . .

There are many low-sodium frostings, the following have less than 70mg per serving.

MIX *(2 TBSP UNLESS NOTED)*

Food	Cal	Fat	Sat	Chol	Carb	Fib	Sug	Sod
*Calorie Control								
Lemon	93	3	1	0	8	0	1	27
Vanilla, Choc, or Cream Cheese	67	3	1	0	8	0	1	27
*Estee, all	67	1	0	0	13	0	0	0
Oetker Simple Organics								
Choc or Vanilla	110	0	0	0	26	0	24	65
*Sweet N'Low								
Choc, 1/14 pkg	60	4	2	0	7	0	0	20
White, 1/14 pkg	60	3	2	0	10	0	0	20

READY-TO-SPREAD *(2 TBSP UNLESS NOTED)*

Food	Cal	Fat	Sat	Chol	Carb	Fib	Sug	Sod
Betty Crocker								
Whipped, Fluffy White or Strawberry	100	5	2	0	15	0	14	25
Whipped, Lemon or Vanilla Cream	100	5	2	0	15	0	14	25
Whipped, Choc	100	5	2	0	14	0	13	45
Whipped, Cream Cheese	100	5	2	0	15	0	14	45
Whipped, Milk Choc	100	5	2	0	14	0	12	50
Coconut Pecan	140	8	3	0	17	0	16	50

Food	Cal	Fat	Sat	Chol	Carb	Fib	Sug	Sod
FROSTING, ICING AND DECORATIONS								
Duncan Hines								
Home-Style Vanilla or French Vanilla	140	5	2	0	22	0	21	60
Strawberries n'Cream or Buttercream	140	5	2	0	22	0	21	60
Caramel or Cream Cheese	140	5	2	0	22	0	21	60
Wild Cherry Vanilla	140	5	2	0	22	0	21	60
Pillsbury Supreme, Hot Fudge	140	6	2	0	21	0	18	55
Creamy Supreme, Milk Choc	140	6	2	0	21	1	19	60

ICING & DECORATIONS

Food	Cal	Fat	Sat	Chol	Carb	Fib	Sug	Sod
Sprinkles, 1 tsp	20	1	1	0	3	0	3	0
Decorating icing, 1 tsp	25	1	1	0	4	0	4	10

BRANDS . . .

Most brands are within the generic range.

LEAVENING AGENTS

Food	Cal	Fat	Sat	Chol	Carb	Fib	Sug	Sod
Yeast, baker's, dry, 1 tbsp	35	1	0	0	5	3	0	0
Cream of tartar, 1 tsp	8	0	0	0	2	0	-	2
Baking powder, 1 tsp	2	0	0	0	1	0	0	488
Baking soda, 1 tsp	0	0	0	0	0	0	0	1259

BRANDS . . . *(1 TSP UNLESS NOTED)*

*Ener-G

Food	Cal	Fat	Sat	Chol	Carb	Fib	Sug	Sod
Baking Powder, SF	0	0	0	0	0	0	0	0
Baking Soda, SF	0	0	0	0	0	0	0	0
*Featherweight Baking Powder, SF	0	0	0	0	0	0	0	0

MARSHMALLOWS

Food	Cal	Fat	Sat	Chol	Carb	Fib	Sug	Sod
Marshmallow creme, 2 tbsp	91	0	0	0	22	0	16	14
Marshmallows, miniatures, 1/2 cup	100	0	0	0	23	0	16	35

BRANDS . . .

Most brands are within the generic range.

MILK & MILK SUBSTITUTES - CANNED & POWDERED

Food	Cal	Fat	Sat	Chol	Carb	Fib	Sug	Sod
Milk, powdered, NF, 1 tbsp	15	0	0	0	2	0	2	23
Buttermilk, powdered, 1 tbsp	20	0	0	1	3	0	3	41
Goat milk, powdered, 1 tbsp	70	4	2	13	6	0	6	58
Canned, 1/2 cup	140	8	6	20	12	0	12	120
Evaporated milk, canned, 1/2 cup	169	10	6	37	13	0	13	133
Skim, canned, 1/2 cup	100	0	0	5	15	0	15	147
Condensed milk, sweetened, canned, 1/2 cup	491	13	8	52	83	0	83	194

Food	Cal	Fat	Sat	Chol	Carb	Fib	Sug	Sod
MILK AND MILK SUBSTITUTES - CANNED AND POWDERED								
BRANDS . . .								
MILK								
Most brands are within the generic range.								
MILK SUBSTITUTES								
Ener-G Soy Quik, powdered, 1/8 cup	50	2	0	0	4	2	2	0
Moo Not Soy Milk Powder, 1 tbsp (makes 8 fl oz)	48	0	0	0	3	2	1	56

(NUTS - BAKING)

(also see Nuts & Seeds, pg 140)

Food	Cal	Fat	Sat	Chol	Carb	Fib	Sug	Sod
Almonds, raw, 1 oz	164	14	1	0	6	3	0	0
Pecans, raw, 1 oz	196	20	2	0	4	3	0	0
Walnuts, raw, 1 oz	185	19	2	0	4	2	0	1

BRANDS . . .
Most brands are within the generic range.

(PASTRY DOUGH)

Food	Cal	Fat	Sat	Chol	Carb	Fib	Sug	Sod
Phyllo (fillo) dough, 1 sheet	57	1	0	0	15	0	0	92
Puff pastry, 1/6 sheet	170	11	3	0	14	1	1	200
Puff pastry shell, 1 shell	150	13	1	0	16	2	4	230
BRANDS . . .								
Athens Mini Fillo Shells, 2 shells	45	2	0	0	5	0	0	20
Shredded Fillo Dough (Kataifi), 2 oz	180	2	0	0	35	4	1	140
Fillo Factory Mini Shells, 3 shells	45	2	0	0	7	0	0	50
Fillo Dough, 3 sheets	190	1	0	0	40	3	0	135
Frieda's French Style Crepes, 1 crepe	30	1	0	5	5	0	2	50
Kineret Puff Pastry, 2 oz sq	250	18	5	0	20	1	0	140
Oronoque Orchards Tart Shell, 3" shell	140	9	2	0	12	0	0	140
Pepperidge Farm Puff Pastry, 1/6 sheet	200	11	3	0	23	3	0	135

(PASTRY FILLINGS)

(also see Pie Fillings, pg 9)

Food	Cal	Fat	Sat	Chol	Carb	Fib	Sug	Sod
Almond paste, 1 oz	130	8	1	0	14	1	11	3
Marzipan, 1 oz	116	4	1	0	18	1	16	5
Fruit filling, all, 1 oz (avg)	80	0	0	0	17	1	13	20
Poppyseed filling, 1 oz	140	4	0	0	24	3	16	30
Date filling, 1 oz	100	0	0	0	22	3	16	40

BRANDS . . .
Most brands are within the generic range.

Food	Cal	Fat	Sat	Chol	Carb	Fib	Sug	Sod

PIE CRUSTS

Food	Cal	Fat	Sat	Chol	Carb	Fib	Sug	Sod
Flour crust, frozen, 1/8	82	5	2	0	8	0	8	104
Mix, prep, 1/8	100	6	2	0	10	0	10	146
Cookie crumb crust, ready-to-eat								
Vanilla, 1/8	117	8	2	9	11	0	11	113
Choc, 1/8	142	9	2	0	15	0	9	188
Graham cracker crust, ready-to-eat, 1/8	145	7	2	0	19	0	19	168

BRANDS . . .

FROZEN/REFRIGERATED *(1/8 SHELL UNLESS NOTED)*

Food	Cal	Fat	Sat	Chol	Carb	Fib	Sug	Sod
Countrys Delight, 9"	80	5	1	0	8	0	1	75
Oronoque Orchards	80	6	2	0	7	0	0	90
Pet-Ritz 9"	80	5	2	5	9	0	0	60
Deep Dish, 9"	100	6	2	5	10	0	0	70
Pillsbury	120	11	3	5	13	0	1	110

MIX *(1/8 SHELL UNLESS NOTED)*

Food	Cal	Fat	Sat	Chol	Carb	Fib	Sug	Sod
Gluten Free Pantry Perfect Pie	75	1	0	0	18	1	0	85
Krusteaz	90	5	0	0	10	0	1	100

SHELF-STABLE *(1/8 SHELL UNLESS NOTED)*

Food	Cal	Fat	Sat	Chol	Carb	Fib	Sug	Sod
Keebler Graham Cracker, Reduced Fat	90	4	1	0	14	0	6	85
Shortbread	100	5	1	0	15	1	6	95
Graham Cracker, 4 oz single shell	120	6	1	0	15	1	6	150
Kemach Graham Cracker	100	4	1	0	14	1	5	50
Mother's Own Graham Cracker	110	6	2	0	12	1	5	115
Nabisco Nilla, 1 oz serv	144	8	1	3	18	0	9	63

PIE FILLINGS

Food	Cal	Fat	Sat	Chol	Carb	Fib	Sug	Sod
Cherry pie filling, 4 oz	130	0	0	0	32	1	31	20
Peach pie filling, 4 oz	120	0	0	0	29	2	26	23
Apple pie filling, 4 oz	114	0	0	0	30	1	29	50
Blueberry pie filling, 4 oz	120	0	0	0	32	1	23	68
Raspberry pie filling, 4 oz	120	0	0	0	32	1	23	68
Lemon pie filling, 4 oz	195	2	0	0	42	0	30	180
Mincemeat pie filling, 4 oz	200	2	0	0	48	0	44	250
Pumpkin pie mix, 4 oz	141	0	0	0	36	11	24	281
Banana cream, choc cream, or coconut								
cream pie fillings, 4 oz (avg)	195	6	2	0	32	0	21	285

BRANDS . . .

FRUIT FILLINGS

Most brands are within the generic range.

PUDDING *(see Puddings & Gelatins, pg 83)*

BAKING & COOKING NEEDS

Salt & Seasonings

Food	Cal	Fat	Sat	Chol	Carb	Fib	Sug	Sod

PIE FILLINGS

VEGETABLE/OTHER FILLINGS (4 OZ UNLESS NOTED)

Libby

Food	Cal	Fat	Sat	Chol	Carb	Fib	Sug	Sod
100% Pumpkin	40	1	0	0	9	5	4	5
Pumpkin Pie, premixed	100	0	0	0	25	2	22	150
Lucky Leaf Mincemeat	190	1	0	0	48	0	44	145

(SALT & SEASONINGS)

SALT & SALT SUBSTITUTES

CAUTION: Salt substitutes often contain high amounts of potassium which may interfere with high blood pressure medications. Check with healthcare provider before using.

Food	Cal	Fat	Sat	Chol	Carb	Fib	Sug	Sod
Salt substitute, 1 tsp	2	0	0	0	0	0	0	0
Lite salt, 1 tsp	0	0	0	0	0	0	0	1160
Seasoned salt, 1 tsp	0	0	0	0	0	0	0	1280
Table salt, 1 tsp	0	0	0	0	0	0	0	2325

BRANDS . . . *(1 TSP UNLESS NOTED)*

Food	Cal	Fat	Sat	Chol	Carb	Fib	Sug	Sod
Estee Seasoned Salt-It	0	0	0	0	0	0	0	0

HERBS, SPICES & SEASONINGS

Food	Cal	Fat	Sat	Chol	Carb	Fib	Sug	Sod
Liquid aminos, all purpose, 1/2 tsp	2	0	0	0	0	0	0	110
MSG, 1 tbsp	0	0	0	0	0	0	0	150
All-purpose seasoning, 1/2 tsp	5	0	0	0	0	0	0	300
Meat tenderizer, 1/2 tsp	0	0	0	0	0	0	0	840

NOTE: Individual herbs & spices have little or no sodium, however, herb and spice blends may contain added salt. Check labels for sodium content or list of ingredients if nutrient values are not listed.

BRANDS . . . *(1 TSP UNLESS NOTED)*

Food	Cal	Fat	Sat	Chol	Carb	Fib	Sug	Sod
Accent Herbal All Purpose	0	0	0	0	0	0	0	0
Flavor Enhancer, 1/8 tsp	0	0	0	0	0	0	0	80
Adolph's Tenderizer, Reg or Seasoned, SF, 1/2 tsp	0	0	0	0	1	0	0	0
Bell's SF Seasoning	0	0	0	0	0	0	0	0
Carmel Spritz, NSA, 1/4 tsp	0	0	0	0	0	0	0	0
Cavender's Greek Seasoning	0	0	0	0	0	0	0	0
Chef Paul Prudhomme, all Magic SF Seasonings, Pizza & Pasta Magic	0	0	0	0	0	0	0	0
Fortner's SF, all	0	0	0	0	0	0	0	0
Graham Kerr's Ethnix, all	0	0	0	0	0	0	0	0
Herbal Bouquet Italian Blend, SF	0	0	0	0	0	0	0	0
Lawry's SF 17	0	0	0	0	0	0	0	0
***Longhorn Grill** Mesquite, 1/4 tsp	0	0	0	0	0	0	0	5

Food	Cal	Fat	Sat	Chol	Carb	Fib	Sug	Sod
HERBS, SPICES AND SEASONINGS								
McCormick Salt Free, all	5	0	0	0	0	0	0	0
Mrs. Dash SF, all	8	0	0	0	0	0	0	4
*****Spice Hunter** SF, all	0	0	0	0	0	0	0	0
Spice Island SF, all	0	0	0	0	1	0	0	0
Spike SF Seasoning	0	0	0	0	0	0	0	0
Sylvia's SF Secret Seasoning	0	0	0	0	0	0	0	0
Tone's LS, all (avg)	0	0	0	0	2	1	0	1
Tony Chachere SF Creole Seasoning	0	0	0	0	0	0	0	0
Vegit All-Purpose Seasoning	0	0	0	0	0	0	0	50

(SWEETENERS)

Food	Cal	Fat	Sat	Chol	Carb	Fib	Sug	Sod
Sugar, powdered, 1/4 cup	117	0	0	0	30	0	30	0
Granulated, 1/4 cup	193	0	0	0	50	0	50	1
Brown, packed, 1/4 cup	207	0	0	0	54	0	54	22
Honey, 1/4 cup	258	0	0	0	70	0	70	3
Rice syrup, brown, 1/4 cup	170	0	0	0	42	0	19	5
Fruit sweetener, 1/4 cup	120	0	0	0	30	2	28	10
Molasses, 1/4 cup	218	0	0	0	57	0	43	30
Blackstrap, 1/4 cup	193	0	0	0	50	0	38	45
Corn syrup, light, 1/4 cup	231	0	0	0	63	0	63	99
Dark, 1/4 cup	231	0	0	0	63	0	63	127

BRANDS . . .

Most brands are within the generic range.

SUGAR SUBSTITUTES

Food	Cal	Fat	Sat	Chol	Carb	Fib	Sug	Sod
Fructose, 1 tsp	15	0	0	0	4	0	4	0
Sweetener w/aspartame, 1 tsp	8	0	0	0	1	0	0	0
Sweetener w/saccharin, 1 tsp	4	0	0	0	1	0	0	0
Sucralose, 1 tsp	0	0	0	0	0	0	0	0

BRANDS . . .

Most brands are within the generic range.

Food	Cal	Fat	Sat	Chol	Carb	Fib	Sug	Sod

BEVERAGES

ALCOHOLIC BEVERAGES

BEER & ALE

Food	Cal	Fat	Sat	Chol	Carb	Fib	Sug	Sod
Beer, regular, 12 fl oz	146	0	0	0	13	1	-	18
Non-alcoholic, 12 fl oz	70	0	0	0	15	0	3	10
Light, 12 fl oz	100	0	0	0	5	0	-	11

BRANDS . . .
Most brands are within the generic range.

LIQUOR & SPIRITS

Food	Cal	Fat	Sat	Chol	Carb	Fib	Sug	Sod
Distilled, all (i.e. gin, rum, vodka, whiskey), 1 fl oz	64	0	0	0	0	0	0	0
Creme de menthe, 1 fl oz	125	0	0	0	14	0	14	2
Coffee liqueur, 1 fl oz	117	0	0	0	16	0	16	3
Daiquiri, canned, 1 fl oz	38	0	0	0	5	0	-	12
Whiskey sour, canned, 1 fl oz	37	0	0	0	4	0	-	14
Tequila sunrise, canned, 1 fl oz	34	0	0	0	4	0	-	18
Pina colada, canned, 1 fl oz	77	3	2	0	9	0	-	23
Coffee liqueur w/cream, 1 fl oz	102	5	3	5	7	0	7	29
Whiskey sour, mix, 1 pkt	64	0	0	0	16	0	-	46

BRANDS . . .
Most brands are within the generic range.

WINE & CHAMPAGNE

Food	Cal	Fat	Sat	Chol	Carb	Fib	Sug	Sod
Table wine, all (includes champagne), 3.5 fl oz	72	0	0	0	1	0	-	8
Dessert wines, 3.5 fl oz	158	0	0	0	12	0	-	9
Cooking wines, 1 fl oz	45	0	0	0	2	0	2	190

NOTE: Instead of cooking wines, use madeira, marsala, sherry, vermouth, etc. from the wine department, which have little or no sodium.

BRANDS . . .
Most brands are within the generic range.

BREAKFAST DRINKS

(see Breakfast Drinks, pg 31)

COCKTAIL MIXERS

(also see Water, Tonic & Seltzers, pg 20)

Food	Cal	Fat	Sat	Chol	Carb	Fib	Sug	Sod
Daiquiri mix, 8 fl oz	140	0	0	0	35	0	33	0
Margarita mix, 8 fl oz	100	0	0	0	25	0	23	0

Food	Cal	Fat	Sat	Chol	Carb	Fib	Sug	Sod
COCKTAIL MIXERS								
Cream of coconut, 1 fl oz	85	2	2	0	18	1	17	45
Collins mix, 8 fl oz	110	0	0	0	25	0	25	55
Pina colada mix, 8 fl oz	360	0	0	0	86	0	80	130
Sweet & sour mix, 8 fl oz	276	0	0	0	70	0	61	131
Bloody mary mix, 8 fl oz	56	0	0	0	11	1	8	1548

BRANDS ...

FROZEN/REFRIGERATED *(8 FL OZ PREP UNLESS NOTED)*

Bacardi Real Fruit Mixers, Pina Colada	170	4	3	0	35	0	35	20

READY-TO-DRINK *(8 FL OZ UNLESS NOTED)*

*Baja Bob's Desert Lime Margarita, Sugar Free	20	0	0	0	2	0	6	90
Bloody Mary Mix	80	0	0	0	8	0	6	840
Major Peters Pina Colada Mix	386	3	0	0	98	0	92	33
Mr. & Mrs. T Sweet & Sour	200	0	0	0	46	0	42	100
Red Eye Bloody Mary Mixes (avg)	47	0	0	0	9	3	1	784

NOTE: Although the Bloody Mary mixes listed above exceed sodium guidelines, they are substantially less than the generic.

COCOA - HOT CHOCOLATE

(see Milk-Based Drinks & Additives, pg 15)

COFFEE

Coffee, brewed, 8 fl oz	5	0	0	0	1	0	0	5
Instant, 8 fl oz	5	0	0	0	1	0	0	7

BRANDS ...
Most brands are within the generic range.

COFFEE CREAMERS & FLAVORINGS

Non-dairy soy creamer, 1 tbsp	20	2	0	0	2	0	1	0
Cream substitute, powder, 1 tsp	11	1	1	0	1	0	0	4
Liquid, 1 tbsp	20	1	0	0	2	0	1	12
Flavored creamer, 1 tbsp	45	2	0	0	7	0	5	5
Cream, liquid, 1 tbsp	29	3	2	10	1	0	0	6
Syrup flavoring, all, 1 oz	85	0	0	0	21	0	20	8

BRANDS ...
Most brands are within the generic range.

COFFEE FLAVORED DRINKS

Mocha-flavor, instant, 2 tsp	51	2	0	0	8	0	6	31
French-flavor, instant, 2 tsp	57	3	1	0	7	0	3	82

BEVERAGES
Coffee Substitutes

Food	Cal	Fat	Sat	Chol	Carb	Fib	Sug	Sod
COFFEE FLAVORED DRINKS								
Cappuccino-flavor, instant, 2 tsp	62	2	0	0	11	0	4	98
Coffee drink, ready-to-drink, 9.5 oz	190	3	2	12	39	0	30	110
BRANDS . . .								
MIX *(8 FL OZ PREP UNLESS NOTED)*								
***Atkins** Cappuccino*	50	2	0	0	3	0	1	70
***Caffe D'Vita** Instant Cappuccino or*								
French Vanilla	60	3	3	0	10	0	7	30
***Caffe D'Amore** Mocha Frappe*	110	3	2	0	22	0	14	35
***Folgers** Cafe Latte, Skinny Vanilla Vibe*	60	3	2	0	8	0	2	35
Mocha Almond Jive, Straight Up Latte,								
or Double Shot Dancin' Java (avg)	100	5	2	5	14	0	7	80
General Foods International								
Cappuccino Cooler, French Vanilla								
or Choc	60	0	0	0	15	0	15	0
Cafe Viennese	50	2	1	0	10	0	9	30
Swiss White Choc	70	3	1	0	12	0	9	30
Suisse Mocha, FF, Sugar Free,								
Decaf	60	2	1	0	9	9	0	35
Suisse Mocha, Sugar Free	25	0	0	0	5	0	0	35
Irish Creme	60	2	1	0	10	0	8	45
Cappuccino Cafe, Mocha	100	3	0	0	18	0	13	45
Italian Cappuccino	60	2	1	0	10	0	8	50
***Maxwell House** Instant Cappuccino,*								
Mocha or Vanilla (avg)	100	3	1	0	17	0	16	65
***Village Inn** French Vanilla*	100	4	3	0	14	0	10	70
READY-TO-DRINK *(8 FL OZ UNLESS NOTED)*								
***Arizona** Iced Coffee (avg)*	110	2	1	6	21	1	16	95
***Folgers** Jakada Latte French Roast,*								
10.5 fl oz	170	4	2	10	31	0	30	70
***Starbucks** Doubleshot Espresso*								
w/Cream, 6.5 fl oz	140	6	4	20	18	0	17	70
Frappuccino Mocha Lite, 9.5 fl oz	100	3	2	13	12	3	11	80

(COFFEE SUBSTITUTES)

Cereal grain, mix, 1 tsp	8	0	0	0	2	0	0	2
Cereal grain, prep w/milk, 6 fl oz	120	6	4	24	10	0	8	91

BRANDS . . .
Most brands are within the generic range.

(EGGNOG)

(see Milk Products & Non-Dairy Alternatives, pg 61)

Food	Cal	Fat	Sat	Chol	Carb	Fib	Sug	Sod

ENERGY DRINKS

(see Sports & Energy Drinks, pg 18)

FLAVORED DRINKS

(see Sodas & Alternative Drinks, pg 16)

FRUIT JUICE & FRUIT-FLAVORED DRINKS

Food	Cal	Fat	Sat	Chol	Carb	Fib	Sug	Sod
Fruit-flavored drink mix, 8 fl oz	60	0	0	0	16	0	16	0
Sugar free, 8 fl oz	5	0	0	0	0	0	0	0
Cranberry juice cocktail, 8 fl oz	144	0	0	0	36	0	34	5
Fruit juice, citrus, 8 fl oz	114	0	0	0	28	0	27	7
Lemonade, 8 fl oz	99	0	0	0	26	0	26	7
Apricot nectar, 8 fl oz	140	0	0	0	36	1	31	8
Fruit punch:								
Frozen, prep, 8 fl oz	113	0	0	0	29	0	29	11
Drink mix, prep, 8 fl oz	97	0	0	0	25	0	25	31
Ready-to-drink, 8 fl oz	116	0	0	0	29	0	29	55
Orange flavor mix, prep, 8 fl oz	114	0	0	0	29	0	29	12
Apple juice, 8 fl oz	110	0	0	0	29	0	23	15
Grape drink, 8 fl oz	113	0	0	0	29	0	29	15
Cranberry apple, 8 fl oz	164	0	0	0	43	0	43	35
Fruit & vegetable drink, 8 fl oz	110	0	0	0	29	0	26	50

BRANDS ...
Most brands are within the generic range. NOTE: Some fruit blends with less than 25% juice may contain as much as 80mg sodium per serving.

MILK-BASED DRINKS & ADDITIVES

(also see Milk Products & Non-Dairy Alternatives, pg 61 and Diet & Nutritional Drinks, pg 88)

Food	Cal	Fat	Sat	Chol	Carb	Fib	Sug	Sod
Drink mixes:								
Strawberry, prep w/milk, 8 fl oz	234	8	5	32	33	0	-	128
Cocoa/hot choc:								
3 tsp mix or 1 envl	101	1	1	1	22	0	21	141
Sugar-free, prep w/water, 1 envl	48	0	0	0	11	1	8	168
Gourmet hot choc, 1 serv	160	0	0	0	28	0	22	240
Milk shake, vanilla, 8 fl oz	254	7	4	27	40	0	-	216
Milk shake, choc, 8 fl oz	270	6	4	25	48	0	-	252
Ready-to-drink:								
Choc, 6 fl oz	130	2	0	0	27	0	26	150

BEVERAGES
Sodas & Alternative Drinks

Food	Cal	Fat	Sat	Chol	Carb	Fib	Sug	Sod
MILK-BASED DRINKS AND ADDITIVES								
Syrup and powder additives:								
Strawberry syrup, 2 tbsp	100	0	0	0	28	0	26	5
Carob flavor, powder, 1 tbsp	458	0	0	0	11	1	-	12
Choc syrup, 2 tbsp	108	0	0	0	25	1	19	28
Malted milk, natural, powder, 4 tbsp	170	0	0	0	17	0	13	65
Malted milk, choc, powder, 4 tbsp	170	0	0	0	18	1	15	115
BRANDS . . .								
DRINK MIXES (*1 ENVL UNLESS NOTED*)								
Ah!Laska Cocoa								
Organic, Non-Dairy	100	0	0	0	23	1	20	4
Organic, Dairy	100	0	0	0	23	1	20	35
Alba Dairy Shake	70	0	0	5	12	2	7	140
*Atkins Hot Cocoa, Sugar Free, 3 tbsp	50	3	0	0	3	0	0	0
*Carbolite Choc Supreme Shake,								
2 tbsp	150	3	0	0	8	5	0	40
Carnation Rich Choc, FF	25	0	0	0	5	1	4	125
Double Choc Meltdown	150	3	3	0	29	1	23	150
Hershey's Goodnight Hugs Hot Cocoa,								
White Choc	150	4	1	0	27	0	22	140
Hot Cocoa Collection, French Vanilla	140	3	0	0	28	0	18	150
Swiss Miss								
Milk Choc w/Marshmallows	120	3	1	0	22	1	17	125
READY-TO-DRINK (*8 FL OZ UNLESS NOTED*)								
SoBe Love Bug Brew	150	3	2	5	33	4	24	75
SYRUPS AND POWDER ADDITIVES								

Most brands are within the generic range.

(RICE BEVERAGES)

(see Non-Dairy Alternatives, pg 62)

(SELTZER)

(see Water, Tonic & Seltzers, pg 20)

(SODAS & ALTERNATIVE DRINKS)

(also see Sports & Energy Drinks, pg 18)

Spritzers w/juice, 12 fl oz	170	0	0	0	42	0	38	25
Ginger ale, 12 fl oz	124	0	0	0	32	0	32	38
Diet, 12 fl oz	0	0	0	0	0	0	0	90
Orange, 12 fl oz	179	0	0	0	46	0	46	45

Food	Cal	Fat	Sat	Chol	Carb	Fib	Sug	Sod

SODAS AND ALTERNATIVE DRINKS

Food	Cal	Fat	Sat	Chol	Carb	Fib	Sug	Sod
Cream soda, 12 fl oz	189	0	0	0	49	0	49	45
Diet, 12 fl oz	0	0	0	0	0	0	0	70
Root beer, 12 fl oz	152	0	0	0	39	0	39	48
Diet, 12 fl oz	0	0	0	0	0	0	0	70
Cola, 12 fl oz	140	0	0	0	39	0	39	50
Diet, 12 fl oz	1	0	0	0	0	0	0	40
Pepper-type, 12 fl oz	151	0	0	0	38	0	38	55
Grape, 12 fl oz	160	0	0	0	42	0	42	56
Lemon-lime, 12 fl oz	147	0	0	0	38	0	38	70
Diet, 12 fl oz	0	0	0	0	0	0	0	35
Lemonade, 12 fl oz	130	0	0	0	35	0	35	130

BRANDS . . . *(12 FL OZ UNLESS NOTED)*

There are many low-sodium sodas, the following have less than 40mg per serving.

Food	Cal	Fat	Sat	Chol	Carb	Fib	Sug	Sod
Barq's Root Beer	186	0	0	0	46	0	46	34
Blue Sky, all (avg)	180	0	0	0	45	0	45	10
Canada Dry Ginger Ale	140	0	0	0	36	0	36	25
Canfield's Diet, all	0	0	0	0	0	0	0	0
Swiss Creme	180	0	0	0	46	0	46	30
Coke Vanilla	150	0	0	0	42	0	42	35
Dad's Diet Root Beer	0	0	0	0	0	0	0	38
Diet Riet, all	0	0	0	0	0	0	0	0
Dr. Brown's Black Cherry	180	0	0	0	45	0	45	25
Fresca	0	0	0	0	0	0	0	35
Green River	180	0	0	0	45	0	45	15
Jones Naturals, all	100	0	0	0	23	0	23	0
Soda, all	170	0	0	0	46	0	46	14
Minute Maid Diet Orange	2	0	0	0	0	0	0	0
Mountain Dew Diet	0	0	0	0	0	0	0	38
Natural Brew Root Beer or Grapefruit	180	0	0	0	44	0	39	0
Vanilla Creme, Outrageous Ginger Ale, or Ginseng Cola	170	0	0	0	42	0	38	18
Orange	150	0	0	0	38	0	34	30
Pepsi Diet or Diet Twist	0	0	0	0	0	0	0	35
Regular, Twist, or Wild Cherry (avg)	150	0	0	0	42	0	42	35
Polar, all (avg)	0	0	0	0	0	0	0	0
Royal Crown RC or Cherry Cola	0	0	0	0	29	0	29	35
Diet, Caffeine-Free	1	0	0	0	0	0	0	0
Santa Cruz Root Beer	140	0	0	0	36	0	32	0
Seagrams Ginger Ale	150	0	0	0	36	0	36	35
Seven-Up Diet	0	0	0	0	0	0	0	35

17

BEVERAGES
Sports & Energy Drinks

Food	Cal	Fat	Sat	Chol	Carb	Fib	Sug	Sod
SODAS AND ALTERNATIVE DRINKS								
Sierra Mist Lemon Lime	150	0	0	0	39	0	39	35
Diet	0	0	0	0	0	0	0	35
Spin Cola	160	0	0	0	43	0	43	35
Diet	0	0	0	0	0	0	0	35
Sprite Diet	0	0	0	0	0	0	0	35
Squirt Diet	0	0	0	0	0	0	0	25
Sterling Ginger Ale	120	0	0	0	30	0	30	38
Diet	0	0	0	0	0	0	0	38
Stewart's Diet	0	0	0	0	0	0	0	25
Original	160	0	0	0	40	0	40	30
Vernors Ginger Ale	150	0	0	0	39	0	39	25
Diet	0	0	0	0	0	0	0	25

ALTERNATIVE DRINKS/SODAS

There are many low-sodium alternative drinks, the following have less than 40mg per serving.

BRANDS . . .

READY-TO-DRINK *(8 FL OZ UNLESS NOTED)*

Food	Cal	Fat	Sat	Chol	Carb	Fib	Sug	Sod
Clearly Canadian Blackberry,	100	0	0	0	24	0	24	10
Raspberry or Strawberry (avg)	80	0	0	0	20	0	20	10
Ginseng Up, all but Apple (avg)	160	0	0	0	41	0	41	10
Apple	160	0	0	0	41	0	41	30
SoBe, Cranberry Grapefuit or Zen Blend (avg)	100	0	0	0	27	0	26	10
Lean Sugar Free, Diet Tropical or Diet Cranberry Grapefruit	5	0	0	0	1	0	0	15
Elixir Orange Carrot	90	0	0	0	24	0	24	15
Dragonfruit, Nirvana, Wisdom, or Lemonade (avg)	115	0	0	0	30	0	29	15
Tsunami, Lizard Lightning, or Lizard Fuel (avg)	120	0	0	0	32	0	31	20
Lizard Lava	120	0	0	0	32	0	31	31
Lean Sugar Free, Diet Peach	5	0	0	0	1	0	0	35

(SOY BEVERAGES)

(see Non-Dairy Alternatives, pg 62)

(SPORTS & ENERGY DRINKS)

(also see Water, Tonic & Seltzers, pg 20)

Food	Cal	Fat	Sat	Chol	Carb	Fib	Sug	Sod
Thirst quencher, 8 fl oz	50	0	0	0	14	0	14	110

Food	Cal	Fat	Sat	Chol	Carb	Fib	Sug	Sod
SPORTS AND ENERGY DRINKS								
BRANDS . . .								
MIX								
Gatorade ReLode, 1 pkt	80	0	0	0	17	-	3	25
*Natural Ovens Alena Energy, 2 tbsp	55	3	0	0	9	6	2	10
READY-TO-DRINK *(8 FL OZ UNLESS NOTED)*								
Biosport	10	0	0	0	2	0	1	20
Elements Energy, canned (avg).........	120	0	0	0	29	0	27	10
Energy, bottled (avg)......................	130	0	0	0	32	0	30	25
Hansen's Energy, 8.3 fl oz	120	0	0	0	32	0	32	25
Smoothies:								
Super Power, Berry Splash, 11 fl oz	170	0	0	0	41	0	40	40
Super Vita, Orange Carrot, 11 fl oz	170	0	0	0	40	0	40	60
KMX Energy, 8.4 fl oz	120	0	0	0	31	0	31	75
Powerade, all	70	0	0	0	19	0	15	55
Power Dream (soy drink) Sky High								
Chai or Java Jolt, 11 fl oz (avg)	245	5	1	0	42	2	25	70
RW Knudsen Recharge	70	0	0	0	18	0	17	25
Slice All Sport Diet Lemon Lime	1	0	0	0	0	0	0	40

TEA

Tea, regular, prep, 8 fl oz	2	0	0	0	0	0	0	2
Ready-to-drink, flavored, 8 fl oz	100	0	0	0	25	0	25	10
Instant, lemon-flavored, prep, 8 fl oz ..	5	0	0	0	1	0	0	14
Chai, mix, prep, 8 fl oz	120	2	0	5	21	0	19	180
BRANDS . . .								
TEA								
Most brands are within the generic range.								
CHAI MIXES *(8 FL OZ PREP UNLESS NOTED)*								
Pacific Chai Decaf Vanilla	120	2	2	0	23	0	14	38
Spice or Vanilla	120	2	1	0	25	0	21	55

VEGETABLE JUICE

Carrot juice, 8 fl oz	80	1	0	0	18	1	9	167
Vegetable juice cocktail, 8 fl oz.............	50	0	0	0	10	2	8	540
Tomato juice, 8 fl oz	50	0	0	0	10	2	7	750
Clam/tomato juice, 8 fl oz	58	0	0	0	12	0	9	885
BRANDS . . . *(8 FL OZ UNLESS NOTED)*								
After The Fall 24 Karrot Orange	120	0	0	0	29	0	23	45
Aylmer Tomato, LS	41	0	0	0	10	-	-	26
Hunt's Tomato, NSA	34	0	0	0	8	2	-	12

19

BEVERAGES
Water, Tonic & Seltzers

Food	Cal	Fat	Sat	Chol	Carb	Fib	Sug	Sod
VEGETABLE JUICES								
RW Knudsen Very Veggie, LS	50	1	0	0	11	0	6	35
Simchan Tomato, 6 fl oz	35	0	0	0	7	2	4	75
Snapple Gravity Carrot Infusion	120	0	0	0	29	0	28	10
SoBe Orange Carrot Elixir	90	0	0	0	24	0	23	20
V8 Vegetable, LS	50	0	0	0	12	2	8	140

(WATER, TONIC & SELTZERS)

(also see Sports & Energy Drinks, pg 18)

Food	Cal	Fat	Sat	Chol	Carb	Fib	Sug	Sod
Water, bottled, 8 fl oz	0	0	0	0	0	0	0	2
Enhanced/fitness, 8 fl oz	10	0	0	0	3	0	2	35
Seltzer, includes fruit-flavored, 8 fl oz (avg)	0	0	0	0	0	0	0	10
Tonic, 8 fl oz	83	0	0	0	22	0	24	10
Diet, 8 fl oz	0	0	0	0	0	0	0	35
Club soda, 8 fl oz	0	0	0	0	0	0	0	50

NOTE: Some fruit-flavored seltzers may contain as much as 46mg sodium per serving.

BRANDS . . . *(8 FL OZ UNLESS NOTED)*

Food	Cal	Fat	Sat	Chol	Carb	Fib	Sug	Sod
Aquafina Essentials	40	0	0	0	11	0	11	15
Canada Dry Club Soda, LS	0	0	0	0	0	0	0	35
Glaceau Vitamin Water, Tropical Citrus or Orange Carrot	50	0	0	0	13	0	13	0
Kiwi Strawberry	40	0	0	0	9	0	8	0
Pulse Heart Health Water (avg)	9	0	0	0	2	0	0	0
Reebok, 24 fl oz	30	0	0	0	10	0	10	0

Food	Cal	Fat	Sat	Chol	Carb	Fib	Sug	Sod

BREAD, ROLLS & BREAD PRODUCTS

BAGELS

Food	Cal	Fat	Sat	Chol	Carb	Fib	Sug	Sod
Cinnamon raisin bagel, med, 2.5 oz	288	2	0	0	58	2	6	338
Egg bagel, med, 2.5 oz	292	2	0	25	56	2	5	530
Oat bran bagel, med, 2.5 oz	268	1	0	0	56	4	5	532
Plain bagel, med, 2.5 oz	289	1	0	0	56	2	5	561
Mini, 1 oz	72	0	0	0	14	3	2	139
Large, 3.9 oz	360	2	0	0	70	3	7	700

BRANDS . . .

FROZEN/REFRIGERATED *(3.3 oz unless noted)*

Food	Cal	Fat	Sat	Chol	Carb	Fib	Sug	Sod
Alvarado St. Bakery Sprouted or Wheat Cinnamon Raisin	280	1	0	0	59	3	28	270
Sprouted Grain Granola	260	2	0	0	51	3	10	280
Lenders Cinnamon Raisin, 2 oz	160	1	0	0	32	1	7	240
Cinnamon Swirl, 2 oz	150	5	1	0	32	1	8	270
Plain Bagelette, 1.8 oz (2)	140	1	1	0	27	1	2	290

MIX

Food	Cal	Fat	Sat	Chol	Carb	Fib	Sug	Sod
Gluten Free Pantry, 1 bagel	150	0	0	0	36	1	-	170

READY-TO-EAT *(3.3 oz unless noted)*

Food	Cal	Fat	Sat	Chol	Carb	Fib	Sug	Sod
Better Bakery, Plain, 2.6 oz	172	4	0	0	17	4	0	156
Earth Grains, all, 3 oz (avg)	245	0	0	0	48	0	-	210
French Meadow Spelt	270	3	0	0	53	0	0	290
Sprouted w/Ezekiel 4:9 Grains	250	1	0	0	51	5	0	290
Natural Ovens Whole Grain, 3 oz	170	2	0	0	37	6	4	200
Blueberry or Raspberry, 3 oz (avg)	185	2	0	0	39	5	10	220
Cinnamon Raisin, 3 oz	180	1	0	0	40	5	6	240
Hearty Grains & Onion, 3 oz	190	4	1	0	37	7	6	250
Brainy, 3 oz	170	2	0	0	38	6	5	270
Pacific Bakery Kamut	190	1	0	0	40	5	0	260
Silver Hills Squirrelly, Sprouted Grain	290	8	2	0	45	10	4	230
Flax, Sprouted Grain	260	4	1	0	42	11	3	260
Trader Joe's Sprouted Wheat Cinnamon Raisin	280	1	0	0	59	3	28	270

NOTE: *Although many of the above bagels exceed sodium guidelines, they are substantially less than the generic.*

BISCUITS

Food	Cal	Fat	Sat	Chol	Carb	Fib	Sug	Sod
Mixed grain biscuit, refrg dough, 1.6 oz	116	2	1	0	21	0	-	295

21

BREAD, ROLLS & BREAD PRODUCTS

Bread

Food	Cal	Fat	Sat	Chol	Carb	Fib	Sug	Sod
BISCUITS								
Plain biscuit, ready-to-eat, 1 oz	103	5	1	0	14	0	-	298
Mix, prep, 1 oz	95	3	1	1	14	1	3	271
Refrg dough, LF, 1 oz	59	1	0	0	11	0	-	287
Refrg dough, 1 oz	90	4	1	0	12	0	-	314

BRANDS ...

MIX

	Cal	Fat	Sat	Chol	Carb	Fib	Sug	Sod
Atkins, 1 biscuit	39	0	0	0	7	2	0	118
Bernard, LS, 1 biscuit	170	4	2	0	30	0	0	10

(BREAD)

(also see Bread Dough & Mixes, pg 25)

	Cal	Fat	Sat	Chol	Carb	Fib	Sug	Sod
Raisin bread, 1 oz slice	78	1	0	0	15	1	5	111
Oat bran bread, 1 oz slice	67	1	0	0	11	1	2	115
Reduced cal, 1 oz slice	57	1	0	0	12	3	-	100
Rice bran bread, 1 oz slice	69	1	0	0	12	1	-	125
Mixed grain bread, 1 oz slice	71	1	0	0	13	2	2	138
Wheat bread, 1 oz slice	69	1	0	0	13	2	2	148
Reduced cal, 1 oz slice	56	1	0	0	12	3	-	145
Cracked wheat bread, 1 oz slice	74	1	0	0	14	2	-	153
White bread, 1 oz slice	76	1	0	0	14	1	1	153
Reduced cal, 1 oz slice	59	1	0	0	13	3	-	128
Protein (gluten) bread, 1 oz slice	70	1	0	0	12	1	-	155
Oatmeal bread, 1 oz slice	76	1	0	0	14	1	-	170
French or sourdough bread, 1 oz slice	78	1	0	0	15	1	1	173
Rye bread, 1 oz slice	73	1	0	0	14	2	1	187
Reduced cal, 1 oz slice	58	1	0	0	12	3	-	115
Pumpernickel bread, 1 oz slice	71	1	0	0	14	2	1	190
Boston brown bread, canned, 1 slice	88	1	0	0	20	2	-	284
Foccacia bread, 1 oz slice	78	1	0	0	15	1	1	308

BRANDS ... *(1 SLICE UNLESS NOTED)*

There are many low-sodium breads, the following have less than 125mg per slice.

	Cal	Fat	Sat	Chol	Carb	Fib	Sug	Sod
Alvarado St. Bakery Multi-Grain, SF	60	1	0	0	11	2	1	0
Arnold Bran'nola Nutty Grain	90	3	0	0	17	3	3	65
Golden Wheat Light	40	0	0	0	10	2	2	68
Bakery Light, Italian or Oatmeal	40	1	0	0	11	3	2	75
Bakery Light, Premium White or Whole Wheat (avg)	40	1	0	0	10	3	2	80
Raisin Cinnamon	70	1	0	0	14	0	3	90
100% Stoneground Whole Wheat	60	1	0	0	12	2	2	115
Bran'nola Country Oat	90	3	1	0	18	3	3	115

Food	Cal	Fat	Sat	Chol	Carb	Fib	Sug	Sod
BREAD								
*Atkins Rye	60	1	1	5	8	5	0	110
Blue Ribbon White, Family	60	1	0	0	13	1	1	115
Breadsmith								
Honey Oat Bran or Honey White (avg)	72	0	0	0	15	1	0	118
Egg Challah, 1 oz	86	2	0	8	15	0	0	123
Brownberry Natural 12 Grain	55	1	0	0	10	1	2	90
Bakery Light, Golden Wheat	40	0	0	0	10	3	2	90
Butternut Small Split-top White	50	1	0	0	10	1	2	85
Small Enriched	50	1	0	0	9	1	1	100
Small Country Wheat	55	1	0	0	10	1	2	115
Honey Wheat	55	1	0	0	10	1	1	115
Jumbo Sandwich	60	1	0	0	11	1	1	120
Countrys Delight Honey Wheat	55	1	0	0	10	1	1	115
Jumbo Sandwich, White	55	1	0	0	11	1	1	115
Damascus Mt. Shepard Lahvash, 1 oz	68	0	0	0	14	1	-	45
D'Italiano Light Italian	40	1	0	0	9	2	1	105
*Ener-G Brown Rice	120	4	0	0	16	1	0	4
Tapioca	140	6	1	0	20	4	2	9
Raisin	182	2	0	0	39	-	20	49
Hi-Fiber	113	3	0	0	21	-	2	66
*Food for Life								
Raisin or Rice Pecan (avg)	130	3	0	0	25	2	6	5
Cinnamon Raisin, 7 Grains	80	0	0	0	18	2	5	65
Ezekiel	80	1	0	0	15	3	0	75
Ezekiel w/Sesame	80	1	0	0	14	3	0	80
Freihofer Low Sodium	130	2	0	0	22	1	2	10
*French Meadow Rye, 100%, SF	103	1	0	0	22	3	0	0
Summer Bread	99	1	0	0	19	-	0	0
Spelt	52	0	0	0	10	1	0	56
Flax & Sunflower Seed	92	2	0	0	18	3	0	90
Giant								
Raisin, NSA	90	1	0	5	19	1	8	0
LS Wheat	55	1	0	0	10	1	1	0
LS White	60	1	0	0	11	0	1	0
Healthy Choice Soft, Multigrain or Honey Wheat	60	1	0	0	12	2	2	120
Healthy Life								
100% Whole Wheat	35	0	0	0	8	3	1	80
White	35	0	0	0	8	2	1	90
Italian or Sourdough	40	0	0	0	9	2	1	100
Iron Kids Crustless White	40	1	0	0	9	1	2	90
Martin Potato	80	1	0	0	15	1	2	115

BREAD, ROLLS & BREAD PRODUCTS

Bread

Food	Cal	Fat	Sat	Chol	Carb	Fib	Sug	Sod
BREAD								
***Montana Mills** Blueberry Cobbler*	79	1	0	5	16	1	-	67
Cranberry Orange or Woodstock (avg)	68	0	0	0	14	1	-	69
Multigrain or Honey Whole Wheat (avg)	67	0	0	0	14	2	-	73
Sticky Bun	70	1	0	5	14	1	-	74
Cinnamon Raisin Walnut	66	1	0	0	13	2	-	85
Sunflower Millet or Garlic Cheddar (avg)	71	1	0	2	14	1	-	86
Apple Raisin Cinnamon Swirl	67	0	0	0	15	0	-	87
Bavarian Rye	61	0	0	0	13	1	-	97
Cinnamon Swirl	66	0	0	0	15	0	-	100
Spinach Feta or Montana Harvest (avg)	67	1	0	3	12	2	-	105
Sourdough or Grandma's White (avg)	65	0	0	0	14	1	-	114
Focaccia	57	1	0	0	10	0	-	116
***Mother's** All Butter, White or Wheat (avg)*	60	1	0	0	12	1	1	113
***Natural Ovens** Mild Rye*	70	1	0	0	13	4	0	70
Whole Grains, all (avg)	70	1	0	0	15	3	1	70
Cinnamon Raisin or Raisin Pecan (avg)	70	1	0	0	15	3	3	70
English Muffin Bread	80	1	0	0	16	3	1	70
***Nature's Path** Manna Bread*								
Millet Rice or Multigrain (avg)	130	0	0	0	28	5	9	3
Sun Seed	160	2	0	0	29	7	11	3
Carrot Raisin or Fruit & Nut	135	0	0	0	27	6	13	6
Whole Rye or Cinnamon Date (avg)	150	0	0	0	30	5	9	13
***Pacific Bakery** Spelt Multigrain*	90	1	0	0	18	2	0	100
Spelt White or Orig Sourdough	90	1	0	0	18	1	0	100
Spelt White Cinnamon Raisin	100	1	0	0	21	1	0	100
Sourdough Rye or Sourdough Multigrain	90	1	0	0	18	2	0	110
Spelt or Ancient Grains (avg)	100	1	0	0	20	3	0	120
***Pepperidge Farm** White, Very Thin*	37	1	0	0	8	1	1	90
Raisin Cinnamon Swirl	80	2	0	0	14	1	6	105
Cinnamon Swirl	80	3	1	0	14	2	4	115
Whole Wheat	60	1	0	0	11	1	1	120
***Pillsbury** Enriched White or Wheat*	70	1	0	0	13	2	2	110
***Rosen** Hawaiian Toaster*	80	1	1	10	15	1	2	120
***Rudolph's** SF Rye*	124	1	-	0	26	4	-	2
Weissbrot	66	0	0	0	14	1	0	46
Ryelite	66	0	0	0	12	1	0	63
Sourdough or 5-Grain	77	1	0	0	16	1	0	76
Volkornbrot	55	0	0	0	13	2	0	87
***Stoehmann** Small Family White*	50	1	0	0	11	1	1	110
***Sunbeam** Sandwich White*	55	1	0	0	11	1	1	90
***Vermont Bread Co.** Wheat, SF*	90	2	0	0	15	2	-	0
Cinnamon Raisin	80	1	0	0	16	0	6	90

Food	Cal	Fat	Sat	Chol	Carb	Fib	Sug	Sod
BREAD								
***Wolferman's** English Muffin Bread*								
Cinnamon Raisin	65	0	0	0	13	1	4	100
Cranberry Citrus	65	0	0	0	14	1	3	100
1910 Original Recipe	65	0	0	0	12	0	1	120
***Wonder** White, High Fiber*	40	0	0	0	9	3	1	80
Whole Wheat, High Fiber	40	0	0	0	6	3	1	80
Cinnamon Raisin	80	2	0	0	15	0	2	110
Thin White	55	1	0	0	10	1	1	110
Light, White, Wheat, or Italian	40	1	0	0	9	3	1	115
Regular White	50	1	0	0	11	1	1	115
Sandwich White	55	1	0	0	11	1	1	120

BREAD DOUGH & MIXES

Food	Cal	Fat	Sat	Chol	Carb	Fib	Sug	Sod
Multigrain, mix, 1/4 cup	130	2	0	0	22	2	-	150
Whole wheat, mix, lowfat, 1/4 cup	120	2	0	0	22	3	-	160
White, mix, 1/4 cup	120	2	0	0	22	3	-	170
Banana, mix, prep, 2.1 oz slice	196	6	1	26	33	1	-	181
Rye, mix, 1/4 cup	120	2	0	0	22	3	-	190
White, bread machine mix, 1/8 pkg	130	2	0	0	25	1	-	250
Cracked wheat, bread machine, 1/12 pkg.	130	2	0	0	25	2	-	260
Cornbread & muffin mix, 1 oz	119	4	1	1	20	2	-	315

BRANDS . . .

Food	Cal	Fat	Sat	Chol	Carb	Fib	Sug	Sod
FROZEN/REFRIGERATED *(1 OZ UNLESS NOTED)*								
***Kineret** Challah*	75	2	1	8	13	1	-	110
***Rhodes** Cracked Wheat*	75	1	0	0	15	0	-	0
Raisin	70	1	0	0	13	0	-	0
MIX *(1 SLICE UNLESS NOTED)*								
***Arrowhead Mills** Seitan Quick*	160	1	0	0	11	2	-	60
Multigrain	160	1	0	0	31	3	1	90
***Atkins** Quick & Easy*								
Caraway Rye	70	0	0	0	8	5	0	150
Country White	70	0	0	0	8	5	0	135
Sourdough	70	0	0	0	8	5	0	170
Carbolite	45	1	0	0	4	2	0	130
***Ener-G** Low-Protein, 1 oz*	109	0	0	0	27	-	2	24
***Gluten Free Pantry** French*	110	0	0	0	25	1	-	115
***Ketogenics**, all (avg)*	80	0	0	0	6	4	1	60
***McCann's** Irish Breakfast, 1/14*	90	1	0	0	17	2	0	100
***Sylvan Border Farm** Dark, White, or Wheat-Free, 2 oz*	140	4	1	35	24	1	6	120
***Wholesome Classics** 9-Grain Beer, 1 oz*	-	0	0	0	20	3	4	160

25

BREAD, ROLLS & BREAD PRODUCTS

Breadsticks

Food	Cal	Fat	Sat	Chol	Carb	Fib	Sug	Sod
BREAD MACHINE								
MIX *(1 SLICE UNLESS NOTED)*								
Betty Crocker Cinnamon Streusel, 1/14	160	5	1	0	28	0	15	150
Bob's Red Mill Rye	150	3	0	0	25	1	0	210
Carbsense Harvest Wheat	60	0	0	0	4	1	0	120
Classic Hearth Hawaiian Royal Sweet, 1/10	160	2	1	5	31	1	9	180
Fleischmann's Sourdough, 2 oz	140	2	1	0	27	1	3	210
SWEET BREADS								
MIX *(1 SLICE UNLESS NOTED)*								
Eagle Mills Choc Nugget Dessert, 1/15	180	4	1	5	25	1	7	160
Lemon Poppy Dessert, 1/15	140	3	0	5	25	1	6	190
Fleischmann's Ice n' Slice Blueberry, Cinnamon, or Pumpkin, 1.6 oz (avg)	160	2	0	0	33	2	11	210
Gluten Free Pantry Cranberry-Orange	150	0	0	0	35	1	-	150
Krusteaz Cinnamon Raisin, 1/12	180	3	0	0	35	2	10	200
Lollipop Tree Summer Berry, 1/16	130	2	1	0	26	1	15	85
Cherry w/Belgian Choc, 1/15	130	2	1	0	27	1	18	105
Pear Spice, 1/15	120	0	0	0	29	1	16	105
Lemon w/Lemon Peel, 1/15	120	0	0	0	28	1	16	115
Cranberry w/Ginger, 1/15	120	0	0	0	28	1	17	150
Pillsbury Cranberry, 1/12	140	2	0	0	30	1	16	150
Date, 1/12	150	2	0	0	32	1	18	150
Cinnamon Streusel, 1/14	160	5	1	0	28	0	15	150
Cinnamon Swirl, 1/12	220	5	2	0	32	0	20	160

BREADSTICKS

	Cal	Fat	Sat	Chol	Carb	Fib	Sug	Sod
Plain, 0.5 oz	60	2	1	0	10	1	0	140
BRANDS . . . *(0.5 OZ UNLESS NOTED)*								
Alessi Sesame	55	1	1	0	11	1	1	105
Angonoa LS	65	2	0	0	10	1	0	33
FF	60	0	0	0	11	1	1	110
Whole Wheat	65	2	0	0	10	2	1	110
Colonna Garlic, 0.6 oz	70	2	0	0	13	0	0	85
Sesame, 0.6 oz	70	2	0	0	13	0	0	90
Plain, 0.6 oz	60	0	0	0	14	0	0	100
Fattorie & Pandea Sesame, 0.6 oz	70	2	0	0	13	1	1	115
Stella D'oro SF, 0.4 oz	45	1	0	0	7	0	1	0
Original, 0.4 oz	40	1	0	0	7	0	0	40
Sesame, 0.4 oz	50	3	1	0	7	1	1	45
Garlic Sesame, 0.5 oz	60	2	0	0	9	1	1	60

BREAD, ROLLS & BREAD PRODUCTS
Buns, Croissants & Rolls

Food	Cal	Fat	Sat	Chol	Carb	Fib	Sug	Sod
BREADSTICKS								
Toufayan Sesame or Whole Wheat, 0.5 oz	45	1	0	0	9	1	1	80

BUNS, CROISSANTS & ROLLS

SANDWICH BUNS
Hot dog or hamburger, whole wheat	114	2	0	0	22	3	-	206
Hot dog or hamburger, white	110	2	0	0	21	1	3	220
Reduced cal	84	1	0	0	18	3	-	190
Hoagie/submarine, small, 2.3 oz	173	3	1	0	33	5	-	311
Large, 4.8 oz	359	6	1	0	69	10	-	645
Hot dog, foot long	258	6	2	1	43	3	-	448

BRANDS ...
MIX *(1 BUN UNLESS NOTED)*

Atkins Bun Mix	26	0	0	0	4	3	0	94

READY-TO-EAT *(1 BUN UNLESS NOTED)*

Arnold Everything Sandwich	190	6	1	0	29	2	7	150
Brownberry Wheat Hot Dog	110	2	0	0	21	1	3	180
Countrys Delight Hamburger, Family Pack	100	2	0	0	18	0	3	190
Food for Life								
Hamburger or Hot Dog (avg)	150	3	0	0	28	5	2	140
Sprouted Ezekiel Hamburger or Hot Dog (avg)	170	2	0	0	34	6	0	170
Sprouted Ezekiel Sesame Hamburger	170	2	0	0	32	5	0	180
Giant Egg	150	3	0	20	28	1	3	135
Martin Potato Rolls, Long	140	2	1	0	24	3	4	190
Natural Ovens Better Buns, Wheat	140	2	0	0	31	7	5	160
Rosen Hamburger w/Sesame Seeds	130	2	0	0	25	1	4	170
Schmidts Sandwich Rolls or Potato Rolls, Long	140	1	0	0	28	2	5	190
Wenner Onion Swirl	150	3	0	20	29	1	4	135

CROISSANTS & ROLLS
Dinner roll, whole wheat, 1 oz	74	1	0	0	14	2	-	134
Brown & serve, 1 oz	84	2	0	0	14	1	-	146
Rye, 1 oz	80	1	0	0	15	1	-	250
Kaiser roll, 1 oz	83	1	0	0	15	1	-	154
French roll, 1 oz	79	1	0	0	14	1	-	173
Croissant, plain, 1 oz	116	6	4	19	13	1	-	212

27

Food	Cal	Fat	Sat	Chol	Carb	Fib	Sug	Sod
CROISSANTS AND ROLLS								
BRANDS . . .								
FROZEN/REFRIGERATED (*1 ROLL UNLESS NOTED*)								
Countrys Delight Crescent	100	6	2	0	11	0	2	150
Brown 'n Serve	80	2	1	0	13	0	1	150
Rhodes White Roll, 1.3 oz	100	2	0	0	17	0	2	140
Rich's Enriched Homestyle Roll, 1	75	2	1	0	14	1	2	140
MIX								
Pillsbury Hot Roll Mix, 1.1 oz	130	1	0	0	21	1	2	200
READY-TO-EAT (*1 ROLL UNLESS NOTED*)								
Arnold Sweet Hawaiian Dinner	110	2	0	0	20	1	6	150
Awrey's Butter Croissant, 1 oz	110	6	4	15	12	0	2	140
Baldwin Hill Organic French	80	0	0	0	18	2	1	85
Giant Mini Egg Twist	90	2	0	10	15	1	2	80
Egg Twist	160	3	0	20	29	1	4	150
King's Hawaiian (avg)	90	2	1	10	15	1	4	80
Martin Potato Rolls	90	1	0	0	17	2	3	120
Potato Rolls, Sliced	100	2	0	0	15	1	3	140
*Natural Ovens Dinner	70	1	0	0	15	4	3	70
Gourmet Dinner	45	1	0	0	15	2	0	140
Wonder Brown N Serve	80	2	1	0	13	0	1	150

SWEET ROLLS (*see Pastries & Coffeecakes, pg 81*)

(COFFEECAKES) ───────────────────────────────

(*see Pastries & Coffeecakes, pg 81*)

(ENGLISH MUFFINS) ─────────────────────────────

Cinnamon-raisin, 2 oz	139	2	0	0	28	2	8	255
Mixed-grain or granola, 2.4 oz	155	1	0	0	31	2	3	275
Plain, 2 oz	134	1	0	0	25	1	2	290
Whole wheat, 2.4 oz	134	1	0	0	27	1	3	420
BRANDS . . . (*1 MUFFIN UNLESS NOTED*)								
Giant Light	90	0	0	0	22	5	1	170
Poi, 2.5 oz	150	0	0	0	32	1	3	210
Thomas Cinnamon Raisin, 1	140	1	0	0	30	1	8	170
Sourdough, 1	120	1	0	0	25	1	2	190
Honey Wheat, 1	110	1	0	0	24	3	2	190
Plain, 1	120	1	0	0	25	1	1	200
*Wolferman's Wild Maine Blueberry	130	1	0	0	28	1	7	170
Cinnamon Raisin	130	1	0	0	29	1	9	180

Food	Cal	Fat	Sat	Chol	Carb	Fib	Sug	Sod

MUFFINS & SCONES

(also see Snack Cakes, Pies & Sweet Snacks, pg 86)

MUFFINS

Food	Cal	Fat	Sat	Chol	Carb	Fib	Sug	Sod
Blueberry muffin, ready-to-eat, 2 oz	158	4	1	17	27	2	-	255
Mix, 2 oz	208	6	2	0	36	0	-	310
Wheat bran muffin, mix, 2 oz	225	7	2	0	41	-	-	397
Corn muffin, mix, prep, 2 oz	182	6	2	35	28	1	-	451

BRANDS . . .

FROZEN/REFRIGERATED *(1.5 OZ UNLESS NOTED)*

Food	Cal	Fat	Sat	Chol	Carb	Fib	Sug	Sod
Awrey's Corn	180	9	2	30	22	0	10	120
Blueberry or Apple/Cranberry Nut	140	7	2	30	18	0	8	125
Banana Nut	170	9	2	30	20	0	10	135

MIX *(1 MUFFIN UNLESS NOTED)*

Food	Cal	Fat	Sat	Chol	Carb	Fib	Sug	Sod
*Atkins Banana Nut	70	2	0	0	6	4	0	135
Corn	60	5	1	0	7	4	0	150
Blueberry	60	5	1	0	9	6	0	160
Lemon Poppy	60	5	1	0	7	4	0	160
Orange Cranberry	60	5	1	0	7	4	0	170
*Authentic Foods Blueberry	140	1	0	0	23	2	3	200
*Bernard Corn	150	2	1	0	31	1	0	20
Betty Crocker Sweet Rewards, Wild Blueberry	110	0	0	0	26	0	14	190
Bob's Red Mill Stone Ground Spice Apple Bran	70	1	0	0	14	0	1	170
*Carbsense, 1.3 oz	120	4	0	0	16	12	0	120
Duncan Hines Bakery Style Blueberry	170	5	1	0	30	0	17	200
Entenmann's Little Bites, Blueberry Mini Muffins, 1.8 oz (4)	95	4	1	15	13	1	8	90
Estee Oat Bran	100	4	0	0	15	-	-	65
*Food for Life Carrot	190	8	1	35	27	1	11	100
*Gluten-Free Pantry Muffin & Scone	100	0	0	0	24	0	7	120
Hodgson Mill Bran, 1/4 cup mix	130	1	0	0	27	3	5	150
Krusteaz Cornbread w/Honey	110	3	1	0	20	1	6	190
*Pantry Shelf								
Cinnamon Fudge, 1.5 oz	150	0	0	0	34	1	21	55
Gingerbread, 1.5 oz	200	0	0	0	48	1	28	95
Pillsbury Blueberry	180	5	2	5	30	0	17	180

READY-TO-EAT *(2 OZ UNLESS NOTED)*

Food	Cal	Fat	Sat	Chol	Carb	Fib	Sug	Sod
*Isabella's Corn	120	0	0	0	27	2	13	80
Chocolate	110	0	0	0	25	3	14	85
Blueberry or Banana Crunch	120	0	0	0	25	2	15	95

29

BREAD, ROLLS & BREAD PRODUCTS
Pita & Pocket Breads

Food	Cal	Fat	Sat	Chol	Carb	Fib	Sug	Sod
MUFFINS AND SCONES								
*Muffin Delight Mini, Sugar Free,								
1 oz (avg)	35	1	0	0	7	0	0	60
*Natural Ovens Raisin Bran LF, 1	130	1	0	0	36	4	10	150
*Our Daily Muffin, 2.8 oz (avg)	120	0	0	0	31	9	16	140
SCONES								
Scone, 1	170	9	2	0	20	1	4	410
BRANDS . . .								
MIX *(1 SCONE UNLESS NOTED)*								
*Bette's Diner Raisin	229	0	0	0	30	1	9	129
*'Cause You're Special English	87	0	0	0	21	1	3	71
*Gluten-Free Pantry Muffin & Scone	100	0	0	0	24	0	7	120
*Lollipop Tree Scones								
Traditional English	140	0	0	0	30	1	6	85
Lemon Poppy Seed	140	1	0	0	30	1	8	135
Apricot Cranberry	130	0	0	0	30	1	10	140
Martha's Cranberry Orange	110	1	0	0	29	1	6	120
Seattle Scone Girl	123	6	4	23	15	0	5	202
READY-TO-EAT *(1 SCONE UNLESS NOTED)*								
Health Valley Scones, all	180	0	0	0	43	5	18	190

PITA & POCKET BREADS

Food	Cal	Fat	Sat	Chol	Carb	Fib	Sug	Sod
Whole Wheat pita, small 4" diam, 1	74	1	0	0	15	2	1	149
Large, 6.5" diam, 1	170	2	0	0	35	5	1	340
BRANDS . . . *(1 PITA UNLESS NOTED)*								
Food for Life Pocket, all, 1.7 oz (avg)	100	1	0	0	21	4	1	120
*Garden of Eatin'								
Bible Bread, LS Pita	160	2	0	0	30	1	1	30
Bible Bread, Whole Wheat Pita	160	2	0	0	31	2	1	115
Giant White Pita, Mini, SF, 2	150	0	0	0	32	1	2	0
White Pita	110	0	0	0	24	1	2	110
Kangaroo Honey & Wheat Pita	90	0	0	0	18	2	1	125
King of Pita Gyros, 3.3 oz	250	4	0	0	45	5	6	110
Trader Joe's Sausage & Hot Dog								
Pita Pockets	90	0	0	0	20	1	0	140
Wenner Onion Pockets	150	2	0	20	25	1	4	130

ROLLS

(see Croissants & Rolls, pg 27)

Food	Cal	Fat	Sat	Chol	Carb	Fib	Sug	Sod

BREAKFAST PRODUCTS

BREAKFAST DRINKS

(also see Diet & Nutritional Drinks, pg 88)

Vanilla drink:

Food	Cal	Fat	Sat	Chol	Carb	Fib	Sug	Sod
Mix, no sugar added, 1 envl	70	0	0	5	12	0	8	80
Mix, 1 envl	220	0	0	5	27	0	17	95
Ready-to-drink, 8 fl oz	220	3	1	10	31	0	29	180

Chocolate drink:

Food	Cal	Fat	Sat	Chol	Carb	Fib	Sug	Sod
Mix, no sugar added, 1 envl	70	1	1	5	12	1	6	95
Mix, 1 envl	220	1	1	5	28	1	20	100
Ready-to-drink, 8 fl oz	220	3	1	10	37	2	34	230
Strawberry drink, mix, 1 envl	130	0	0	5	27	0	19	160

BRANDS . . .
Most brands are within the generic range.

CEREAL, GRANOLA & BREAKFAST BARS

Food	Cal	Fat	Sat	Chol	Carb	Fib	Sug	Sod
Cereal bar, 1 oz	140	3	1	0	27	2	13	110
Granola bar, soft, plain, 1 oz	124	5	2	0	19	1	-	78
Peanut butter, choc coated, 1 oz	144	9	5	3	15	1	-	55
Choc chip, choc coated, 1 oz	130	7	4	1	18	1	-	56
Choc chip, 1 oz	118	5	3	0	19	1	-	76
Peanut butter, 1 oz	119	4	1	0	18	1	-	115
Granola bar, hard, plain, 1 oz	132	6	1	0	18	1	12	82
Peanut, 1 oz	136	6	1	0	18	1	-	79
Peanut butter, 1 oz	135	7	1	0	18	1	-	80
Choc chip, 1 oz	124	5	3	0	20	1	-	98

BRANDS . . . *(1 OZ BAR UNLESS NOTED)*
There are many low-sodium cereal and granola bars, the following have less than 95mg per serving.

Barbara's Bakery

Granola Bars, 0.8 oz:

Food	Cal	Fat	Sat	Chol	Carb	Fib	Sug	Sod
Peanut Butter or Cinnamon & Raisin (avg)	80	2	0	0	16	3	7	5
Oats 'n' Honey or Carob Chip (avg)	80	2	0	0	16	3	7	5
Cereal Bars, all, 1.3 oz	110	2	0	0	27	2	11	75

Breadshop Granola Bars

Food	Cal	Fat	Sat	Chol	Carb	Fib	Sug	Sod
Blueberry 'n Cream or Raspberry & Cream, 1.8 oz	220	8	1	0	32	4	7	0
Crunchy Oat Bran, 1.8 oz	210	9	1	0	31	5	9	0

31

BREAKFAST PRODUCTS
Cereal, Granola & Breakfast Bars

Food	Cal	Fat	Sat	Chol	Carb	Fib	Sug	Sod
CEREAL, GRANOLA AND BREAKFAST BARS								
Carnation Chewy Choc Chip, 1.3 oz.	150	6	3	0	22	0	10	80
Chewy Peanut Butter Choc Chip, 1.3 oz	140	5	2	0	21	0	9	90
Entenmann's Multi-Grain, 1.3 oz	140	3	1	0	25	1	15	90
Giant Fruit & Grain, all, 1.3 oz	140	3	1	0	27	13	1	60
Chewy Choc Chip	120	4	2	0	21	1	9	70
LF Chewy Granola Choc Chunk	110	2	1	0	22	1	10	80
Health Valley Moist & Chewy								
Granola, Berry, 1.5 oz	100	1	0	0	22	2	10	5
FF Fruit or FF Granola, all, 1.5 oz (avg)	140	0	0	0	35	3	14	10
Moist & Chewy Granola, Apple,1.5 oz	100	1	0	0	22	2	12	15
FF Marshmallow, all, 1.5 oz (avg)	100	0	0	0	24	1	11	20
Breakfast Bakes, FF, all, 1.5 oz	110	0	0	0	26	3	13	25
LF Cereal, all, 1.5 oz (avg)	130	2	0	0	27	1	13	50
Cobbler Bars, FF, all, 1.3 oz	130	2	0	0	27	1	13	50
Cafe Creations Pastry, 1.4 oz (avg)	130	3	0	0	27	2	17	70
Kellogg's								
Fruit Loops Cereal & Milk, 0.8 oz	100	3	2	0	16	1	10	75
Rice Krispies Treats:								
Double Choclatey Chunk, 0.8 oz	100	4	2	0	15	1	9	75
Rainbow, 0.8 oz	100	3	1	0	17	0	9	85
Frosted Flakes Cereal & Milk, 0.9 oz	110	3	3	0	19	1	11	90
Kudos Choc Chip	130	5	3	0	20	1	13	85
Peanut Butter	130	6	2	0	18	1	13	90
Nature's Choice, all, 0.7 oz (avg)	120	2	0	0	25	2	13	65
Nutri-Grain Twists, Cappuccino &								
Creme, 1.3 oz	140	3	1	0	26	1	15	90
Quaker								
Chewy Granola Bars:								
Trail Mix, 1.3 oz	150	5	1	0	24	2	13	55
Choc Chip or Nestle Crunch (avg)	120	4	2	0	21	1	10	70
Oatmeal Raisin, LF	110	2	1	0	22	1	10	70
Butterfinger	120	3	1	0	22	1	10	75
Cookies & Cream or S'mores (avg)	110	3	1	0	22	1	10	80
Choc Chunk	110	2	1	0	22	1	10	80
Wholesome Favorites, Cinnamon								
Sugar or Oatmeal Raisin	110	2	1	0	22	1	9	65
Chewy Graham Slam, Choc Chip	110	2	1	0	22	1	10	75
Chewy Dipps, Choc Fudge or								
Caramel Nut, 1.1 oz	140	6	4	0	21	1	10	80
Fruit & Oatmeal Bites, Apple Crisp,								
1.1 oz	140	3	0	0	27	1	15	85
Sunbelt, most, 1.5 oz (avg)	120	5	2	0	19	1	9	65

32

Food	Cal	Fat	Sat	Chol	Carb	Fib	Sug	Sod

CEREALS

HOT CEREAL

Food	Cal	Fat	Sat	Chol	Carb	Fib	Sug	Sod
Farina, cooked w/o salt, 1 cup	117	0	0	0	25	3	0	0
Oat cereal, reg or quick, cooked, 1 cup	145	2	0	0	25	4	1	1
Instant, flavored, cooked, 1 cup	138	2	0	0	24	4	15	377
Rice cereal, cooked, 1 cup	127	0	0	0	28	0	0	2
Wheat cereal, reg, cooked, 1 cup	133	0	0	0	28	2	0	3
Instant, cooked, 1 serv	130	0	0	0	30	1	14	210
Grits, instant, cooked, 1 serv	100	0	0	0	22	1	0	300

BRANDS . . .

INSTANT

Food	Cal	Fat	Sat	Chol	Carb	Fib	Sug	Sod
Mother's Instant, all, 1 cup	150	3	1	0	27	4	1	0
Stone-Buhr 7-Grain, 1/3 cup	140	2	0	0	31	7	0	0

REGULAR/COOKED

Most brands are within the generic range.

READY-TO-EAT CEREAL

Food	Cal	Fat	Sat	Chol	Carb	Fib	Sug	Sod
Puffed rice, 1 cup	56	0	0	0	13	0	0	0
Puffed wheat, 1 cup	44	0	0	0	10	1	0	1
Granola, LF, 2/3 cup	210	3	0	0	44	3	13	150
Crispy rice, 1 cup	111	0	0	0	25	0	3	206
Bran flakes, 3/4 cup	100	1	0	0	24	5	5	210
Corn flakes, 1 cup	110	0	0	0	26	1	2	330
Wheat & barley, 1/2 cup	210	1	0	0	47	5	5	340
Bran & raisins, 1 cup	190	1	0	0	46	8	13	360

BRANDS . . . *(1 CUP UNLESS NOTED)*

There are many low-sodium ready-to-eat cereals, the following have less than 65mg per serving.

Food	Cal	Fat	Sat	Chol	Carb	Fib	Sug	Sod
Alpen Swiss Style, LF, NSA, 2 oz	200	3	0	0	40	4	7	30
American Prairie Museli, 1/2 cup (avg)	210	3	1	0	37	6	10	15
*Arrowhead Mills Amaranth Flakes	130	2	0	0	25	3	3	0
Nature-O's, Buckwheat, Oat, or Wheat (avg)	130	2	1	0	24	3	1	5
*Atkins Nutlettes To Go, 1/3 cup	133	2	0	0	12	7	6	43
Back to Nature Granola, 1/2 cup (avg)	170	3	1	0	34	4	11	10
The Baker Forest Berry Muesli	340	5	1	0	64	7	20	0
Nut & Berry Muesli	380	12	2	0	54	8	12	0
Honey Crunch Muesli	290	13	2	0	59	9	15	0
*Barbara's Shredded Wheat, 2 biscuits	140	1	0	0	31	5	0	0
Honey Crunch Stars	110	1	0	0	26	2	5	55

BREAKFAST PRODUCTS
Cereals

Food	Cal	Fat	Sat	Chol	Carb	Fib	Sug	Sod
CEREAL								
*Breadshop								
Granola, most, 1/2 cup (avg)	220	8	1	0	32	4	7	0
Triple Berry Crunch, 2/3 cup	220	7	0	0	36	4	9	35
Granola, Pralines 'n Cream or Mocha								
Almond Crunch, 1/2 cup	210	7	0	0	34	4	8	40
Sierra Crunch Museli, 3/4 cup	190	3	1	0	38	3	10	60
Butte Creek Mill Ten Grain High Fiber,								
1/4 cup	100	1	0	0	20	4	0	0
*Ener-G Crisp Rice, 1.7 oz	183	2	1	0	40	0	3	5
*Erewhon Banana O's, Crispy Brown								
Rice, or Super O's (avg)	110	0	0	0	24	4	1	10
Natural Corn Flakes or Kamut								
Flakes, 3/4 cup (avg)	100	0	0	0	22	2	1	55
Galaxy or Raisin Grahams, 3/4 cup	100	0	0	0	22	2	1	55
Perfect Harvest Multigrain	140	2	0	0	25	5	2	60
Estee Corn Flakes, 1 oz	90	0	0	0	24	4	0	50
*Grainfields Corn Flakes or Crispy								
Rice, LS, low sugar	110	0	0	0	26	0	1	20
Health Valley, all, 1 oz (avg)	100	0	0	0	24	4	5	10
Kashi Heart to Heart or Honey								
Puffed (avg)	120	1	0	0	25	2	7	6
Go Lean, 3/4 cup	120	1	0	0	28	10	7	35
Medley, 1/2 cup	100	1	0	0	20	2	5	50
Kellogg's Mini-Wheats, 2 oz (avg)	190	1	0	0	41	5	10	5
Smacks, 1 oz	100	1	0	0	24	1	15	50
*LifeStream								
Multigrain Honey Puffs, 3/4 cup	120	3	0	0	24	3	12	0
8 Grain Synergy, 3/4 cup	130	1	0	0	27	5	3	12
Malt-O-Meal Puffed, all, 1 oz (avg)	100	0	0	0	25	1	15	40
Michaelene's Gourmet Granola, 1 oz								
(avg)	103	2	0	0	18	3	5	11
Nabisco Apple Fruit Wheats, 1 oz	90	0	0	0	23	3	-	15
*Natural Ovens Great Granola, 1/4 cup	110	4	0	0	18	5	3	10
*Nature's Path								
Puffed Cereals, 1 cup (avg)	55	0	0	0	12	1	0	0
Organic Ginger Zing Granola, 2/3 cup	270	11	1	0	37	4	12	25
Organic Hemp Plus Granola, 2/3 cup	260	9	1	0	37	7	11	38
Multigrain Oatbran Flakes, 2/3 cup	110	1	0	0	24	3	3	40
Organic Soy Plus Granola	260	9	1	0	38	3	11	50
Kamut Crisp, 3/4 cup	115	1	0	0	23	2	3	53
Northern Gold Cashews & Raisins								
Granola, 1/2 cup	240	8	1	0	38	5	11	5

Food	Cal	Fat	Sat	Chol	Carb	Fib	Sug	Sod
CEREAL								
Nu-World Foods Cinnamon Snaps ..	145	2	0	0	26	4	6	1
Cocoa Cereal Snaps	128	2	0	0	25	4	7	2
Berry Delicious Puffed	91	1	0	0	16	3	2	9
Post Shredded Wheat, 1 oz	96	0	0	0	23	3	3	0
Shredded Wheat 'N Bran, 2 oz	200	1	0	0	48	8	1	0
Frosted Shredded Wheat, Bite Size, 2 oz.	190	1	0	0	44	5	12	10
Golden Crisp, 1 oz	110	0	0	0	25	0	15	40
Quaker 100% Natural Granola, Oats,								
Honey & Raisins, 1/2 cup	220	9	4	0	31	3	13	0
Puffed Rice or Wheat	50	0	0	0	12	0	0	0
Sun Country Granola/Almonds, 1/2 cup	266	10	1	0	38	3	12	19
Soy-N-Ergy, all, 3/4 cup	120	2	0	0	19	3	4	40
Trader Joe's Soy Granola	220	3	1	0	39	4	15	0
Soy Oat Flakes, 3/4 cup	110	1	0	0	22	3	6	0
Oat Bran Flakes w/Raisins	200	1	0	0	45	5	15	20
Whole Foods Market 365								
Honey Puffed Wheat, 3/4 cup	130	3	0	0	25	2	11	0

FRENCH TOAST

French toast, 2.1 oz pc	126	4	1	48	19	1	-	292

BRANDS . . .
No low-sodium alternatives

FRENCH TOAST MEALS *(see Breakfast Meals, pg 93)*

GRANOLA BARS

(see Cereal, Granola & Breakfast Bars, pg 31)

PANCAKES & WAFFLES

Pancake, plain, 4" diam, frozen, 1.3 oz	82	1	0	3	16	1	15	183
Waffle, 4" diam, frozen, 1.3 oz	88	3	1	11	14	1	13	262
Potato pancake, mix, 1 tbsp	50	0	0	0	12	1	0	270
Pancake or waffle, plain, 1.4 oz mix	130	1	0	0	28	3	4	550

BRANDS . . .

FROZEN/REFRIGERATED *(1 WAFFLE UNLESS NOTED)*

Eggo Banana Bread	95	3	1	0	15	1	3	140
Special K, FF	60	0	0	0	13	1	2	140
Buttermilk or Strawberry (avg)	100	4	1	10	15	1	2	210
Whole Wheat, LF	70	1	0	0	14	2	2	215
Van's Gourmet Original, Blueberry	79	2	0	0	12	1	2	76
Organic Blueberry or Original (avg)	101	3	0	0	17	3	3	115

BREAKFAST PRODUCTS
Pancake & Waffle Syrup

Food	Cal	Fat	Sat	Chol	Carb	Fib	Sug	Sod
PANCAKES AND WAFFLES								
MIX *(1/3 cup mix unless noted)*								
*Arrowhead Mills Pancake Mixes								
Wild Rice	140	1	0	0	30	0	-	65
Blue Corn	150	2	0	0	28	3	-	130
Oat Bran	140	2	0	0	25	6	-	160
*Atkins Quick & Easy Pancake & Waffle, 1/4 cup mix	80	2	1	5	6	3	0	120
Aunt Candice Old Fashioned, 1 pancake	64	0	0	0	15	1	0	150
*Authentic Foods Pancake & Baking, 1/4 cup mix	130	2	0	0	24	0	1	170
*'Cause You're Special Hearty Pancake-Waffle, 1 pancake	52	0	0	0	12	0	1	153
Estee, prep, 4" pancake	44	0	0	0	9	0	-	57
Featherweight, prep, 4" pancake	47	1	0	0	8	0	-	30
Krusteaz Oat Bran, LF, 1 pancake	115	2	1	0	23	2	6	190
Martha's Southern Pecan Pancake & Waffle	86	4	1	0	13	1	3	84
*Natural Ovens Pancake, 3 tbsp mix	90	1	0	0	17	4	2	75
*Orgran Apple Cinnamon, 1.4 oz	136	0	0	0	34	-	3	164
Buckwheat, 1.4 oz	160	0	0	0	30	2	1	180
*Sweet N'Low Pancake	150	0	0	0	36	1	0	20

PANCAKE & WAFFLE MEALS *(see Breakfast Meals, pg 93)*

PANCAKE & WAFFLE SYRUP

Food	Cal	Fat	Sat	Chol	Carb	Fib	Sug	Sod
Maple syrup, 1/4 cup	206	0	0	0	52	0	26	8
Fruit syrup, 1/4 cup	210	0	0	0	52	0	50	50
Pancake syrup, 1/4 cup	226	0	0	0	60	0	38	66
Sugar free, 1/4 cup	30	0	0	0	12	0	0	115
Lite, 1/4 cup	100	0	0	0	26	0	25	160
BRANDS . . . *(1/4 cup unless noted)*								
*Atkins (avg)	0	0	0	0	0	0	0	20
Featherweight, 2 tbsp	32	0	0	0	8	0	-	50
Knott's Berry Farm Fruit (avg)	100	0	0	0	25	0	25	20
New Organics, 2 tbsp	105	0	0	0	27	-	-	0
Smucker's Fruit Syrup (avg)	210	0	0	0	52	0	50	0
Spring Tree Sugar Free	30	0	0	0	11	0	0	35
*Steel's Fruit, No Sugar Added (avg)	60	0	0	0	20	0	0	20
*Wax Orchards Fruit, Fruit Sweetened (avg)	120	0	0	0	30	4	28	10

Food	Cal	Fat	Sat	Chol	Carb	Fib	Sug	Sod

TOASTER FOODS & PASTRIES

Food	Cal	Fat	Sat	Chol	Carb	Fib	Sug	Sod
Toaster pastry, fruit, frosted, 1.8 oz	200	5	1	0	37	1	16	210
Toaster hash browns, 3.5 oz	190	12	2	0	24	1	1	550

BRANDS . . .

FROZEN/REFRIGERATED (*1 SERVING UNLESS NOTED*)

Amy's Toaster Pops

Food	Cal	Fat	Sat	Chol	Carb	Fib	Sug	Sod
Apple	140	3	0	0	26	1	6	130
Strawberry	140	3	0	0	26	1	6	130

Pillsbury

Food	Cal	Fat	Sat	Chol	Carb	Fib	Sug	Sod
Toaster Strudel, Fruit, all, 1.9 oz (avg)	190	8	2	5	26	1	10	190
Toaster Strudel, Cream Cheese Strawberry	200	10	3	10	24	1	9	220
Toaster Scrambles, Cheese/Egg/ Bacon, 1.7 oz	180	12	4	25	14	0	1	360
Toaster Scrambles, Cheese/Egg/ Sausage, 1.7 oz	180	12	4	25	14	0	1	370

PACKAGED (*1 SERVING UNLESS NOTED*)

Kellogg's Pop Tarts

Frosted:

Food	Cal	Fat	Sat	Chol	Carb	Fib	Sug	Sod
Fruit, all (avg)	210	5	1	0	39	1	20	170
Brown Sugar Cinnamon	210	7	2	0	34	1	17	180
S'mores	200	6	2	0	36	1	18	200

Pastry Swirls:

Food	Cal	Fat	Sat	Chol	Carb	Fib	Sug	Sod
Strawberry	260	11	3	0	38	1	17	170
Apple Cinnamon	260	11	3	0	38	11	1	190
Cheese Danish or Cheese & Cherry	260	11	3	0	37	0	12	200

Food	Cal	Fat	Sat	Chol	Carb	Fib	Sug	Sod
Pillsbury Toaster Bagel, Strawberry & Cream Cheese, 1.7 oz	130	2	1	0	24	1	8	190

Food	Cal	Fat	Sat	Chol	Carb	Fib	Sug	Sod

CONDIMENTS & SAUCES

CAPERS

	Cal	Fat	Sat	Chol	Carb	Fib	Sug	Sod
Capers, 1 tbsp	2	0	0	0	0	0	0	255

BRANDS ...
No low-sodium alternatives.

CHUTNEYS & FRUIT RELISHES

(see Chutneys & Fruit Relishes, pg 43)

COOKING WINES

(see Wine & Champagne, pg 12)

HORSERADISH

	Cal	Fat	Sat	Chol	Carb	Fib	Sug	Sod
Horseradish, 1 tsp	22	3	0	3	1	0	0	50
BRANDS ... *(1 TSP UNLESS NOTED)*								
Beano's	19	2	0	0	1	0	0	28
Beaver Cream Style	10	1	0	0	1	0	0	20
Boar's Head	45	0	0	0	0	0	0	30
Heluva Good	0	0	0	0	0	0	0	6
Inglehoffer Thick & Creamy	10	1	0	0	0	0	0	15
Kraft	20	2	0	5	1	0	1	35
Reese Prepared	0	0	0	0	1	0	0	40
Tulkoff Extra Hot	0	0	0	0	1	0	0	40

JAMS, JELLIES & FRUIT SPREADS

	Cal	Fat	Sat	Chol	Carb	Fib	Sug	Sod
Jam or jelly, 1 tbsp	56	0	0	0	14	0	10	6
Fruit butter, 1 tbsp	40	0	0	0	10	0	9	10

BRANDS ...
Most brands are within the generic range.

KETCHUP

	Cal	Fat	Sat	Chol	Carb	Fib	Sug	Sod
Ketchup, 1 tbsp	16	0	0	0	4	0	4	178
BRANDS ... *(1 TBSP UNLESS NOTED)*								
*Chef Allen Mango	20	0	0	0	5	0	4	25
Estee Imitation, SF	15	0	0	0	3	0	2	0
Hain Natural NSA	16	0	0	0	4	0	-	5
Heinz NSA	20	0	0	0	5	0	4	0
Hunt's NSA	15	0	0	0	3	0	4	6

Food	Cal	Fat	Sat	Chol	Carb	Fib	Sug	Sod
KETCHUP								
Featherweight	6	0	0	0	0	0	0	20
McIlhenny Spicy	20	0	0	0	5	0	3	115
***Steel's** Rocky Mountain	5	0	0	0	0	0	0	20
***Tree of Life**	10	0	0	0	3	0	3	25
***Westbrae Natural**								
Fruit Sweetened, NSA	10	0	0	0	3	0	2	5
Unsweetened Un-Ketchup	5	0	0	0	1	0	0	60

MARASCHINO CHERRIES

	Cal	Fat	Sat	Chol	Carb	Fib	Sug	Sod
Cherries, 1	10	0	0	0	2	0	1	0

BRANDS . . .

Most brands are within the generic range.

MAYONNAISE & SANDWICH SPREADS

	Cal	Fat	Sat	Chol	Carb	Fib	Sug	Sod
Mayonnaise, 1 tbsp	100	11	2	5	0	0	0	80
Light, 1 tbsp	50	5	1	5	1	0	0	120
FF, 1 tbsp	10	0	0	0	2	0	1	120
Mayonnaise-type salad dressing, 1 tbsp	60	6	1	5	2	0	1	100
Light, 1 tbsp	35	3	0	5	2	0	2	130
Sandwich Spread, 1 tbsp	50	5	1	5	2	0	2	180

BRANDS . . .

MAYONNAISE AND MAYONNAISE-TYPE DRESSINGS (1 TBSP UNLESS NOTED)

	Cal	Fat	Sat	Chol	Carb	Fib	Sug	Sod
Arise Cajun Mayo	100	11	2	10	0	0	0	65
Duke's	100	12	-	-	0	-	0	75
Featherweight Soyamaise	100	1	0	5	0	0	0	35
Hain Eggless, NSA	100	11	2	0	1	0	1	0
Hellman's Dijonnaise, 1 tsp	5	0	0	0	1	0	1	70
Nalley Light	60	6	1	10	1	0	0	95
Saffola	100	11	1	10	0	0	0	70
Spectrum Lite Canola	35	3	0	0	1	0	0	60
Organic	100	11	2	5	0	0	0	90
Trader Joe's Dressing	35	3	0	0	1	0	0	75
Lemon Mayo	40	4	0	0	1	0	0	105
Roasted Garlic Mayo	35	3	0	0	1	0	0	110
Soyonaise	30	3	0	0	1	0	0	110
Weight Watchers Light, 1 tbsp	25	2	1	5	1	0	0	40
FF	10	0	0	0	3	0	2	105
Whole Foods Market 365	110	12	1	10	0	0	0	85

SANDWICH SPREADS (1 TBSP UNLESS NOTED)

	Cal	Fat	Sat	Chol	Carb	Fib	Sug	Sod
Beano's All American	50	4	1	5	3	0	2	105
Kroger	50	4	1	5	3	1	2	125

Food	Cal	Fat	Sat	Chol	Carb	Fib	Sug	Sod
MUSTARD								
Yellow mustard, 1 tsp	3	0	0	0	0	0	0	56
Dijon-type mustard, 1 tsp	5	0	0	0	0	0	0	120
BRANDS . . . *(1 TSP UNLESS NOTED)*								
Bee Maid Honey, Hot N' Spicy	20	0	0	0	5	0	4	10
Boar's Head Honey	10	0	0	0	2	0	1	25
*Brad's Gourmet Spicy	20	1	0	0	2	0	0	0
Zesty Pretzel Dip	10	0	0	0	2	0	0	0
East Shore, all	15	0	0	0	2	0	0	0
Featherweight Yellow	0	0	0	0	0	0	0	0
Grey Poupon Honey Dijon	10	0	0	0	2	0	2	5
Hain Stone Ground NSA	14	1	0	0	1	0	0	10
Haus Barkyte Sweet & Sour	15	0	0	0	3	0	3	20
Hickory Farms Honey	15	0	0	0	2	0	2	15
HoneyCup Uniquely Sharp or Stone Ground	15	1	0	0	3	0	1	0
Inglehoffer Sweet Hot Mustard	15	1	0	0	2	0	0	30
Plochman's Honey Dijon	3	0	0	0	1	0	1	0
*Westbrae Natural Stone Ground NSA	0	0	0	0	0	0	0	0
NUT BUTTERS								
Tahini, 2 tbsp	178	16	2	0	6	2	0	34
Almond butter, 2 tbsp	203	19	2	0	7	1	0	144
Peanut butter, 2 tbsp	200	16	3	0	7	2	3	150
Cashew butter, 2 tbsp	188	16	3	0	9	1	2	196
BRANDS . . .								
PEANUT BUTTER *(2 TBSP UNLESS NOTED)*								
Adams Natural, Unsalted	200	16	3	0	7	2	2	5
*Arrowhead Mills								
Creamy or Crunchy	200	15	3	0	6	1	1	0
*Atkins Nut Butter	230	24	4	0	3	0	1	0
Crazy Richard's Natural Creamy	200	17	-	0	6	-	2	0
Eastwind, all (avg)	200	15	3	0	9	2	3	10
Estee SF	180	16	3	0	6	2	2	0
*Fifty50, No Sugar Added	220	18	4	0	6	2	2	15
Hollywood Unsalted	70	6	0	0	2	2	-	0
Kettle Chips Organic	166	14	2	0	5	0	0	2
North Farm, all (avg)	180	15	3	0	5	2	2	5
Peter Pan LS	190	17	3	0	5	2	2	10
Simply Jif	190	16	3	0	6	2	2	65
Smucker's Natural NSA	200	16	3	0	6	0	2	10

Food	Cal	Fat	Sat	Chol	Carb	Fib	Sug	Sod
OTHER NUT BUTTERS *(2 TBSP UNLESS NOTED)*								
Marantha Tahini	190	16	2	0	9	3	0	5
Cashew	190	15	3	0	11	2	2	5
Almond, Unsalted	220	18	1	0	6	3	0	20
Nutella	200	11	2	0	23	2	20	15
*Peanut Wonder Choc, 85% Less Fat	100	2	0	0	17	1	10	35
Seed Butters Sesame or Hazelnut (avg)	164	14	2	0	5	0	0	2

OLIVES

Food	Cal	Fat	Sat	Chol	Carb	Fib	Sug	Sod
Black, small, 0.5 oz	25	3	0	0	1	0	0	115
Kalamata, 0.5 oz	35	3	0	0	1	0	0	220
BRANDS . . . *(0.5 OZ UNLESS NOTED)*								
Black Pearl Black	23	2	0	0	1	0	0	88
Kalamata Gold Organic Kalamata	45	4	1	0	2	0	0	100

PATÉS & SPREADS

(also see Cream Cheese Spreads, pg 60 and Sandwich Spreads, pg 131)

Food	Cal	Fat	Sat	Chol	Carb	Fib	Sug	Sod
Chicken liver paté, 1 oz	57	4	1	111	2	0	0	109
Goose liver paté, smoked, 1 oz	131	12	4	43	1	0	0	198
BRANDS . . .								
MIX *(1 TSP MIX UNLESS NOTED)*								
*The Original Bagel Spreads (avg)	10	0	0	0	3	0	1	10
READY-TO-EAT *(1 OZ UNLESS NOTED)*								
Bonavita Vegetarian Paté	60	4	0	0	4	0	0	140
Cowboy Vegetable Caviar								
Red Bell Pepper, 1 tbsp	10	1	0	0	2	0	1	100
Black Olive, 1 tbsp	10	1	0	0	2	0	0	110
California Caponata, 1 tbsp	10	1	0	0	2	0	1	125
Loma Linda Bean & Peanut Spread	40	2	1	0	4	2	0	130
Native South Black-Eyed Pea Paté	19	0	0	0	4	0	0	88
Oasis Hommus, Mediterranean Medley	180	0	0	3	1	0	37	
Baba Ghannouj	31	2	0	0	3	1	0	73
Hommus, Roasted Garlic, Spinach, or Roasted Red Pepper (avg)	32	1	0	0	4	1	0	76
Hommus Spread, Original	34	1	0	0	4	1	0	81
Sabra Vegetarian Liver	70	7	1	14	1	1	1	87
Simcha Classic Bruschetta, 2 oz	10	0	0	0	2	1	1	75
Tartex Patés, 0.9 oz								
Olive	59	5	3	0	2	1	0	110
Herb Meadow or Original Veg	57	5	1	0	2	1	0	125
Mushroom Veg	58	5	1	0	2	1	0	130
Pesto Veg	45	4	3	0	2	1	0	140

CONDIMENTS & SAUCES
Pickled Vegetables

Food	Cal	Fat	Sat	Chol	Carb	Fib	Sug	Sod
PATÉS AND SPEADS								
*Walden Farms Bruschetta Pesto, 1 tsp	10	1	0	0	0	0	0	20
Bruschetta Original, 1 tsp	35	3	0	0	0	0	0	90

PICKLED VEGETABLES

(also see Chili Peppers, pg 111)

Food	Cal	Fat	Sat	Chol	Carb	Fib	Sug	Sod
Giardiniera, 1/4 cup	5	0	0	0	0	0	1	170
Cocktail onions, 0.5 oz	5	0	0	0	0	0	0	220
Hot banana peppers, 1 oz	5	0	0	0	1	1	0	378
Jalapeños, 1 oz	18	0	0	0	4	0	0	441
Pepperoncini, 1 oz	8	0	0	0	2	1	0	453
Red peppers, 1 oz	10	0	0	0	2	1	0	480
BRANDS . . . *(1 OZ UNLESS NOTED)*								
Aunt Nellie's Sliced Pickled Peppers .	15	0	0	0	4	0	4	56
B&G Hot Chopped Sandwich Peppers,								
1 tbsp..	5	0	0	0	1	0	1	120
Gaea Roasted Red Peppers, 1/2 cup ...	10	0	0	0	2	0	1	120

PICKLES

Food	Cal	Fat	Sat	Chol	Carb	Fib	Sug	Sod
Bread & butter pickles, 1 oz	17	0	0	0	4	0	4	106
Sweet pickles, 1 oz	33	0	0	0	9	0	9	263
Dill pickles, 1 oz	5	0	0	0	1	0	0	359
BRANDS . . .								
BREAD AND BUTTER PICKLES								
Most brands are within the generic range.								
DILL PICKLES *(1 OZ UNLESS NOTED)*								
Ba Tampte Half Sour	0	0	0	0	1	0	0	135
*Cascadian Farm Kosher Dill, LS	5	0	0	0	1	0	0	135
Featherweight Dill, Whole, 1 pc	4	0	0	0	1	0	0	5
SWEET PICKLES *(1 OZ UNLESS NOTED)*								
Carrara Sweet Baby Gherkins	25	0	0	0	11	0	11	25
Farman's Sweet	25	0	0	0	7	0	7	70
Sweet Gherkins	30	0	0	0	7	0	7	90
Featherweight Sweet, Sliced, 3.5 pcs	24	0	0	0	6	0	6	5
Giant Sweet Spears...........................	15	0	0	0	4	0	4	120
Heinz Sweet Gherkins	23	0	0	0	5	0	5	129
Sweet Cucumber Stix......................	25	0	0	0	6	0	4	150
Mt Olive Sweet, Sweet Gerkins, or								
Midgets..	35	0	0	0	8	0	7	100
Sweet Cucumber Strips	20	0	0	0	6	0	4	105

PICKLE RELISH *(see Pickle Relishes, pg 43)*

Food	Cal	Fat	Sat	Chol	Carb	Fib	Sug	Sod

PIMIENTO

Food	Cal	Fat	Sat	Chol	Carb	Fib	Sug	Sod
Pimiento, 1 oz	10	0	0	0	2	0	0	5

BRANDS . . .
Most brands are within the generic range.

RELISHES

CHUTNEYS & FRUIT RELISHES

Food	Cal	Fat	Sat	Chol	Carb	Fib	Sug	Sod
Chutney, 1 tbsp	60	0	0	0	14	0	9	170

BRANDS . . . *(1 TBSP UNLESS NOTED)*

Food	Cal	Fat	Sat	Chol	Carb	Fib	Sug	Sod
American Spoon Cherry Gooseberry	35	0	0	0	10	0	9	35
Busha Browne's Banana	40	0	0	0	10	0	9	0
Crosse & Blackwell Apple Curry	100	0	0	0	7	0	5	20
Floribbean Papaya w/Rum	38	0	0	0	10	0	9	0
Fox's Fine Foods Cranberry Apple	33	0	0	0	9	0	8	0
Gloria's Depoe Bay Cranberry	50	0	0	0	14	0	-	0
Kozlowski Farms Apple Chutney	35	0	0	0	9	0	4	0
Peach Chutney	30	0	0	0	7	0	3	0
Major Grey's	60	0	0	0	14	0	9	170
Neera's, all (avg)	20	0	0	0	5	0	2	26
Prairie Thyme Raspberry Jalapeño Ambrosia or Peach Habanero	35	0	0	0	9	0	8	5
Roasted Tomato	20	0	0	0	5	0	5	38
Roland Mango	50	0	0	0	12	0	9	70
Steel's Mango Ginger	5	0	0	0	1	0	1	2
Susan's Gourmet Foods Cranberry	40	0	0	0	11	0	7	5
Tuscan Tepenade w/Sun-Dried Tomatoes	17	1	0	0	3	1	1	46
Wild Thymes Chutneys (avg)	14	0	0	0	6	0	5	0

CRANBERRY SAUCE & RELISH

Food	Cal	Fat	Sat	Chol	Carb	Fib	Sug	Sod
Cranberry sauce, whole or jellied, 1/4 cup	80	0	0	0	21	0	26	10
Cranberry/orange relish, 1/4 cup	122	0	0	0	31	0	27	22

BRANDS . . .
Most brands are within the generic range.

PICKLE RELISH

Food	Cal	Fat	Sat	Chol	Carb	Fib	Sug	Sod
Sweet pickle relish, 1 tbsp	20	0	0	0	4	0	2	125
Hamburger relish, 1 tbsp	10	0	0	0	3	0	2	180
Dill pickle relish, 1 tbsp	5	0	0	0	1	0	1	240

BRANDS . . . *(1 TBSP UNLESS NOTED)*

Food	Cal	Fat	Sat	Chol	Carb	Fib	Sug	Sod
B&G SF Sweet	20	0	0	0	5	0	4	0
Cascadian Farm Sweet Pickle	20	0	0	0	5	0	4	75
Claussen Sweet Pickle	10	0	0	0	3	0	2	85

CONDIMENTS & SAUCES
Salad Dressings

Food	Cal	Fat	Sat	Chol	Carb	Fib	Sug	Sod
PICKLE RELISH								
Farman's Sweet Pickle	15	0	0	0	3	0	2	80
Heinz Hot Dog	20	0	0	0	5	0	3	95
Sweet Relish	20	0	0	0	5	0	3	95
Mt Olive Sweet Pickle	20	0	0	0	4	0	2	80

VEGETABLE RELISHES

Food	Cal	Fat	Sat	Chol	Carb	Fib	Sug	Sod
Corn relish, 1 tbsp	20	0	0	0	5	0	2	40

BRANDS . . . *(1 TBSP UNLESS NOTED)*

Food	Cal	Fat	Sat	Chol	Carb	Fib	Sug	Sod
Best South Vidalia Sweet Onion	15	0	0	0	4	0	4	85
***Fox's Fine Foods** Pepper	23	0	0	0	6	0	5	1
***Jok 'n' Al** Tomato Relish	8	0	0	0	2	0	1	53

SALAD DRESSINGS

Food	Cal	Fat	Sat	Chol	Carb	Fib	Sug	Sod
Vinegar & oil, 2 tbsp	144	16	3	0	1	0	0	0
Thousand island dressing, 2 tbsp	120	11	2	8	5	0	5	224
LF, 2 tbsp	48	3	0	4	5	1	4	300
Italian dressing, 2 tbsp	137	14	2	0	3	0	2	231
LF, 2 tbsp	31	3	0	2	2	0	2	236
Mix, prep, 2 tbsp	140	15	2	0	2	0	2	300
FF, 2 tbsp	20	0	0	0	4	0	2	430
Zesty Italian, 2 tbsp	110	11	1	0	2	0	1	510
Buttermilk dressing, mix, prep, 2 tbsp	115	12	2	10	2	0	1	250
Russian dressing, 2 tbsp	148	15	2	5	3	0	2	260
Ranch dressing, 2 tbsp	148	16	2	8	1	0	1	287
Mix, prep, 2 tbsp	120	12	2	10	2	0	1	210
Lite, 2 tbsp	80	7	1	10	3	0	1	300
FF, 2 tbsp	50	0	0	10	11	1	2	350
Caesar dressing, 2 tbsp	110	11	2	10	1	0	0	290
FF, 2 tbsp	30	0	0	0	5	0	2	330
Blue cheese or roquefort dressing, 2 tbsp	151	16	3	3	2	0	1	328
French dressing, 2 tbsp	138	13	3	0	5	0	4	438
LF, 2 tbsp	43	2	0	0	7	0	5	252

BRANDS . . .

MIX

Bear Creek Dip & Dressing Mix

Food	Cal	Fat	Sat	Chol	Carb	Fib	Sug	Sod
Veg or Sesame Garlic, 1 tbsp	5	0	0	0	1	0	1	5
Cajun, 1 tbsp	5	0	0	0	1	0	1	25

READY-TO-USE *(2 TBSP UNLESS NOTED)*

There are many low-sodium salad dressings, the following have less than 95mg per serving.

Food	Cal	Fat	Sat	Chol	Carb	Fib	Sug	Sod
***American Spoon** Raspberry Dazzler	30	0	0	0	7	0	7	0

Food	Cal	Fat	Sat	Chol	Carb	Fib	Sug	Sod
SALAD DRESSINGS								
Anne's Original Cranberry & Honey	15	0	0	0	4	0	3	0
Lemon & Pepper	20	0	0	0	3	0	3	10
Daddy JJ's Pineapple & Ginger Dijon	15	0	0	0	3	0	1	50
Honey Mustard	25	0	0	0	6	0	5	75
Dijon & Garlic	15	0	0	0	2	0	1	80
***Annie's Naturals** Balsamic Vinaigrette	100	10	1	0	3	0	3	75
LF Raspberry Vinaigrette	35	2	0	0	5	0	4	75
Cilantro Lime Vinaigrette	100	10	1	0	2	0	2	90
Cary Randall's								
Roasted Garlic Vinaigrette	5	0	0	0	1	0	1	55
Roasted Pepper Vinaigrette	10	0	0	0	2	0	2	60
Sun-Dried Tomato	10	0	0	0	2	0	1	70
Chelton House Raspberry Vinaigrette	60	6	1	0	3	0	2	70
***Consorzio** Raspberry & Marinade,								
Mango, or Raspberry & Balsamic (avg)	24	0	0	0	6	0	4	0
***Diet Source** Italian or French,								
1 pkt (avg)	15	1	0	0	2	0	1	15
Emeril's House Herb Vinaigrette	170	19	2	0	2	0	0	40
Estee, all (avg)	5	0	0	0	1	0	0	40
The Ginger People Ginger Lemon								
Grass Dressing & Cooking	90	9	1	0	3	0	3	90
Girard's Raspberry Vinaigrette	120	10	2	0	9	0	9	65
***Gloria's** Caribbean Sunshine	45	1	0	0	9	0	0	0
Raspberry Poppyseed	140	9	0	0	16	0	0	0
Raspberry Poppyseed, Oil Free	60	0	0	0	15	0	0	0
Roasted Red Pepper Vinaigrette, LS	65	7	0	0	2	0	0	70
Island Grove Garlic Marinade/Dressing	70	7	-	-	-	-	-	5
LF Raspberry Poppy	40	3	-	-	-	-	-	40
LF Vadalia Onion	35	2	-	-	-	-	-	55
Johnny Fleeman's 3 Pepper Vinaigrette	25	3	1	0	0	0	0	3
Basil Dijon Vinaigrette	76	8	1	0	1	0	0	44
Honey Mustard	80	8	1	5	2	0	2	85
Knott's Honey Dijon	130	13	2	5	4	0	4	90
Maple Grove Farms Poppyseed, FF	50	0	0	0	11	0	8	80
Balsamic Vinaigrette, FF	10	0	0	0	2	0	2	90
Marzetti Wilde Raspberry	150	12	2	0	12	0	11	65
***Miko**, Ginger Dressings, all	70	6	-	0	4	-	-	50
***Minnesota Wild** Sweet Blackberry								
or Cranberry Peppercorn	150	15	-	0	4	0	3	0
Blueberry Poppyseed	140	14	-	0	3	0	2	35
Raspberry Balsamic	130	14	-	0	1	0	1	45

CONDIMENTS & SAUCES
Salad Toppings

Food	Cal	Fat	Sat	Chol	Carb	Fib	Sug	Sod
SALAD DRESSINGS								
Naturally Fresh Lemon Vinaigrette ...	25	0	0	0	7	1	6	0
Poppyseed	140	13	2	0	6	0	6	60
*****Olde Cape Cod** Poppyseed	80	4	0	0	11	0	10	6
Raspberry Vinaigrette	70	3	0	0	12	0	11	30
Balsamic Vinaigrette	25	0	0	0	6	0	6	60
Paula's Lemon & Dill or Lime & Cilantro	15	0	0	0	4	0	4	40
Tangerine & Mint	15	0	0	0	4	0	4	57
Orange & Basil	15	0	0	0	4	0	4	64
Honey Mustard Seed	80	6	0	0	7	0	7	70
Roasted Garlic or Toasted Onion	10	0	0	0	3	0	3	80
*****Pritikin** Zesty Italian	30	0	0	0	7	0	4	70
Raspberry Vinaigrette	35	0	0	0	11	0	9	75
*****Rising Sun Farms** Pesto Parmesan	80	7	1	0	3	0	3	65
Pesto Dried Tomato	5	0	0	0	2	0	1	75
*****Steel's** Sweet Ginger Lime	136	14	0	0	2	2	0	0
Trader Giotto's Balsamic Vinaigrette	70	6	1	0	5	0	5	60
Tree of Life Frisco's Raspberry	120	11	1	0	5	0	3	80

SALAD TOPPINGS

Food	Cal	Fat	Sat	Chol	Carb	Fib	Sug	Sod
Croutons, plain, 0.5 oz	58	1	0	0	10	1	0	100
Croutons, seasoned, 0.5 oz	66	3	1	1	9	1	0	175
Bacon bits, 1 tbsp	25	2	0	5	0	0	0	220
BRANDS . . .								
BACON BITS *(1 TBSP UNLESS NOTED)*								
Betty Crocker Bac'Os	20	1	0	0	1	0	0	80
Schilling Imitation, 1 tsp	26	0	0	0	2	0	0	51
Ultra Soy Imitation	25	1	0	0	2	1	0	105
CROUTONS *(0.5 OZ UNLESS NOTED)*								
Arnold Cheese Garlic	60	2	0	0	10	1	2	110
Seasoned	60	2	0	0	10	1	2	150
Brownberry Homestyle Caesar	60	3	0	0	8	0	0	140
Classic Seasoned	60	2	0	0	8	0	0	140
Homestyle Seasoned	60	2	0	0	10	2	0	150
Chatham Village Caesar	70	3	0	0	8	0	0	100
Devonsheer Italian	60	1	0	0	10	0	0	130
Fresh Gourmet Seasoned, all (avg)	50	3	0	0	6	0	0	110
Giant Homestyle Caesar	60	2	0	0	10	0	2	140
Seasoned	60	2	0	0	10	0	2	150
*****Heaven Sent** Onion & Garlic	26	0	0	0	20	0	0	80
Marzetti Caesar	70	3	0	0	8	0	2	100
Butter & Garlic	70	3	0	0	8	0	2	110
Cheese & Garlic	80	5	0	0	6	0	2	120

Food	Cal	Fat	Sat	Chol	Carb	Fib	Sug	Sod
CROUTONS								
Old London Toastettes								
Toasted Onion	50	2	0	0	6	0	0	100
Cheese-Garlic, Caesar, Buttermilk-Ranch, or Herb Seasoned	50	2	0	0	6	0	0	110
Osem Onion Garlic	50	2	0	0	8	0	0	45
Savion Toastettes Gourmet Round, Natural Herb Seasoning	50	2	0	0	6	0	0	130
OTHER TOPPINGS								
Durkee Salad Sensations Garden Style, 1 tbsp	35	2	0	0	3	1	1	70
McCormick Garden Veg, 1 1/3 tbsp	35	2	0	0	3	0	1	60

(SAUCES)

BBQ/GRILLING SAUCES & MARINADES *(also see Asian Sauces, pg 108)*

Food	Cal	Fat	Sat	Chol	Carb	Fib	Sug	Sod
Barbecue sauce, 2 tbsp	44	0	0	0	9	0	8	416
BRANDS . . .								
MIX *(2 TBSP UNLESS NOTED)*								
Bernard BBQ, LS, prep	40	0	0	0	10	0	6	5
READY-TO-USE *(2 TBSP UNLESS NOTED)*								
Annie Chun's Lemongrass Herb Marinade, 1 tbsp	30	2	0	0	3	0	3	38
Annie's Naturals Smokey Maple or Original	45	0	0	0	11	0	9	65
Billy Bee Honey Garlic	80	0	0	0	20	0	20	30
Blue Crab Bay Co.								
Seafood Marinade & Grilling	120	12	2	0	6	0	6	40
Bobby Flay's Glazes, 1 tbsp (avg)	40	0	0	0	11	0	11	0
Bronco Bob's Roasted Chipotle, 1 tbsp	30	0	0	0	7	0	7	40
Chef Allen Orange Chipotle, 1 tbsp	5	0	0	0	10	0	0	20
Papaya Pineapple BBQ	30	0	0	0	8	0	2	50
Key Lime Mojo Marinade, 1 tbsp	5	0	0	0	2	0	1	55
Emeril's Orange Herb w/Poppy Seeds Marinade, 1 tbsp	80	8	1	1	2	0	1	85
Roasted Veg Marinade, 1 tbsp	70	7	1	0	1	0	0	90
Enrico's, all	36	2	0	0	6	0	-	8
Figaro Liquid Smoke & Hickory Marinade, 1 tbsp	0	0	0	0	0	0	0	55
Fischer & Wieser								
Charred Pineapple Bourbon	70	0	0	0	16	0	16	0
Seville Orange Cranberry Horseradish	50	0	0	0	14	0	12	0
Mango Ginger Habanero	80	0	0	0	22	0	20	0
Hot Plum Chipotle	80	0	0	0	22	0	20	30

47

CONDIMENTS & SAUCES
Sauces - BBQ/Grilling Sauces & Marinades

Food	Cal	Fat	Sat	Chol	Carb	Fib	Sug	Sod
BBQ/GRILLING SAUCES AND MARINADES								
Fischer & Wieser *(cont'd)*								
Sweet, Sour & Smokey Mustard	60	0	0	0	12	0	12	90
Original Roasted Raspberry Chipotle	80	0	0	0	20	2	18	130
Floribbean Goombay Mango	40	0	0	0	10	0	8	5
Key Lime w/Ginger	40	0	0	0	10	0	7	5
Garlic Survival Co.								
Roasted Garlic Marinade, 1 tbsp	5	0	0	0	1	0	0	0
Garlic Lemon Marinade, 1 tbsp	5	0	0	0	1	0	0	5
Jim Beam Kentucky Bourbon	20	0	0	0	5	0	2	110
Lea & Perrins Original	50	0	0	0	13	0	11	125
Lollipop Tree Mango Garlic	60	0	0	0	14	0	13	10
Apple Chipotle	60	0	0	0	14	0	13	120
Sweet Pepper	60	0	0	0	14	0	13	135
Lum Taylor's Barbeque	110	0	0	0	27	0	27	15
Med-Diet Bar-B-Q	35	0	0	0	8	-	-	35
Mr. Spice Honey	60	0	0	0	14	0	7	0
Honey Mustard	30	0	0	0	7	0	7	0
Hot Wing	24	0	0	0	6	0	3	0
Nantucket Off-Shore, all (avg)	40	0	0	0	9	0	8	30
Natural Exotic								
Mango Ginger Marinade, 1 tbsp	0	0	0	0	6	0	6	0
Chipotle BBQ	45	0	0	0	12	0	11	125
Nellie & Joe's Key West Style								
Traditional Marinade, 1 tbsp	80	8	1	0	2	0	0	40
Oasis Foods Papaya Serrano, 1 tbsp	40	0	0	0	10	0	9	0
Honey Mango Ginger Grilling, 1 tbsp	40	0	0	0	11	0	10	0
Smokin' Sweet Mustard, 1 tbsp	10	0	0	0	2	0	2	15
Hot Plum Chipotle Grilling, 1 tbsp	50	0	0	0	13	0	13	35
Roasted Raspberry Chipotle, 1 tbsp	40	0	0	0	10	1	9	65
Olde Cape Cod								
Lemon or Oriental BBQ & Grilling	25	0	0	0	5	0	4	10
Cranberry BBQ & Grilling	70	0	0	0	18	0	17	75
Orange BBQ & Grilling	70	0	0	0	18	0	17	75
Private Harvest Mango Lime	30	0	0	0	6	1	5	95
Robbies Hot or Mild	25	0	0	0	5	0	5	30
Rustler's Pit Style	48	0	0	0	12	0	0	135
Sal's Hot Sassy	40	0	0	0	10	0	9	105
Steel's Rocky Mt BBQ	40	0	0	0	10	0	0	25
Tom Douglas Redhook Blackhook								
Porter w/Poblano Chiles & Molasses	20	0	0	0	4	0	2	60
Spicy Blonde Ale w/Jalapeño & Mango	20	1	0	0	4	0	2	100
w/ESB Smoked Chiles & Maple	20	1	0	0	6	0	4	120

Food	Cal	Fat	Sat	Chol	Carb	Fib	Sug	Sod
BBQ/GRILLING SAUCES AND MARINADES								
Uncle Fred's Tongue Slapping BBQ .	25	0	0	0	6	0	6	110
Vonn's Superior Choice All-Purpose ...	25	0	0	0	6	0	0	10
***Wax Orchards** Smokey Barbecue ..	30	0	0	0	7	1	5	60
World Harbors Acadia Maine's Lemon Pepper Garlic Marinade, 1 tbsp	18	0	0	0	4	0	4	70
Blue Mt Jamaican Style Jerk, 1 tbsp .	35	0	0	0	9	0	8	100
BEARNAISE SAUCE								
Bearnaise sauce, mix, 1 tsp	20	1	0	0	3	0	0	210
BRANDS ...								
Trader Joe's French, 1 tbsp	90	10	1	10	0	0	0	60
BROWNING & SEASONING SAUCE								
Browning & seasoning sauce, 1 tsp	15	0	0	0	3	0	0	10
BRANDS ...								
Most brands are within the generic range.								
CHEESE SAUCE								
Cheese sauce, ready-to-serve, 14 cup	110	8	4	18	4	0	0	522
Mix, prep, 1/4 cup	123	5	2	6	17	0	3	897
BRANDS ...								
MIX *(1/4 CUP PREP UNLESS NOTED)*								
***Bernard** Diet	25	1	0	0	5	0	2	70
***Med-Diet** Cheddar Cheese	20	0	0	0	3	-	-	115
READY-TO-USE								
No low-sodium alternatives.								
CLAM SAUCE								
Red clam sauce, 1/2 cup	60	1	0	10	8	1	4	350
White clam sauce, 1/2 cup	140	10	2	15	5	0	1	510
BRANDS ...								
No low-sodium alternatives.								
COCKTAIL SAUCE								
Cocktail sauce, 1 tbsp	20	0	0	0	5	0	-	210
BRANDS ... *(1 TBSP UNLESS NOTED)*								
Great Impressions LS	21	0	0	0	5	0	-	6
***Steel's**	8	0	0	0	0	0	0	40
Stokely	18	0	0	0	5	0	-	90
Uncle Dave's Kickin'	5	0	0	0	2	0	1	60
CURRY SAUCE								
Curry sauce, ready-to-use, 2 tbsp	15	1	0	0	2	0	-	144
Mix, prep w/milk, 2 tbsp	34	2	1	5	4	0	-	155

CONDIMENTS & SAUCES

Sauces - Gourmet Sauce

Food	Cal	Fat	Sat	Chol	Carb	Fib	Sug	Sod
CURRY SAUCE								
BRANDS . . . *(2 TBSP UNLESS NOTED)*								
Atkins Mango Curry	260	0	0	0	6	0	0	0
Mr. Spice Indian	30	0	0	0	6	0	6	0
Rising Sun Farms Cafe Yumm Creamy	140	14	2	0	2	0	0	90
TAJ Cuisine of India Bombay	23	1	0	0	3	1	-	118
GOURMET SAUCE								
BRANDS . . . *(1 TBSP UNLESS NOTED)*								
Rising Sun Farms Cafe Yumm, all	70	7	1	0	1	0	0	45
GRAVY								
Au jus, canned, 1/4 cup	10	0	0	0	2	0	0	30
Mix, 1 tsp	9	0	0	0	1	0	0	348
Onion gravy, mix, prep, 1/4 cup	19	0	0	0	4	0	1	251
Brown gravy, mix, prep, 1/4 cup	22	1	0	0	4	0	0	291
Beef gravy, canned, 1/4 cup	31	3	1	4	6	0	0	326
Mushroom gravy, canned, 1/4 cup	30	2	0	0	3	0	0	340
Mix, prep, 1/4 cup	18	0	0	0	3	0	0	350
Chicken gravy, canned, 1/4 cup	47	3	1	1	3	0	0	343
Mix, prep, 1/4 cup	30	1	0	2	5	0	0	332
Turkey gravy, canned, 1/4 cup	30	1	0	1	3	0	0	344
Mix, prep, 1/4 cup	26	1	0	1	5	0	1	307
BRANDS . . .								
MIX								
Med-Diet Premium Mushroom, Chicken, or Brown (avg)	15	0	0	0	3	-	-	40
Tony Chachere's								
Cream of Mushroom, 0.3 oz	25	0	0	0	5	0	0	5
Brown, 0.1 oz	10	0	0	0	2	0	0	160
READY-TO-USE								
Hain Brown, 1/4 cup	15	0	0	0	3	0	1	125
HARD SAUCE								
Plum pudding hard sauce, 1 tbsp	180	8	5	15	26	0	25	65
BRANDS . . .								
Most brands are within the generic range.								
HOLLANDAISE SAUCE								
Hollandaise sauce, mix, 1 tsp	20	1	1	0	3	0	1	170
BRANDS . . . *(1 TSP UNLESS NOTED)*								
Durkee, mix	10	0	0	5	1	0	0	45
French's, prep, 2 tbsp	10	0	0	0	2	0	0	75
Wagner's, mix	15	1	0	10	2	0	0	75

Food	Cal	Fat	Sat	Chol	Carb	Fib	Sug	Sod
HOT SAUCE *(also see Mexican Sauces, pg 113)*								
Hot sauce, 1 tsp	1	0	0	0	0	0	0	124
BRANDS . . . *(1 TSP UNLESS NOTED)*								
McIlhenny Tabasco (red)	1	0	0	0	0	0	0	30
Mezette California	0	0	0	0	0	0	0	70
*Mr. Spice Tangy Bang	2	0	0	0	0	0	0	0
Phamous Phloyd's	15	0	0	0	4	1	0	2
Pickapeppa	5	0	0	0	1	0	1	40
Watkins Calypso Hot or Caribbean Red	10	0	0	0	0	0	2	25
The Wizard's Hot Stuff	0	0	0	0	0	0	0	65
MINT SAUCE								
Mint sauce, 1 tsp	5	0	0	0	1	0	1	0
BRANDS . . .								
Most brands are within the generic range.								
PASTA SAUCE								
Marinara, ready-to-eat, 1/2 cup	71	3	0	0	10	2	8	515
Cheese, 1/2 cup	320	28	14	65	7	0	-	650
Pesto, sun-dried tomato, 1/4 cup	110	8	2	5	8	2	4	710
Pesto, basil, 1/4 cup	240	23	4	5	5	2	2	730
Spaghetti sauce, mix, prep, 1/2 cup	28	0	0	0	6	0	-	848
Alfredo sauce, 1/2 cup	340	30	12	80	10	0	-	1080
BRANDS . . .								
ALFREDO SAUCE *(1/4 CUP UNLESS NOTED)*								
Contadina Light Alfredo, refrg	80	5	3	20	5	0	2	330
*Walden Farms Calorie Free	0	0	0	0	0	0	0	20
PASTA/SPAGHETTI SAUCE								
FROZEN/REFRIGERATED *(1/2 CUP UNLESS NOTED)*								
Di Giorno Marinara	70	0	0	0	15	2	10	220
Plum Tomato/Mushroom	60	0	0	0	13	2	10	260
MIX *(1/2 CUP UNLESS NOTED)*								
*Bernard LS, prep	55	0	0	0	14	0	4	140
Durkee American, prep	15	0	0	0	6	0	1	170
French's All American, prep	20	0	0	0	7	0	1	200
Uncle Dave's								
Pasta Primavera, prep	120	0	0	0	24	1	1	260
READY-TO-USE *(1/2 CUP UNLESS NOTED)*								
Buitoni Garden Veg Marinara	60	2	0	0	9	-	-	260
*Casa Visco FF	30	0	0	0	6	1	3	110
Colavita Marinara	70	3	0	0	9	2	6	220
Classic Hot	80	3	0	0	12	3	6	250
Garden Style	60	3	0	0	12	3	0	290

CONDIMENTS & SAUCES
Sauces - Pasta Sauce

Food	Cal	Fat	Sat	Chol	Carb	Fib	Sug	Sod
PASTA/SPAGHETTI SAUCE								
*Eden Organic Spaghetti, NSA	80	3	0	0	12	3	6	10
*Enrico's Organic, NSA	45	0	0	0	11	1	10	20
Traditional, NSA	70	0	0	0	13	4	9	55
FF Organic Basil	50	0	0	0	8	4	8	220
FF Organic Traditional	45	0	0	0	4	6	7	280
Francesco Rinaldi NSA	90	4	0	0	11	3	6	30
Mama Rizzo's								
Primavera Veg (avg)	50	2	0	0	8	2	3	220
Mushroom Onion or Pepper								
Mushroom Onion	60	2	0	0	9	1	6	290
Manischewitz Pasta, NSA	70	1	0	0	12	2	8	45
*Med-Diet Spaghetti	20	0	0	0	3	-	-	100
*Melissa's Chicago Style Veg &								
Pasta	60	4	1	0	8	2	4	300
Mom's Spaghetti	60	4	-	-	6	-	0	280
*Muir Glen Italian Herb	55	1	0	0	10	0	5	320
Balsamic Roasted Onion	50	1	0	0	10	0	4	320
Chunky Tomato Herb	50	1	0	0	10	0	5	320
Garlic & Onion	55	1	0	0	10	0	5	320
Garlic Roasted Garlic	50	1	0	0	10	0	4	320
Mushroom Marinara	45	0	0	0	10	0	4	320
Cabernet Marinara	50	1	0	0	10	0	4	330
Portabello Mushroom	50	0	0	0	10	0	4	330
Patsy's Puttanesca	100	6	1	0	8	2	3	315
Pomodoro Fresca Solo	50	0	0	0	6	1	3	10
*Pritikin Traditional	30	0	0	0	6	1	3	110
Tomato Basil	30	0	0	0	6	1	3	110
Rao's Homemade Marinara	80	6	1	0	6	1	3	320
Savion Marinara, NSA	60	2	0	0	9	-	-	50
Steff Gourmet Traditional	35	1	0	0	-	-	-	190
Testo's Gourmet Pasta	110	10	2	5	6	1	2	320
Timpone's Spaghetti	80	3	-	-	7	-	4	310
Trader Giotto's								
Caponata Marinara	80	2	0	0	16	3	4	320
Marinara di Napoli	70	2	0	0	12	2	8	340
*Tree of Life NSA	50	2	0	0	9	0	8	0
Pasta Sauce Plus, Onion & Garlic, FF	30	0	0	0	7	0	6	240
Classic Tomato, FF	40	0	0	0	8	0	6	250
Sweet Pepper, FF	30	0	0	0	7	0	6	280
Original	50	2	0	0	9	0	8	290
Pasta Sauce Plus, Mushroom								
& Basil, FF	30	0	0	0	7	0	6	300

Food	Cal	Fat	Sat	Chol	Carb	Fib	Sug	Sod
PASTA/SPAGHETTI SAUCE								
Uncle Dave's Excellent Marinara....	80	3	0	0	13	2	1	280
Mushroom Marinara	80	3	0	0	11	2	1	280
Walnut Acres Tomato & Basil, LS ..	45	0	0	0	9	0	0	80

NOTE: Although many of the pasta sauces listed above exceed sodium guidelines, they are substantially less than the generic.

PESTO

READY-TO-EAT *(1/4 CUP UNLESS NOTED)*

Food	Cal	Fat	Sat	Chol	Carb	Fib	Sug	Sod
Candoni Sun Dried Tomato Pesto ...	190	17	3	5	9	2	5	95
***Melissa's** Basil Pesto	340	34	6	10	3	0	1	230
***Rising Sun Farms**								
The Ultimate Classic, 2 tbsp	100	10	-	5	1	-	-	115
Pesto Pronto, 2 tbsp	100	10	-	0	1	-	-	120
Dried Tomato, 2 tbsp	100	10	-	0	3	-	-	130
Garlic Galore, 2 tbsp	100	10	-	0	3	-	-	130
Artichoke & Lemon, 2 tbsp	100	9	-	5	2	-	-	150

PIZZA SAUCE

Food	Cal	Fat	Sat	Chol	Carb	Fib	Sug	Sod
Pizza sauce, ready-to-eat, 1/4 cup	40	2	0	0	9	1	-	410
BRANDS . . . *(1/4 CUP UNLESS NOTED)*								
Cento	30	0	0	0	5	1	3	140
***Enrico's** All Natural	35	2	0	0	6	0	5	150
Furmano's Pizza Sauce	25	1	0	0	4	1	2	190
Chunky	25	1	0	0	5	1	3	220
***Muir Glen**	40	0	0	0	6	2	3	230
Progresso	35	1	0	0	5	1	2	140

SLOPPY JOE SAUCE

Food	Cal	Fat	Sat	Chol	Carb	Fib	Sug	Sod
Sloppy joe sauce, canned, 1/4 cup	30	0	0	0	6	1	5	360
Mix, 1/8 pkg	15	0	0	0	3	0	1	360
BRANDS . . .								

No low-sodium alternatives.

STEAK SAUCE

Food	Cal	Fat	Sat	Chol	Carb	Fib	Sug	Sod
Steak sauce, 1 tbsp	14	0	0	0	4	0	2	262
BRANDS . . . *(1 TBSP UNLESS NOTED)*								
Angostura Salsa Flavored	8	0	0	0	2	0	2	85
Regular	12	0	0	0	3	0	3	90
***Busha Browne's** Planters	5	0	0	0	2	0	1	10
Earp's Western	30	0	0	0	10	0	10	55
Lea & Perrins Original	20	1	0	0	5	0	-	110
Sweet 'n Spicy	25	0	0	0	6	0	6	140
McIlhenny Caribbean Style	15	0	0	0	4	0	3	135
***Mr. Spice**	15	0	0	0	4	0	2	0

CONDIMENTS & SAUCES

Vinegar

Food	Cal	Fat	Sat	Chol	Carb	Fib	Sug	Sod
STEAK SAUCE								
Newman's Own	20	1	0	0	4	0	1	85
Southern Comfort	15	0	0	0	3	0	3	60
STROGANOFF SAUCE								
BRANDS . . .								
Durkee Stroganoff, mix, 1 tbsp	20	0	0	0	5	0	1	180
TARTAR SAUCE								
Tartar sauce, 1 tbsp	70	8	2	5	0	0	0	130
BRANDS . . .								
No low-sodium alternatives.								
WHITE SAUCE								
White sauce, mix, prep, 1/4 cup	23	1	0	0	2	0	-	171
Ready-to-eat, 1/4 cup	92	7	2	4	6	0	-	221
BRANDS . . .								
Tony Chachere's Instant Roux, 0.1 oz	10	0	0	0	2	0	0	80
WORCESTERSHIRE SAUCE								
Worcestershire sauce, 1 tsp	5	1	0	1	0	0	0	55
BRANDS . . . *(1 TSP UNLESS NOTED)*								
Angostura	5	0	0	0	1	0	1	20
Life All Natural	3	1	0	1	0	0	0	1
Robbie's	0	0	0	0	1	0	1	15

VINEGAR

Food	Cal	Fat	Sat	Chol	Carb	Fib	Sug	Sod
Vinegar, 1 tbsp	2	0	0	0	1	0	0	0
Balsamic vinegar, 1 tbsp	5	0	0	0	2	0	2	0
Rice vinegar, 1 tbsp	0	0	0	0	0	0	0	0

BRANDS . . .
Most brands are within the generic range. NOTE: Some rice vinegars may contain as much as 180mg per tbsp.

Food	Cal	Fat	Sat	Chol	Carb	Fib	Sug	Sod

DAIRY PRODUCTS & ALTERNATIVES

BUTTER, MARGARINE & SPREADS

Food	Cal	Fat	Sat	Chol	Carb	Fib	Sug	Sod
Margarine, unsalted, 1 tbsp	100	11	2	0	0	0	0	0
Butter, unsalted, 1 tbsp	102	12	8	31	0	0	0	2
Butter spray, 2 sprays	0	0	0	0	0	0	0	5
Butter, whipped, salted, 1 tbsp	70	7	5	2	0	0	0	55
Margarine, salted, 1 tbsp	100	11	2	0	0	0	0	105
Butter, salted, 1 tbsp	102	12	8	31	0	0	0	117

BRANDS . . .

BUTTER (1 TBSP UNLESS NOTED)

Food	Cal	Fat	Sat	Chol	Carb	Fib	Sug	Sod
Breakstone Unsalted	100	11	7	30	1	0	1	0
Horizon Organic Unsalted	100	11	7	30	1	0	1	0
Land O Lakes Whipped, Unsalted	70	7	5	20	0	0	0	0
Stick, Unsalted	100	11	8	30	0	0	0	0
Ultra Creamy, Unsalted	110	12	8	30	0	0	0	0
Honey	90	8	4	15	4	0	3	35

MARGARINE, UNSALTED

Most brands are within the generic range. NOTE: Unsalted margarine brands include Fleischman's, Mother's and Smart Beat.

BUTTER SUBSTITUTES

Food	Cal	Fat	Sat	Chol	Carb	Fib	Sug	Sod
Butter sprinkles, 1 tsp	5	0	0	0	2	0	0	120

BRANDS . . .
Most brands are within the generic range.

CHEESE

DELI & PACKAGED CHEESES (also see Shredded & Grated Cheeses, pg 57 and Sliced Cheeses, pg 58)

BLUE, GORGONZOLA, ROQUEFORT AND STILTON

Food	Cal	Fat	Sat	Chol	Carb	Fib	Sug	Sod
Stilton, 1 oz	110	9	5	30	0	0	0	220
Gorgonzola, 1 oz	100	8	5	20	1	0	0	350
Blue, 1 oz	100	8	5	21	1	0	0	396
Roquefort, 1 oz	105	9	6	26	1	0	0	513

BRANDS . . . (1 OZ UNLESS NOTED)

Food	Cal	Fat	Sat	Chol	Carb	Fib	Sug	Sod
Denmark's Finest Blue	100	8	6	15	0	0	0	310
Rosenborg Danish Blue	100	8	5	15	0	0	0	310
Treasure Cave Gorgonzola, Crumbled	100	8	5	20	1	0	0	310

Although the cheeses listed above exceed sodium guidelines, they are less than the generic.

55

DAIRY PRODUCTS & ALTERNATIVES
Cheese

Food	Cal	Fat	Sat	Chol	Carb	Fib	Sug	Sod
BRIE, CAMEMBERT AND LIMBURGER								
Brie, 1 oz	95	8	5	28	0	0	0	178
Limburger, 1 oz	93	8	5	26	0	0	0	227
Camembert, 1 oz	85	7	4	20	0	0	0	239
BRANDS . . .								
No low-sodium alternatives.								
CHEDDAR AND COLBY								
Colby, 1 oz	112	9	6	27	1	0	0	171
Cheddar, 1 oz	114	9	6	30	0	0	0	176
BRANDS . . . *(1 OZ UNLESS NOTED)*								
Organic Valley Slim Line, Reduced Sodium Cheddar	90	6	4	15	1	0	0	135
*Papa Cheese Cheddar, LF, LS	100	7	4	20	0	0	0	100
Tillamook Cheddar, LS	120	10	6	25	1	0	0	55
Tree of Life Cheddar, Natural, LS	110	9	6	24	0	0	0	110
EDAM, FONTINA AND GOUDA								
Fontina, 1 oz	110	9	5	33	0	0	0	227
Gouda, 1 oz	101	8	5	32	1	0	0	232
Edam, 1 oz	101	8	5	25	0	0	0	274
BRANDS . . .								
No low-sodium alternatives.								
FETA AND GOAT								
Goat, 1 oz	76	6	4	13	0	0	0	104
Feta, 1 oz	75	6	4	25	1	0	0	316
BRANDS . . . *(1 OZ UNLESS NOTED)*								
Athenos Basil & Tomato Feta, Crumbled	80	6	4	20	1	0	1	220
*Mozzarella Co. Goat	63	5	–	–	1	0	0	50
Although the feta cheese listed above exceeds sodium guidelines, it is substantially less than the generic.								
HAVARTI AND BRICK								
Brick, 1 oz	105	8	5	27	1	0	0	159
Havarti/tilsit, 1 oz	96	6	5	29	1	0	0	214
BRANDS . . .								
Denmark's Finest								
Havarti w/Caraway	120	10	7	25	0	0	0	140
Havarti	120	10	7	25	0	0	0	150
Tilsit	90	7	5	20	1	0	0	160
MONTEREY JACK AND MUENSTER								
Monterey jack, 1 oz	106	9	5	25	0	0	0	152
Muenster, 1 oz	104	9	5	27	0	0	0	178

Food	Cal	Fat	Sat	Chol	Carb	Fib	Sug	Sod
MONTERY JACK AND MUENSTER								
BRANDS . . . *(1 OZ UNLESS NOTED)*								
Boar's Head Muenster, LS	100	8	5	20	0	0	0	75
MOZZARELLA AND PROVOLONE								
Mozzarella, 1 oz	90	7	4	25	1	0	0	118
Part-skim, low moisture, 1 oz..........	79	5	3	15	1	0	0	150
Provolone, 1 oz	100	8	5	20	1	0	0	248
BRANDS . . . *(1 OZ UNLESS NOTED)*								
Calabro, FF Mozzarella	40	0	0	0	1	0	1	110
Mozzarella Co. Mozzarella	87	7	-	-	1	-	-	70
PARMESAN, ROMANO AND ASIAGO *(also see Shredded & Grated Cheeses below)*								
Romano, 1 oz	110	8	5	30	1	0	0	340
Asiago, 1 oz	110	9	5	0	1	0	1	400
Parmesan, 1 oz	111	7	5	19	1	0	0	454
BRANDS . . .								
No low-sodium alternatives.								
QUESO (MEXICAN CHEESES)								
Chihuahua, 1 oz	106	8	5	30	2	0	0	175
Asadero, 1 oz	101	8	5	30	1	0	0	186
Anejo, 1 oz	106	8	5	30	1	0	0	321
BRANDS . . .								
No low-sodium alternatives.								
SWISS, GRUYERE AND JARLSBERG								
Swiss, 1 oz	107	8	5	26	1	0	0	74
Gruyere, 1 oz	117	9	5	31	0	0	0	95
BRANDS . . . *(1 OZ UNLESS NOTED)*								
Boar's Head Swiss, NSA	110	8	5	25	1	0	0	10
Lacey Swiss, Reduced Fat/Sodium	90	6	4	15	0	0	0	15
Gold Label Premium Imported Swiss .	110	8	5	20	1	0	0	65
Dietz & Watson Swiss	110	8	5	28	0	0	0	30
Emmentaler Swiss	120	9	6	25	0	0	0	50
SHELF-STABLE CHEESES								
Processed, boxed	80	6	4	25	3	0	2	410
Processed spread, jar............................	90	7	3	15	4	0	3	490
BRANDS . . .								
No low-sodium alternatives.								
SHREDDED & GRATED CHEESES								
Swiss, shredded, 1/4 cup	100	8	5	25	0	0	0	40
Romano, grated, 1 tbsp	19	2	1	5	0	0	0	70
Parmesan, grated, 1 tbsp	23	2	1	4	0	0	0	93

DAIRY PRODUCTS & ALTERNATIVES
Cheese - Cottage Cheese

Food	Cal	Fat	Sat	Chol	Carb	Fib	Sug	Sod
SHREDDED AND GRATED CHEESES								
Cheddar, shredded, 1/4 cup	100	8	6	30	0	0	0	170
Mozzarella, part skim, shredded, 1/4 cup ..	90	6	4	20	0	0	0	220
BRANDS . . . *(1/4 CUP UNLESS NOTED)*								
CHEDDAR								
No low-sodium alternatives.								
MOZZARELLA								
Maggio Mozzarella	100	8	5	30	2	0	2	50
Sargento Fancy Swiss	110	8	5	25	1	0	1	60
Light Mozzarella, 50% Less Fat	70	3	2	10	1	0	0	140
Sorrento Whole Milk Mozzarella	90	7	5	25	1	0	0	120
Part Skim Mozzarella	80	6	4	15	1	0	0	150
PARMESAN AND ROMANO *(1 TBSP UNLESS NOTED)*								
Kraft Romano/Parmesan, Reduced Fat	20	1	0	1	2	0	0	75
Weight Watchers FF Grated Italian Topping, 1 tbsp	20	0	0	0	0	2	0	60
SWISS								
Most brands are within the generic range.								
SLICED CHEESES								
American/Processed, 1 oz	106	9	6	27	1	0	2	406
BRANDS . . . *(1 SLICE UNLESS NOTED)*								
Alpine Lace								
Swiss, Reduced Fat, 50% Less Sodium	110	7	5	25	0	0	0	75
Cheddar, Reduced Sodium	110	9	5	25	1	0	0	85
Provolone, Reduced Fat	70	5	3	15	1	0	0	120
Lorraine Cheese Premium Sandwich .	110	9	5	25	1	0	1	15
Pinata Swiss, Reduced Sodium	110	8	5	25	1	0	1	45
Sara Lee Swiss, 0.8 oz	80	6	4	20	1	0	0	45
Swiss	100	8	5	25	1	0	0	60
Hot Pepper Monterey Jack & Jalapeño	80	6	4	20	0	0	0	125
Sargento Swiss, Light Deli Style	70	4	2	15	1	0	0	40
Swiss, Deli Style, Aged or Thin Sliced	70	5	3	20	0	0	0	40
Jarlsberg	120	9	5	20	1	0	0	50
SUBSTITUTE CHEESES								
Soy-based, mozzarella or american, 1 slice (avg)	20	0	0	0	3	0	1	220
Soy-based, parmesan, grated, 2 tsp	15	1	0	0	1	0	0	85
BRANDS . . .								
Most brands are within the generic range.								

Food	Cal	Fat	Sat	Chol	Carb	Fib	Sug	Sod
CHEESE - COTTAGE CHEESE								
Dry curd cottage cheese, 4 oz	96	1	0	8	2	0	0	15
Creamed cottage cheese, 4 oz	120	5	3	25	4	0	3	430
LF, 4 oz	90	1	0	10	4	0	3	360
FF, 4 oz	80	0	0	0	4	0	3	380
BRANDS . . .								
COTTAGE CHEESE *(4 OZ UNLESS NOTED)*								
Friendship Creamed, LF, NSA	90	1	1	5	4	0	3	50
Giant 1% Milkfat, NSA	80	1	1	10	6	0	5	60
Hood Creamed, LF, NSA	80	1	1	10	6	0	5	60
Lucerne Creamed, NSA	80	1	1	5	4	0	3	40
HOOP AND FARMER CHEESES *(4 OZ UNLESS NOTED)*								
Friendship Hoop, 2 tbsp	20	0	0	0	0	0	0	10
Farmer, NSA, 2 tbsp	50	3	2	10	0	0	0	10
CHEESE - RICOTTA								
Ricotta cheese, 1/4 cup	108	8	5	31	2	0	2	52
Part skim, 1/4 cup	86	5	3	19	3	0	3	78
BRANDS . . . *(1/4 CUP UNLESS NOTED)*								
Calabro FF	25	0	0	0	1	0	1	30
Giant Part Skim	90	6	4	25	2	0	1	50
Whole Milk	100	8	5	30	2	0	1	50
NF	60	0	0	5	4	0	3	60
Maggio Whole Milk	100	8	5	30	2	0	2	50
Part Skim	80	5	4	30	2	0	2	65
*Mozzarella Co.	74	5	-	-	2	0	0	36
Precious LF	70	3	2	15	3	0	3	45
Sargento Light	60	3	2	15	3	0	3	55
FF	50	0	0	10	5	0	2	65
Sorrento FF	60	0	0	5	5	0	4	60

CHEESE SAUCE

(see Cheese Sauce, pg 49)

COFFEE CREAMERS & FLAVORINGS

(see Coffee Creamers & Flavorings, pg 13)

CREAM

Food	Cal	Fat	Sat	Chol	Carb	Fib	Sug	Sod
Light whipping cream, 1 tbsp	44	5	3	17	0	0	0	5
Half & half, 1 tbsp	20	2	1	6	1	0	1	6

DAIRY PRODUCTS & ALTERNATIVES
Cream - Sour

Food	Cal	Fat	Sat	Chol	Carb	Fib	Sug	Sod
CREAM								
Light cream, 1 tbsp	29	3	2	10	1	0	1	6
Heavy whipping cream, 1 tbsp	52	6	4	21	0	0	0	6

BRANDS . . .
Most brands are within the generic range.

(CREAM - SOUR)

Sour cream, regular, 2 tbsp	51	5	3	11	1	0	1	15
Reduced fat, 2 tbsp	40	3	2	11	1	0	1	25
FF, 2 tbsp	35	0	0	5	6	0	1	40

BRANDS . . . *(2 TBSP UNLESS NOTED)*
Most brands are within the generic range.

SOUR CREAM ALTERNATIVES
Imitation sour cream, 2 tbsp	59	6	5	0	2	0	2	29

BRANDS . . .
Most brands are within the generic range.

(CREAM CHEESE & ALTERNATIVE SPREADS)

CREAM CHEESE
Cream cheese, 2 tbsp	99	10	6	31	1	0	1	84
FF, 2 tbsp	25	0	0	5	2	0	1	135
Light, 2 tbsp	100	5	-	15	2	0	1	150
Neufchatel, 2 tbsp	148	13	8	43	2	0	2	226

BRANDS . . . *(2 TBSP UNLESS NOTED)*

PLAIN
Most brands are within the generic range.

FLAVORED
Philadelphia Flavors, Strawberry	100	9	6	30	5	0	3	65
Flavors, Chive & Onion	110	10	7	30	2	0	1	110
Neufchatel	70	6	4	20	0	0	0	120
Ultra Delight Mixed Berry	70	4	3	20	5	1	-	70
Strawberry	60	4	3	20	4	1	-	80

CREAM CHEESE ALTERNATIVES
BRANDS . . . *(2 TBSP UNLESS NOTED)*
Soya Kaas	100	9	2	0	0	0	0	115
Tofutti Better Than Cream Cheese	80	8	2	0	1	0	0	135

CREAM CHEESE SPREADS
BRANDS . . . *(2 TBSP UNLESS NOTED)*
Alouette Spinach Artichoke	60	6	4	15	1	0	1	80
Savory Vegetable	60	6	4	15	1	0	1	85

60

Food	Cal	Fat	Sat	Chol	Carb	Fib	Sug	Sod
CREAM CHEESE SPREADS								
Alouette (cont'd)								
Spinach Cheese	60	6	4	25	1	0	0	85
Salmon	60	5	3	15	1	0	0	95
Light Spring Vegetable	50	4	3	20	1	0	0	110
***Rising Sun Farms** Cheese Tortas*								
Marionberry	120	11	5	20	5	0	3	45
Mild Curry w/Apricots, Cranberries & Cashews	110	9	5	20	7	0	3	45
Key Lime w/Cranberries	110	10	5	0	5	0	3	50
Roasted Garlic	100	8	5	20	6	1	2	70
Mediterranean	90	7	5	20	5	0	3	85
Pesto Dried Tomato	100	9	5	25	3	0	2	90
Gorgonzola	110	9	5	20	4	0	3	100
Rondele Strawberry	90	8	5	30	4	0	3	75
Bagel Spread Original Plain	110	10	7	35	1	0	1	115
Vita Cream Cheese & Smoked Salmon	100	9	6	25	1	0	1	80

EGGS & EGG SUBSTITUTES

Food	Cal	Fat	Sat	Chol	Carb	Fib	Sug	Sod
Egg, whole, small, 1	55	4	1	157	0	0	0	47
Medium, 1	66	4	1	187	1	0	0	55
Large, 1	75	5	2	213	1	0	0	63
Egg white, large, 1	17	0	0	0	0	0	0	55
Egg substitute, 1/4 cup (1 egg)	25	0	0	0	1	0	1	115
BRANDS . . . *(1/4 CUP UNLESS NOTED)*								
Kroger Break-Free, 1/4 cup	30	0	0	0	1	0	1	80
Morningstar FF Scramblers, 1/4 cup	35	0	0	0	2	0	2	95

MILK PRODUCTS & NON-DAIRY ALTERNATIVES

(also see Milk-Based Drinks & Additives, pg 15)

Food	Cal	Fat	Sat	Chol	Carb	Fib	Sug	Sod
Milk, whole, 1 cup	149	8	5	34	11	0	11	120
2%, 1 cup	122	5	3	20	12	0	12	122
1%, 1 cup	102	3	2	10	12	0	12	123
NF, 1 cup	86	0	0	5	12	0	12	127
Goat milk, 1 cup	168	10	7	27	11	0	11	122
Buttermilk, LF, 1 cup	98	2	1	10	11	0	-	157
BRANDS . . . *(1 CUP UNLESS NOTED)*								
Friendship Buttermilk, LF	120	4	3	15	12	0	12	125
Knudsen Buttermilk, 2%	120	5	-	0	12	0	-	140

DAIRY PRODUCTS & ALTERNATIVES
Whipped Toppings

Food	Cal	Fat	Sat	Chol	Carb	Fib	Sug	Sod
FLAVORED DRINKS *(also see Milk-Based Drinks & Additives, pg 15)*								
Eggnog, ready-to-drink, 1 cup	342	19	11	149	34	0	21	138
Mix, prep w/milk, 1 cup	261	8	5	33	39	1	-	163
Choc milk, ready-to-drink, 1 cup	208	8	5	30	26	2	24	150
LF, 1 cup	158	3	2	8	26	1	25	153

BRANDS . . .
Most brands are within the generic range.

	Cal	Fat	Sat	Chol	Carb	Fib	Sug	Sod
NON-DAIRY ALTERNATIVES *(also see Diet & Nutritional Drinks, pg 88)*								
Rice milk, 1 cup	100	3	0	0	24	0	18	70
Soy milk, 1 cup	80	5	1	0	15	0	13	85
BRANDS . . . *(1 CUP UNLESS NOTED)*								
Westsoy Soy Drink								
Plain, Unsweetened	90	5	0	0	5	4	0	30
Vanilla, Unsweetened	100	5	1	0	5	4	0	30

(WHIPPED TOPPINGS)

	Cal	Fat	Sat	Chol	Carb	Fib	Sug	Sod
Whipped topping, ready-to-eat, 1 tbsp	13	1	1	0	1	0	1	1
Powder, prep, 1 tbsp	8	0	0	0	1	0	1	3
Pressurized, 1 tbsp	8	0	0	2	0	0	0	4

BRANDS . . .
Most brands are within the generic range.

(YOGURT)

	Cal	Fat	Sat	Chol	Carb	Fib	Sug	Sod
Yogurt, plain, whole milk, 8 oz	151	8	5	31	11	0	11	114
LF, 8 oz	155	4	2	15	17	0	17	172
FF, 8 oz	137	0	0	4	19	0	19	187
Yogurt, fruit, LF, 8 oz	250	3	2	10	47	0	47	143
BRANDS . . . *(8 OZ UNLESS NOTED)*								
Axelrod Fruit, 6 oz (avg)	70	0	0	0	12	0	7	95
Blue Bunny Lite85, 6 oz (avg)	80	0	0	5	13	0	8	90
Brown Cow Cream at the Top (avg)	230	8	5	30	34	0	32	100
Cascade Fresh Whole Milk, Vanilla	200	7	4	25	24	0	24	90
FF, Plain	110	0	0	0	16	0	10	120
FF, Vanilla	160	0	0	5	27	0	22	120
Colombo Classic Fruit on the Bottom,								
Strawberry or Banana	230	2	2	15	47	0	42	90
Light, most (avg)	120	0	0	5	21	0	15	110
Dannon Light NF, most (avg)	120	0	0	5	23	0	17	130
LaCreme, all, 4 oz	140	5	3	20	20	0	18	75
Horizon Organic Fruit on the Bottom,								
all, 6 oz	140	0	0	5	27	1	26	105

Food	Cal	Fat	Sat	Chol	Carb	Fib	Sug	Sod
YOGURT								
La Yogurt French Style, NF, all, 6 oz .	70	0	0	5	12	0	-	90
Light N' Lively Free, all, 4.4 oz	70	0	0	5	13	0	10	55
Mountain High FF, Plain	110	0	0	5	19	0	15	150
LF, Plain	150	2	1	15	22	0	15	150
LF, Vanilla	200	2	1	15	34	0	33	150
Stonyfield Farm								
YoSelf Organic LF, 4 oz (avg)	110	1	1	5	21	2	19	70
Whole Milk Organic, 6 oz (avg)	170	6	4	25	24	2	22	90
Organic LF, most (avg)	140	2	1	5	25	2	23	100
Organic NF, most (avg)	200	0	0	0	46	1	44	135
Tillamook Cranberry Raspberry, FF, 6 oz	180	0	0	5	37	0	34	105
Wallaby Organic, all, 6 oz	140	3	2	15	24	0	21	105
Yoplait Expresse, Strawberry, 1 tube .	70	2	1	5	11	0	10	40
Whips, all, 4 oz	140	3	2	10	25	0	21	75
Light, most, 6 oz	90	0	0	5	16	0	8	85

NON-DAIRY YOGURT ALTERNATIVES
BRANDS . . .

Food	Cal	Fat	Sat	Chol	Carb	Fib	Sug	Sod
Silk Soy, 6 oz (avg)	170	2	0	0	32	1	25	20
Stir Fruity Blueberry, 6 oz	140	1	0	0	26	0	-	72
All (except Pina Colada & Tropical Fruit), 6 oz (avg)	155	2	0	0	29	0	-	110
White Wave Silk Dairyless Soy, all, 6 oz (avg)	110	2	0	0	23	0	16	10

⬭ YOGURT - FROZEN ⬭

(see Frozen Yogurt, pg 76)

Food	Cal	Fat	Sat	Chol	Carb	Fib	Sug	Sod

DESSERTS & SWEETS

BROWNIES & DESSERT BARS

Food	Cal	Fat	Sat	Chol	Carb	Fib	Sug	Sod
Lemon bar, ready-to-eat, 1 oz	130	5	1	3	21	1	12	63
Mix, 1 oz	150	4	1	0	29	0	24	90
Brownie, ready-to-eat, 1 oz	150	6	1	15	23	0	21	115
Mix, 1 oz	123	4	1	0	22	0	17	100

BRANDS . . .

BROWNIES

FROZEN/REFRIGERATED

Food	Cal	Fat	Sat	Chol	Carb	Fib	Sug	Sod
Pillsbury One Step, 1.6 oz	180	8	2	0	25	1	16	105
Sara Lee Brownie Bites, 1.4 oz	170	8	4	10	24	1	16	60

MIX (1 OZ UNLESS NOTED)

Food	Cal	Fat	Sat	Chol	Carb	Fib	Sug	Sod
*Arrowhead Mills Wheat Free	90	2	1	0	21	1	13	40
Brownie	90	2	1	0	21	1	14	45
*Atkins Kitchen, Fudge, 0.8 oz	60	0	0	0	17	4	0	80
*Bernard Butterscotch or Choc, 2.5" sq	70	0	0	0	20	0	7	10
Betty Crocker Choc Chunk	130	3	2	0	24	0	18	90
Walnut Supreme	120	4	2	0	22	0	15	90
Turtle Supreme	120	3	1	0	23	0	16	95
Fudge, Traditional Chewy	170	2	1	0	23	0	17	100
*'Cause You're Special Choc Fudge, 1 brownie	62	0	0	0	15	1	11	50
Duncan Hines Walnut	130	5	1	0	22	1	16	100
Choc Lovers, Chewy Fudge, or Butterfinger (avg)	150	7	2	20	21	0	15	100
Estee Lite, 1 brownie	50	2	1	0	12	0	1	0
Firenza Triple Choc	160	2	1	0	23	1	17	70
Greenfield Home Style, 1 brownie	120	0	0	0	29	1	21	65
*Hol-grain Wheat Free, Choc	90	0	0	0	22	1	17	70
*No Pudge, 1/15 pkg (avg)	90	0	0	0	21	0	13	90
Oetker Choc, 1.5 oz	160	1	0	0	36	0	26	90
Choc Chip, 1.5 oz	120	2	0	0	24	0	13	110
Pillsbury								
Thick 'n Fudgy Cheesecake Swirl	110	3	1	0	19	1	13	80
Rich & Moist Fudge	130	3	1	0	26	1	18	85
Thick 'n Fudgy Double Choc	150	3	1	0	23	1	15	90
Caramel Swirl	160	3	1	0	23	1	16	95
*Wholesome Classics, 0.8 oz	0	0	0	0	21	0	10	90

READY-TO-EAT

Food	Cal	Fat	Sat	Chol	Carb	Fib	Sug	Sod
*Golden Star Frosted, 2.5 oz	107	0	0	0	24	0	16	30

Food	Cal	Fat	Sat	Chol	Carb	Fib	Sug	Sod
DESSERT BARS								
MIX (1 OZ UNLESS NOTED)								
Betty Crocker Sunkist Lemon Bars	130	4	1	0	24	0	17	80
Krusteaz Lemon Bars, 2" bar	150	3	0	0	29	0	24	80
READY-TO-EAT								
Health Valley Pastry Bar								
Choc Espresso, 1.4 oz	130	3	0	0	27	2	17	60
Cafe Creations, 1.4 oz	130	3	0	0	27	2	17	80

CAKES

(also see Cheesecakes, pg 66 and Snack Cakes, Pies & Sweet Snacks, pg 86)

Food	Cal	Fat	Sat	Chol	Carb	Fib	Sug	Sod
Sponge cake, 1 oz	82	1	0	29	17	0	-	69
Fruitcake, 1 oz	92	3	0	1	18	1	-	77
Chocolate cake, w/o frosting, 1 oz	100	3	1	1	16	0	-	92
Mix, 1 oz	121	4	1	0	21	1	-	234
Mix, pudding-type, 1 oz	112	3	1	0	22	1	-	253
German, pudding-type, mix, 1 oz	114	3	1	0	23	1	-	182
Yellow cake, w/o frosting, 1 oz	100	3	1	1	16	0	-	92
Mix, light, 1 oz	115	2	0	0	24	0	-	171
Mix, 1 oz	123	3	1	1	22	0	-	186
Mix, pudding-type, 1 oz	120	3	1	0	23	0	-	195
White cake, w/o frosting, 1 oz	100	3	1	1	16	0	-	92
Mix, 1 oz	121	3	1	0	22	0	-	188
Pound cake w/butter, 1 oz	116	6	4	66	15	0	13	119
Marble cake, pudding-type, mix, 1 oz	118	3	1	0	23	1	-	147
Carrot cake, pudding-type, mix, 1 oz	118	3	0	0	23	1	-	161
Gingerbread, mix, 1 oz	124	4	1	0	21	1	-	186
Angel food cake, 1 oz	73	0	0	0	16	0	15	212
Mix, 1 oz	106	0	0	0	24	0	-	209
BRANDS . . .								
FROZEN/REFRIGERATED								
Awrey's Raspberry Nut, 2.8 oz	320	18	4	30	35	2	26	110
Pepperidge Farm								
3-Layer Golden, 2.5 oz	250	12	0	25	33	1	21	120
3-Layer Devil's Food, 2.5 oz	250	13	3	25	31	1	20	140
MIX *(1 OZ UNLESS NOTED)*								
*Atkins Devils Food, 2 oz	35	0	0	0	5	1	3	146
*Authentic Foods Lemon	110	1	0	0	24	1	14	45
Choc	100	1	0	0	23	1	14	105
*'Cause You're Special Choc or								
Golden Pound, 1.3 oz (avg)	144	0	0	0	34	1	21	2
Yellow or Choc (avg)	97	0	0	0	23	0	14	118

65

DESSERTS & SWEETS
Cakes - Cheesecakes

Food	Cal	Fat	Sat	Chol	Carb	Fib	Sug	Sod
CAKES								
***Diet Source** Choc or White, 1/20 pkg .*	90	1	0	0	19	2	6	95
***Gluten Free Pantry** Angel Food, 1.4 oz*	140	0	0	0	32	0	2	90
Old Fashioned Cake & Cookie, 1.3 oz .	130	0	0	0	31	0	13	130
***Martha's** Choc Killer, 1/12 pkg*	105	1	0	0	28	0	13	122
***Sweet 'N Low**, all, 1/5 pkg*	160	3	1	0	36	1	1	30
***Sylvan Border Farm** Lemon, 2.9 oz .*	280	11	1	55	42	1	19	95
READY-TO-EAT *(1 OZ UNLESS NOTED)*								
***Atkins** Cake Roll, Carrot, 2.6 oz*	220	18	11	75	5	1	1	180
Choc Cake Roll, 2.6 oz	230	20	12	70	6	1	1	200
***Entenmann's** Light Golden Loaf*								
Pound, 1.7 oz	120	0	0	0	28	1	17	160
Milk Chocolatey, 2.4 oz	310	19	5	15	35	1	25	190
Light Loaf, 1.7 oz	120	0	0	0	28	0	16	190
Light Marble Loaf, 1.7 oz	130	0	0	0	29	1	18	190
Kuchen Meister								
Marzipan Stollen, 1.8 oz	203	9	3	3	29	1	16	60
Cakes, all, 1.8 oz (avg)	220	10	5	35	29	14	12	100
***Wolferman's** Pound, all, 2.5 oz (avg)*	260	13	4	80	33	0	21	120
CHEESECAKES								
Cheesecake, ready-to-eat, 2 oz	182	12	6	32	14	0	12	118
No-bake, mix, prep, 2 oz	155	7	4	16	20	1	-	215
BRANDS . . .								
FROZEN/REFRIGERATED								
***Atkins**, all, 3 oz (avg)*	250	24	14	95	3	0	1	180
***David Glass** Ultimate, 2.2 oz*								
Milk Choc Mousse	270	20	10	27	20	1	11	76
Choc Covered	217	14	8	65	19	0	15	86
New York	203	13	8	60	18	0	14	91
Key Lime Mousse	200	13	6	21	18	1	13	140
***Sara Lee** Choc-Dipped Bar, 2.8 oz ...*	190	14	11	20	14	0	12	50
Choc Mousse, 2.2 oz	200	13	10	15	19	1	14	95
***Unbelievable**, 2.3 oz*	100	0	0	0	19	0	17	70
***Weight Watchers** Smart Ones*								
New York Style w/Black Cherry								
Swirl, 1 cheesecake	150	5	3	15	21	1	18	140
MIX								
***Atkins** Cheesecake, mix only*	11	0	0	0	2	1	0	23
***Carbolite** Vanilla, 1/8 slice*	260	25	14	280	2	0	0	80

CAKE FROSTING, ICING & DECORATIONS

(see Frosting, Icing & Decorations, pg 6)

Food	Cal	Fat	Sat	Chol	Carb	Fib	Sug	Sod

CANDY & CHEWING GUM

Food	Cal	Fat	Sat	Chol	Carb	Fib	Sug	Sod
Breath savers, 1 pc	10	0	0	0	2	0	0	0
Lollipop, 1	22	0	0	0	6	0	17	2
Gumdrops, 1 oz	34	0	0	0	9	0	21	4
Sweet choc candy, 1 oz	143	10	6	0	15	2	-	5
Sugar-coated almonds, 1 oz	128	5	0	0	20	1	-	6
Jelly beans, 1 oz	104	0	0	0	26	0	18	7
Choc coated fondant, 1 oz	102	3	2	0	22	0	-	7
Choc coated raisins, 1 oz	109	4	2	1	19	1	17	10
Hard candy, 1 oz	106	0	0	0	28	0	20	11
Butterscotch, 1 oz	112	1	0	3	2	0	24	12
Choc coated peanuts, 1 oz	145	9	4	3	14	1	-	12
Caramels, choc-flavored roll, 1 oz	103	2	0	0	22	0	19	24
Carob, 1 oz	153	9	8	1	19	1	-	30
Caramel, 1 oz	108	2	2	2	22	0	24	70

BRANDS . . .

Most brands are within the generic range.

CANDY BARS

Food	Cal	Fat	Sat	Chol	Carb	Fib	Sug	Sod
Sweet choc bar, 1 oz	143	10	6	0	17	0	16	5
Milk choc bar w/almonds, 1 oz	147	10	5	5	15	2	12	21
Milk choc bar, 1 oz	147	9	5	7	17	0	16	23
Milk choc w/rice cereal, 1 oz	130	7	4	5	18	1	15	41

BRANDS . . . *(1 CANDY BAR UNLESS NOTED)*

Food	Cal	Fat	Sat	Chol	Carb	Fib	Sug	Sod
3 Muskateers, 2.1 oz	260	8	5	5	46	1	40	110
Almond Joy, 1.6 oz	220	12	8	0	27	2	22	65
Baby Ruth, 2.1 oz	280	13	9	0	37	2	31	130
Butterfinger, 2.1 oz	270	11	6	0	44	1	30	120
Estee Sugar Free								
Rice Crunchy Bars	60	1	0	0	15	0	8	40
Milk Choc or Milk Choc w/Almonds,								
1.4 oz (avg)	220	16	9	20	18	0	15	65
Milk Choc w/Fruit & Nuts, 1.4 oz	220	16	9	20	18	0	15	65
***Fifty50** Almond Choc, 1.4 oz	210	15	8	10	20	1	4	35
***Glutano**								
Choc Covered Hazelnut, 0.9 oz	141	9	5	3	13	1	3	20
Big-Break Choc Bar, 1.8 oz	258	15	7	10	28	1	22	45
Break Bar, 1.6 oz	247	14	8	10	26	0	22	45
Heath, 1.4 oz	210	12	5	10	24	1	23	135
Hershey's Milk Choc, 1.2 oz	180	11	7	5	20	1	17	30
Milky Way, 2.1 oz	270	10	5	5	41	1	35	95
Snickers, 2.1 oz	280	14	5	5	35	1	30	140

DESSERTS & SWEETS

Cookies

Food	Cal	Fat	Sat	Chol	Carb	Fib	Sug	Sod
CANDY BARS								
Tofutti Soy Good Choc or Choc								
w/Crisp Rice, 1.5 oz (avg)	170	5	1	0	30	2	27	100
Twix, 2 oz	280	14	5	5	37	1	27	115
Yamate Chocolatier								
Dark Choc, Sugar Free, 1.5 oz	220	16	10	0	21	4	0	25
Milk Choc, Sugar Free, 1.5 oz	210	16	10	5	20	2	0	50
Weight Watchers LF, 1.2 oz (avg)	130	2	1	0	27	2	18	85
CHEWING GUM								
Chewing gum, 1 stick	5	0	0	0	1	0	1	0

BRANDS . . .

Most brands are within the generic range.

PEANUT BARS *(see peanut bars, pg 141)*

(COFFEECAKES)

(see Pastries & Coffeecakes, pg 81)

(COOKIES)

Food	Cal	Fat	Sat	Chol	Carb	Fib	Sug	Sod
Sugar wafers w/creme filling, 1 oz	145	7	1	0	20	0	13	42
Ladyfingers, 1 oz	103	3	1	103	17	0	11	42
Marshmallow, choc coated, 1 oz	119	5	1	0	19	1	16	48
Coconut macaroons, 1 oz	115	4	3	0	21	1	8	70
Wafers, vanilla, 1 oz	134	6	1	0	20	1	11	87
Choc, 1 oz	123	4	1	1	21	1	11	164
Chocolate chip cookies, 1 oz	136	6	2	0	19	1	8	89
Mix, 1 oz	141	7	2	0	19	0	14	82
Refrg dough, 1 oz	140	7	2	5	17	1	10	100
LF, 1 oz	128	4	1	0	21	1	-	107
Fig Bar, 1 oz	99	2	0	0	20	1	14	99
Sandwich, vanilla w/creme filling, 1 oz	137	6	1	0	20	0	13	99
Choc w/creme filling, 1 oz	134	6	1	0	20	1	-	171
Butter cookies, 1 oz	132	5	3	33	20	0	-	100
Sugar cookies, 1 oz	136	6	2	15	19	0	13	101
Refrg dough, 1 oz	124	6	2	8	17	0	-	120
Prep w/margarine, 1 oz	134	7	1	7	16	0	-	139
Oatmeal cookies, 1 oz	128	5	1	0	20	1	9	109
Refrg dough, 1 oz	120	5	1	7	17	1	-	83
Mix, 1 oz	131	5	1	0	19	-	-	134
Prep, w/o raisins, 1 oz	127	5	1	10	19	-	-	170
Animal crackers, 1 oz	126	4	1	0	21	0	8	111

Food	Cal	Fat	Sat	Chol	Carb	Fib	Sug	Sod
COOKIES								
Peanut butter, 1 oz	135	7	1	0	17	1	5	118
Refrg dough, 1 oz	130	6	2	5	16	0	9	130
Prep from recipe, 1 oz	135	7	1	9	17	0	-	147
Shortbread, 1 oz	142	7	2	6	18	1	6	129
Molasses, 1 oz	122	4	1	0	21	0	12	130
Gingersnaps, 1 oz	118	3	1	0	22	1	10	185
BRANDS . . .								
FROZEN/REFRIGERATED *(1 OZ UNLESS NOTED)*								
Nestle Toll House Choc Chip, 0.9 oz	110	5	2	10	16	1	9	90
Pillsbury Cookie Dough								
Choc Chip	120	6	2	5	15	1	9	80
Choc Chip w/Walnuts	130	7	2	5	16	1	9	90
MIX *(1 OZ UNLESS NOTED)*								
Betty Crocker Choc Chip, prep	160	3	2	0	21	0	14	55
Double Choc Chunk, prep	170	3	2	0	21	0	13	55
Rainbow Choc Candy, prep	150	2	1	0	22	0	14	65
Sugar, prep	160	3	1	0	22	0	13	65
***'Cause You're Special**								
Classic Sugar, 1	51	0	0	0	12	0	4	27
Choc Chip, 1	66	1	0	0	14	0	7	56
***Gluten Free Pantry** Choc Chip, 0.5 oz	60	1	0	2	-	4	4	50
Sweet 'N Low Choc Chip, prep	110	3	1	0	22	0	0	30
READY-TO-EAT *(1 OZ UNLESS NOTED)*								
There are many low-sodium cookies, the following have less than 70mg per serving.								
Archway Coconut Macaroon	106	6	5	0	12	1	10	38
Raisin Oatmeal	130	5	1	5	19	1	9	40
Wedding Cakes, 1.1 oz	160	8	2	0	20	0	9	45
Shortbread, Sugar Free	107	5	1	0	16	0	0	47
Choc Chip Ice Box	117	6	2	8	15	0	8	59
Choc Chip, Sugar Free	110	5	2	0	16	0	0	65
Rocky Road, Sugar Free	100	5	1	0	15	1	0	65
***Atkins** Meringues, all, 1	1	0	0	0	1	0	0	0
Gourmet Choc Chip, 1	140	10	4	25	11	1	1	40
Gourmet Coconut or Lemon, 1 (avg)	140	11	4	30	9	1	1	50
Gourmet Peanut Butter, 1	140	11	4	25	9	1	1	50
Bakery Wagon Cobbler FF Apple, Apple Cranberry, Raspberry, or Mixed Fruit, 1 (avg)	70	0	0	0	1	-	15	60
Baking on the Lite Side Raspberry Linzer or Crunchy Oatmeal, 1.2 oz	60	0	0	0	13	0	2	20

DESSERTS & SWEETS
Cookies

Food	Cal	Fat	Sat	Chol	Carb	Fib	Sug	Sod
COOKIES								
***Barbara's Bakery** Fig Bars, all, 1 (avg)*	60	0	0	0	13	1	6	20
Choc Chip Crisp or Double Dutch Choc	60	3	2	5	10	1	5	30
Tradtional Shortbread Cookie, 1	80	4	3	10	10	1	3	40
Vanilla Snackimals, 8	120	5	0	0	19	1	7	55
Barry's Bakery								
Merangos, Choc Chip, 11	108	1	1	0	24	0	23	18
Merangos, Choc, French Vanilla, or								
Mocha, 11	99	0	0	0	24	1	22	22
French Twists, 1 (avg)	40	2	0	0	7	0	4	25
Choc Creme, Sugar Free, 2	110	5	2	0	17	0	1	20
Almond, Sugar Free, 6	110	4	1	0	17	0	0	60
***BP Gourmet** Meringues (avg)*	90	0	0	0	27	0	0	0
Dreams (avg)	100	0	0	0	25	0	25	35
***Carr's** Chococcines*	150	9	6	0	16	1	12	20
Dark Choc Imperials	150	7	5	5	18	2	10	40
Petits Bijoux	140	5	2	0	21	1	9	40
Milk Choc Imperials	150	7	5	5	18	1	12	50
***Cathy's** Fig Bars (avg)*	90	0	0	0	18	2	12	15
Cookies M&Ms, 1.1 oz	170	9	3	0	20	1	13	50
Country Choice Soft-Baked								
Rocky Road, 1	90	4	1	5	13	1	8	30
Double Fudge Brownie, 1	80	3	1	5	14	1	9	35
Oatmeal Raisin, 1	100	4	0	5	15	1	9	65
Oatmeal Choc Chip, 1	100	4	1	5	15	1	8	65
Choc Chip Walnut, 1	100	4	2	5	15	1	10	65
DeBenkelaer Pirouline	130	4	3	15	23	1	13	50
Delacre Matadi Creme-Filled Wafers .	190	11	7	5	20	1	15	15
Marquisettes	140	7	4	5	17	1	7	45
***Ener-G** Coconut Macaroon, 1*	80	5	3	0	8	1	7	10
White Choc Macadamia, 1	90	5	1	0	11	0	6	16
Almond Butter, 1	56	3	0	5	6	0	3	30
French Almond, 1	71	4	0	0	18	0	15	32
Potato Choc Chip, 1	80	4	1	5	11	0	6	32
Lemon Vanilla Cream, 1	147	6	3	0	21	0	11	39
Vanilla Cream, 1	147	6	3	0	22	0	12	39
Ginger, 1	64	2	0	0	10	0	5	45
Lemon Sandwich, 1	163	6	2	0	28	1	15	45
Vanilla Choc Sandwich, 1	154	7	3	0	22	1	11	48
Choc Sandwich, 1	200	9	4	0	29	1	14	55
Estee Creme Wafers, Vanilla	175	9	2	0	22	0	0	20
Creme Wafers, Choc	170	9	2	0	22	0	0	30
Choc Sandwich	133	5	1	0	20	1	9	31

70

Food	Cal	Fat	Sat	Chol	Carb	Fib	Sug	Sod
COOKIES								
Fifty/50 Strawberry Vanilla Creme Wafer	150	9	2	1	20	1	0	15
Peanut Butter	160	7	2	0	19	1	8	25
Choc Chip	170	9	3	0	20	1	6	35
Coconut	160	10	3	0	18	1	6	45
Choc Creme-Filled Wafers	160	9	2	0	20	1	0	45
Hearty Oatmeal	160	7	2	0	21	1	8	55
Glenny's Noah 'n Friends Animal Crackers	90	4	0	0	15	5	1	30
Glutano Wafers, 3	35	0	0	0	8	0	0	24
Choc Creme Wafer, 3	150	9	6	0	16	1	8	25
Choc Chip Biscuit, 4	126	6	3	1	17	0	6	26
Tarteletts, 0.9 oz	122	6	3	0	17	1	4	29
Half-covered Choc, 6	134	7	4	1	17	1	3	44
Hazelnut, 4	111	7	2	0	12	1	5	45
Apricot Biscuit, 9	250	10	5	0	38	1	13	55
Biscuit, 4	112	4	2	0	18	0	5	55
CoCo, 4	99	6	3	0	11	0	6	57
Choc O's, 3	148	8	4	0	19	1	7	58
Lemon Creme-Filled Wafers, 3	150	9	6	0	16	0	7	61
Golden Batch Creme Wafer, 1.1 oz	150	7	0	0	20	0	0	45
Golden Fruit, all, 1 (avg)	75	2	0	0	15	0	7	55
Golden Star Celebration, 2 oz	75	0	0	0	16	0	7	37
Black & White, 2.5 oz	173	0	0	0	38	0	18	53
Health Valley								
Cobbler Bites, all, 0.9 oz (avg)	100	2	0	0	21	1	10	40
Choc Chip, Wheat-Free, 0.8 oz	100	4	0	0	14	1	7	50
Peanut, Wheat-Free, 0.8 oz	100	4	0	0	14	1	6	60
Heavenly Desserts Meringues, 1 (avg)	0	0	0	0	1	0	0	0
Joseph's Sugar Free								
Almond, 0.9 oz	100	5	1	0	13	0	0	20
Lemon, 0.9 oz	95	4	1	0	15	0	0	30
Coconut, Choc Walnut, or Peanut Butter, 0.9 oz (avg)	105	5	1	0	14	0	0	40
Pecan Shortbread, Oatmeal, or Choc Chip, 0.9 oz (avg)	100	5	1	0	14	0	0	40
Keebler Sugar Wafers, Creme-Filled	130	6	1	0	19	0	14	20
Peanut & Caramel Cluster, 0.8 oz	100	6	3	0	12	0	7	35
Fudge Sticks	150	8	4	0	19	0	15	55
E.L. Fudge Sandwich, 0.9 oz	120	5	1	5	17	1	8	60
Fudge Shoppe Clusters, 1.1 oz	140	7	4	0	20	1	12	65
Danish Wedding	130	6	3	0	19	1	11	65
Frosted Animal Crackers	130	6	4	0	18	0	10	65

DESSERTS & SWEETS
Cookies

Food	Cal	Fat	Sat	Chol	Carb	Fib	Sug	Sod
COOKIES								
Lance Strawberry or Vanilla Creme-filled Sugar Wafers, 1.1 oz	150	8	2	0	18	0	14	20
Lenell Family Favorites	150	8	2	0	18	2	6	53
Pinwheels	135	8	2	0	17	2	6	53
Lor Ladyfingers, 1 oz	119	1	0	18	26	0	19	10
Lu Le Chocolatier	150	8	7	0	17	1	11	10
Le Truffe, Praline/Choc, 1.2 oz	170	9	7	0	20	2	15	15
Le Petit Ecolier, Dark Choc	120	6	4	5	17	1	9	50
Le Petit Ecolier, Milk Choc	120	6	4	5	17	1	10	55
Mallopuffs, 1	70	2	2	0	12	0	-	35
*Miss Meringue Choc, Vanilla, or Cappuccino, 1.1 oz (avg)	80	0	0	0	20	0	20	15
Triple Choc Chip, 1.1 oz	90	2	1	0	20	0	18	15
Strawberry Meringue, 1.3 oz	100	0	0	0	24	0	24	20
Lemon Meringue, 1.1 oz	80	0	0	0	20	0	19	25
Mother's Wafers	140	8	2	0	18	0	9	20
Mrs. Dennison's Choc, 0.9 oz	80	0	0	0	17	1	9	47
*Murray Sugar Free Vanilla Wafers	130	10	2	0	19	0	0	15
Nabisco Mallomars, 0.9 oz	120	5	3	0	19	1	12	35
Biscos Waffle Cremes, 1.1 oz	180	9	2	0	24	0	17	35
Biscos Sugar Wafers	140	6	2	0	21	0	13	40
Pecanz Shortbread, 0.6 oz	90	5	1	5	9	0	3	50
Iced Oatmeal, 0.6 oz	80	3	0	0	12	0	6	55
Family Favorites Iced Oatmeal, 1	80	3	0	0	12	0	-	55
Fruit 'n Grain Bars, Blueberry, 1	130	3	0	0	25	1	-	60
Apple Cinnamon, 1	130	3	0	0	25	1	-	60
Family Favorites Oatmeal, 1	80	3	1	0	12	0	-	65
Oatmeal, 0.6 oz	80	3	1	0	12	0	5	65
*Natural Ovens Carob Chip, 1.3 oz	90	4	0	0	16	3	6	15
Oatmeal Raisin, 1	90	3	0	0	15	3	6	15
Newman's Own Organic Dark Choc Peppermint Cups, 1.2 oz	180	12	6	5	20	1	18	0
Champion Chip, 0.7 oz	90	5	0	0	11	0	6	40
Choc Bars, all, 1.5 oz (avg)	215	14	8	10	24	1	22	45
Dark Choc Peanut Butter Cups, 1.2 oz	180	12	6	0	18	1	14	50
Newtons Cobblers Apple & Cinnamon, FF, 0.8 oz	70	0	0	0	17	1	10	40
Cobblers Peach Apricot, FF, 0.8 oz	70	0	0	0	17	0	10	55
Tropical Newton's Strawberry Kiwi	90	2	0	0	19	0	10	55
Apple	100	0	0	0	21	1	12	65

Food	Cal	Fat	Sat	Chol	Carb	Fib	Sug	Sod
COOKIES								
Pamela's Ginger, 0.8 oz	110	5	0	0	14	1	4	35
Lemon Shortbread, 0.8 oz	120	6	4	15	16	0	3	60
Chunky Choc, 0.8 oz	120	6	1	10	16	0	8	60
Pecan Shortbread, 0.8 oz	130	8	4	20	15	1	4	65
Papadopoulos Caprice Creme-Filled								
Wafers, 1.1 oz (avg)	150	7	3	0	20	1	15	40
Parmalat Bed & Breakfast								
Choc Chunk Pecan or Chunky								
Choc, 0.9 oz	130	8	3	6	14	1	7	40
Pecan Shortbread, 0.9 oz	140	9	2	6	13	1	6	45
Pepperidge Farm								
Spritzers, 1.1 oz (avg)	140	7	2	5	21	0	9	60
Creme Magnifique, 1.1 oz	150	7	3	5	21	1	10	60
Pirouettes, 0.9 oz (avg)	130	6	5	10	19	1	11	60
Brussels, 1 oz	150	7	3	5	20	1	11	65
Milano Orange or Mint, 2	130	7	4	5	16	1	8	65
Salzburg, 2	150	6	2	0	21	1	9	65
Sargento S'mores	110	6	3	0	14	0	10	35
Strawberry & Sprinkles	130	5	1	0	19	0	12	65
Choc Chip	30	6	2	0	18	1	12	65
Snackwell's								
Golden Devil's Food, 0.6 oz	50	1	0	0	11	0	7	25
Devil's Food FF, 0.6 oz	50	0	0	0	12	0	7	30
Caramel Delights, 0.6 oz	70	2	1	0	13	0	8	35
Stella D'oro Anginetti, 1.1 oz	140	4	2	40	23	1	17	10
Swiss Fudge, 0.9 oz	130	7	2	5	16	1	9	55
Choc Castelets	130	6	2	5	19	1	-	55
Trader Joe's								
Cappuccino Meringues, 1.1 oz	80	0	0	0	20	0	20	15
Chocolate Meringues, 1.1 oz	100	2	1	0	20	0	16	15
Mint Meringues, 1.1 oz	90	2	1	0	20	0	19	15
Lemon Meringues, 1.3 oz	100	0	0	0	24	0	24	20
Shortbread Cookies, 1.1 oz	70	8	5	15	17	1	5	20
Gingeroos, 0.9 oz	100	3	1	10	16	0	9	60
***Tree of Life**								
Toasted Almond Butter, 0.9 oz	70	0	0	0	16	1	7	35
Oatmeal, 0.9 oz	70	0	0	0	16	1	7	40
Carrot Cake, 0.9 oz	50	0	0	0	13	1	6	50
Twix Caramel Bars	140	7	3	0	19	0	14	60
Walker's Shortbread, 0.7 oz (avg)	100	6	3	15	11	0	3	65
Weight Watchers Fruit, 1 (avg)	70	0	0	0	16	0	8	50

Food	Cal	Fat	Sat	Chol	Carb	Fib	Sug	Sod
COOKIES								
Whole Foods Market 365								
Vanilla Twists	120	4	1	0	19	0	6	40
Vanilla Sandwich Cremes	130	6	0	0	19	1	10	45
Lemon Twists	110	4	1	0	18	1	6	50
Oatmeal Raisin	110	5	1	0	17	1	7	50
Choc Twists	120	5	1	0	18	0	6	60
BISCOTTI								
Biscotti, 1 oz	110	0	0	0	24	0	15	95
BRANDS . . . *(1 OZ UNLESS NOTED)*								
Alex & Dani's Totally Choc	130	5	3	28	20	1	12	55
Amazing Almond	130	6	3	25	17	1	8	55
***Aunt Gussie's** Organic Wheat*								
Orange Biscottini, 0.8 oz	90	0	0	0	14	0	6	65
Sugar Free, 0.8 oz	60	0	0	0	15	1	0	65
***Bake Boy** (avg)*	80	0	0	0	18	0	6	25
Belletieri Cherry Choc	150	5	3	20	18	1	10	60
***Bon Appetito**, 0.6 oz (avg)*	85	0	0	0	14	0	6	30
***BP Gourmet** (avg)*	110	0	0	0	24	0	15	75
Burns & Ricker Biscotti	130	5	1	20	19	1	10	30
Biscotti Decadence, 1.2 oz	130	5	3	25	19	1	11	65
***Freida's Kitchen** (avg)*	80	0	0	0	18	0	6	25
Health Valley Amaretto or Choc, 1.1 oz	120	3	0	0	23	3	7	50
***Irene's**, 0.4 oz (avg)*	21	0	0	0	7	1	3	0
Nonni's Biscottini, 0.5 oz	60	3	2	10	9	0	6	35
Original, 1.2 oz	100	4	2	25	19	0	11	65
San Anselmos, 1.1 oz (avg)	80	0	0	5	16	0	7	30
***Scotto's** (avg)*	110	0	0	0	23	0	6	25
Stella D'oro Hazelnut	100	4	1	10	15	0	8	60
***Upper Crust** all (avg)*	110	4	0	19	15	1	7	41

DOUGHNUTS

Food	Cal	Fat	Sat	Chol	Carb	Fib	Sug	Sod
French cruller, glazed, 1.5 oz	169	8	2	5	24	0	-	141
Cake doughnuts:								
Choc, sugar or glazed, 1.5 oz	175	8	2	24	24	1	-	143
Plain, sugar or glazed, 1.5 oz	192	10	3	14	23	1	9	181
Choc-coated or frosted, 1.5 oz	204	13	3	26	21	1	-	184
Plain, 1.5 oz	198	11	2	17	23	1	-	257
Yeast doughnuts:								
Glazed, 1.5 oz	169	10	2	3	19	1	-	144
Jelly-filled, 3 oz	289	16	4	22	33	1	-	249
Creme-filled, 3 oz	307	21	5	20	26	1	-	263

DESSERTS & SWEETS
Ice Cream, Ices & Frozen Yogurt

Food	Cal	Fat	Sat	Chol	Carb	Fib	Sug	Sod
DOUGHNUTS								
Honeybun, 2.3 oz	262	15	4	4	29	1	-	222
BRANDS . . .								
FROZEN/REFRIGERATED								
Tio Pepe's Cinnamon Churros, 1 oz	110	5	2	15	14	2	5	100
READY-TO-EAT								
Hostess Donut Bites, 1.9 oz	250	15	8	10	27	0	23	160
Glazed Donut Holes, 1 oz	125	8	4	5	14	0	12	80
Rich's Glazed Donuts, 1	130	7	2	0	-	-	-	40
Svenhard's Variety, 1	190	10	2	1	14	2	10	180

FROZEN DESSERTS

(also see Pastries & Coffeecakes, pg 81)

BRANDS . . .

Food	Cal	Fat	Sat	Chol	Carb	Fib	Sug	Sod
***Barbara's Bakery** Dipped Desserts*								
Coconut Almond Chocolately, 1	120	5	3	0	20	1	8	10
Espresso Bean Chocolately, 1	120	3	3	0	22	1	9	10
Lemon Yogurt, 1	120	4	3	0	22	1	9	10
Roasted Peanut Chocolately, 1	130	5	2	0	20	1	8	30
Breyer's Ice Cream Cake, Vanilla Viennetta, 2.5 oz	190	11	7	40	19	0	16	40
Weight Watchers Smart Ones Choc Chip Cookie Dough Sundae, 2.7 oz	190	5	2	5	35	1	15	120

GELATIN

(see Puddings & Gelatins, pg 83)

ICE CREAM, ICES & FROZEN YOGURT

Food	Cal	Fat	Sat	Chol	Carb	Fib	Sug	Sod
Sherbet, orange, 1/2 cup	102	2	1	4	23	0	20	34
Sorbet, fruit flavored, 1/2 cup	120	2	1	5	26	0	26	35
Ice cream:								
Strawberry, 1/2 cup	127	6	3	19	18	1	15	40
Choc, 1/2 cup	143	7	4	22	19	1	15	50
Light, 1/2 cup	104	2	1	7	20	1	5	46
Vanilla, 1/2 cup	133	7	5	29	16	0	13	53
Light, 1/2 cup	92	3	2	9	15	0	5	56
Sugar-free, 1/2 cup	99	4	2	11	12	0	0	58
Soft-serve:								
French vanilla, 1/2 cup	185	11	6	78	19	0	15	52
Vanilla, light, 1/2 cup	111	2	1	11	19	0	-	62

75

DESSERTS & SWEETS
Ice Cream, Ices & Frozen Yogurt

Food	Cal	Fat	Sat	Chol	Carb	Fib	Sug	Sod
ICE CREAM, ICES AND FROZEN YOGURT								
Frozen yogurt, soft-serve, vanilla, 1/2 cup	114	4	2	2	17	0	14	63
Choc, 1/2 cup	115	4	3	4	18	2	-	71

BRANDS . . .

Most ice cream, ices and frozen yogurt are low sodium, the following flavors are the lowest of each brand.

FROZEN YOGURT *(1/2 CUP UNLESS NOTED)*

Food	Cal	Fat	Sat	Chol	Carb	Fib	Sug	Sod
Ben & Jerry's Cherry Garcia	170	3	2	20	32	0	27	80
Blue Bunny FF, Homemade Choc	100	0	0	10	19	0	16	60
Brownie Fudge Fantasy	120	0	0	5	26	0	19	70
Breyer's, most (avg)	150	5	3	15	23	1	17	50
Cascadian Farm Double Choc	170	7	4	24	25	1	21	15
Choc	105	2	1	7	20	1	18	54
Vanilla	109	2	1	7	20	0	19	65
Dreyer's/Edy's Raspberry	90	3	2	10	16	0	13	25
Vanilla	100	3	2	10	17	0	13	30
Choc Decadence, Heath Toffee Crunch, or Cookies 'n Cream (avg)	120	4	2	10	19	0	14	45
FF, Vanilla, Vanilla Choc Swirl, or Black Cherry Vanilla Swirl (avg)	90	0	0	0	19	0	13	45
Elan Strawberry or Choc (avg)	125	3	2	10	22	0	18	48
Andes Mint	160	5	2	10	24	0	20	50
Black Raspberry, Coffee, or Vanilla (avg)	130	3	2	10	23	0	18	55
Häagen-Dazs Vanilla Raspberry Swirl	170	3	2	30	31	1	24	30
Strawberry	140	0	0	5	30	0	20	40
Peach Melba	210	4	2	50	37	0	29	45
Coffee	200	5	3	65	31	0	20	50
Choc Choc Chip	230	7	4	60	32	2	26	55
Hood, all (avg)	110	0	0	0	27	0	25	50
Sealtest, all (avg)	120	2	1	10	24	0	17	45
Turkey Hill FF Choc Marshmallow	130	0	0	0	30	0	21	40
FF Orange Swirl	100	0	0	0	22	0	20	40
FF Neapolitan	100	0	0	0	22	0	19	50
Black Raspberry or Peach Raspberry	110	3	2	10	20	0	20	60

GELATO *(1/2 CUP UNLESS NOTED)*

Food	Cal	Fat	Sat	Chol	Carb	Fib	Sug	Sod
Häagen-Dazs Hazelnut	260	12	4	75	33	1	23	55
Chocolate	240	8	5	80	37	2	26	70
Raspberry	240	7	4	80	40	1	25	75

ICE CREAM *(1/2 CUP UNLESS NOTED)*

Food	Cal	Fat	Sat	Chol	Carb	Fib	Sug	Sod
Ben & Jerry's Pistachio Pistachio	240	15	10	40	20	0	18	50
Chunky Monkey	310	19	11	55	32	3	24	55
New York Super Fudge Chunk	290	20	11	50	28	2	25	55

Food	Cal	Fat	Sat	Chol	Carb	Fib	Sug	Sod
ICE CREAM								
Ben & Jerry's (cont'd)								
Cherry Garcia	260	16	11	70	26	0	23	60
World's Best Vanilla	250	16	11	75	22	0	23	60
Blue Bunny								
Premium:								
Bordeaux Cherry Choc or Double Strawberry (avg)	170	8	6	30	22	0	18	45
French Vanilla, Homemade Choc, or Choc Chip, (avg)	160	8	5	45	18	0	16	50
Triple Raspberry Temptation	160	7	5	25	24	0	21	55
Hi Lite:								
Cherry Nut or Homemade Vanilla	120	4	3	15	19	0	16	55
Choc Chip or Mint Chip	120	4	3	10	18	0	15	55
Original:								
Banana Split or Vanilla (avg)	145	8	5	25	18	0	14	50
French or Neapolitan (avg)	140	7	5	28	16	0	13	60
Homemade Vanilla, Strawberry, or Strawberry Cheesecake (avg)	140	7	5	30	18	0	16	60
FF, No Sugar Added:								
Burgundy Cherry	90	0	0	0	22	0	4	60
Mint Fudge Swirl or Choc	80	0	0	0	19	0	5	70
Brownie Sundae or Vanilla (avg)	85	0	0	0	22	0	5	70
LF, No Sugar Added;								
Double Strawberry or Exquisite Mint (avg)	120	5	4	15	19	0	3	60
Banana Split, Cherry Vanilla, or Rocky Road (avg)	125	5	3	15	20	0	3	65
Neapolitan or Vanilla	110	5	3	20	16	0	4	65
Breyer's								
Fresa Banana or Creamsicle (avg)	135	5	4	15	20	0	16	35
Extra Creamy Choc	140	7	5	20	18	1	15	35
Strawberry Shortcake	160	6	4	15	23	0	18	40
Extra Creamy Vanilla	150	8	5	20	17	0	14	45
All Natural Light:								
Mint Choc Chip	130	5	3	10	20	0	18	45
Natural Vanilla	110	3	2	10	17	0	15	50
Vanilla/Choc/Strawberry	110	3	2	10	18	0	14	50
No Sugar Added:								
Vanilla	100	5	3	15	15	0	4	45
Vanilla/Choc/Strawberry	100	4	3	10	15	0	4	45
Vanilla Fudge Twirl	110	4	3	10	19	1	4	50
Cascadian Farm Organic Vanilla	160	8	5	30	20	1	19	15

DESSERTS & SWEETS
Ice Cream, Ices & Frozen Yogurt

Food	Cal	Fat	Sat	Chol	Carb	Fib	Sug	Sod
ICE CREAM								
Dreyer's								
Grand:								
Real Strawberry	130	6	4	20	16	0	15	30
Toasted Almond	150	9	5	25	15	0	12	30
Vanilla Choc	150	8	5	25	16	0	4	30
Rocky Road	170	10	5	25	17	0	13	30
Choc or Neapolitan (avg)	150	7	3	25	16	0	15	35
Vanilla or Vanilla Bean (avg)	145	9	5	30	16	0	13	35
Triple Choc Thunder	160	9	6	25	18	0	15	35
Coffee or French Vanilla (avg)	150	9	5	38	16	0	12	40
Andes Cool Mint	170	9	6	25	19	0	16	40
Grand Light:								
Strawberry Shortcake	110	4	2	20	18	0	14	40
Rocky Road	120	4	2	20	17	0	12	40
Vanilla	100	4	2	20	15	0	11	45
Mocha Almond Fudge	120	5	2	20	16	0	12	45
Mint Choc Chips! or French Silk (avg)	125	5	3	18	18	0	14	50
Crazy for Caramel	110	3	2	15	18	0	15	50
Choc Fudge Chunk	120	4	3	15	19	0	14	50
Fudge Tracks	120	4	3	15	18	0	13	50
Vanilla Raspberry Escape	120	3	2	15	18	0	15	50
No Sugar Added:								
Neapolitan or Strawberry	90	3	2	10	13	0	4	45
Mint Choc Chips!	110	5	3	10	15	0	3	45
Vanilla	90	3	2	10	13	0	4	50
FF, Raspberry Vanilla Swirl	80	0	0	0	19	0	4	50
FF, Vanilla Choc Swirl or Vanilla (avg)	95	0	0	0	19	0	4	50
Chips 'N Swirls or Triple Choc (avg)	90	3	2	10	16	0	3	58
Godiva Belgian Dark Choc	280	17	10	65	26	2	23	40
White Choc Raspberry	260	12	7	55	32	0	28	65
Häagen-Dazs Belgian Choc	330	21	12	85	29	3	26	50
Mango or Pineapple Coconut (avg)	240	14	8	85	27	1	25	53
Choc Choc Chip or Tres Leches (avg)	295	20	12	105	26	1	24	55
Healthy Choice Mint Choc Chip	110	2	1	10	18	1	4	50
In the Beginning	110	2	1	5	21	1	20	50
Choc Choc Chunk	120	2	1	5	21	1	17	60
Choc Fudge Brownie, No Sugar	120	2	1	5	21	1	4	60
Rocky Road or Brownie Bliss (avg)	130	2	1	8	25	1	17	60
Vanilla or Tin Roof Sundae (avg)	115	2	1	10	20	1	15	60
Hood LF, No Sugar Added	100	3	2	10	14	0	5	50
Regular, most (avg)	140	6	4	25	20	0	19	60
Light, most (avg)	140	5	3	10	22	0	20	60
Peak Treasures, most (avg)	180	9	6	25	21	1	18	60

Food	Cal	Fat	Sat	Chol	Carb	Fib	Sug	Sod
ICE CREAM								
Starbucks Classic Coffee	230	12	7	65	26	0	24	50
Java Chip	250	13	8	60	29	0	26	55
LF Latte	170	3	2	10	30	0	23	60
Turkey Hill Premium, Black Cherry or Black Raspberry (avg)	160	9	5	45	19	0	17	35
Philadelphia Style, all (except Butter Almond & Caramel Pecan) (avg)	180	11	6	35	18	0	12	50
Light, Vanilla & Choc or Vanilla Bean (avg)	110	3	2	15	18	0	17	65
FF, no sugar, Dutch Choc or Vanilla Bean (avg)	90	0	0	0	20	0	6	65
SHERBET AND SORBET *(1/2 CUP UNLESS NOTED)*								
Blue Bunny Sherbet (avg)	110	0	0	0	24	0	20	30
Breyer's Rainbow or Orange Sherbet	120	2	1	5	26	0	20	35
Choc Rainbow	140	7	5	20	15	0	14	40
Cascadian Farm Sorbet (avg)	80	0	0	0	20	2	18	5
Ciao Bella Sorbet (avg)	150	0	0	0	38	0	38	0
Häagen-Dazs Sorbet								
Tropical, Orange, or Zesty Lemon (avg)	120	0	0	0	30	1	27	0
Strawberry, Raspberry, or Mango (avg)	120	0	0	0	31	1	28	0
Orchard Peach	130	0	0	0	33	1	29	0
Howler Organic Sorbet (avg)	110	0	0	0	27	1	26	10
Luigi's Italian Ice (avg)	110	0	0	0	27	0	22	20
Turkey Hill Sherbet, all	120	1	0	0	26	0	21	20
BARS, POPS & SANDWICHES								
Bar, fruit & juice, 1 bar	63	0	0	0	16	0	16	10
Yogurt bar, choc, 1 bar	120	0	0	0	22	0	15	45
Bar, choc covered, 2.2 oz bar	220	15	11	15	18	0	15	55
Bar, drumstick, 3.4 oz	340	20	11	20	34	1	23	85
Sandwich, 2.3 oz	180	7	4	20	26	0	12	160
BRANDS . . .								
FRUIT AND JUICE BARS *(1 BAR UNLESS NOTED)*								
Most brands are within the generic range.								
ICE CREAM AND YOGURT BARS *(1 BAR OR UNLESS NOTED)*								
Blue Bunny Root Beer Float	80	2	2	10	14	0	11	25
Star Bar	110	7	6	5	11	0	9	30
Health Smart FF Creme Bar	70	0	0	0	18	0	2	35
Homemade Vanilla Bar	150	11	8	10	20	13	0	35
Heath Ice Cream Bar	190	13	10	20	16	0	13	40
Fruitfull Cream-Based Bars (avg)	130	5	3	15	24	-	-	25

DESSERTS & SWEETS
Ice Cream, Ices & Frozen Desserts

Food	Cal	Fat	Sat	Chol	Carb	Fib	Sug	Sod
ICE CREAM AND YOGURT BARS								
Häagen-Dazs Raspberry Sorbet &								
Vanilla Yogurt Frozen Yogurt	90	0	0	0	21	1	15	15
Vanilla & Dark Choc Ice Cream	280	20	12	70	22	1	20	40
Choc & Dark Choc Ice Cream	350	24	15	85	28	2	24	45
Choc Sorbet	80	0	0	0	20	1	14	50
Hood Orange Cream	90	2	1	5	18	0	18	30
LF Ice Cream	90	6	5	5	9	0	3	30
Sweet Nothings Fudge	100	0	0	0	23	0	12	5
SANDWICH AND DRUMSTICKS *(1 SANDWICH OR DRUMSTICK UNLESS NOTED)*								
Nestle 1880 Ice Cream Sandwich	200	7	3	15	31	0	17	30
NON-DAIRY ALTERNATIVES								
BRANDS . . . *(1/2 CUP UNLESS NOTED)*								
Soy Delicious Choc Velvet	130	4	0	0	23	2	13	25
Mint Marble Fudge or Strawberry (avg)	140	3	0	0	25	1	15	35
Neapolitan	130	4	0	0	23	1	13	40
Choc Peanut Butter	150	5	0	0	23	1	12	65
Sweet Nothings FF Tiger Stripes	120	0	0	0	28	0	15	45
FF Vanilla	120	0	0	0	28	0	16	45
FF Choc	110	0	0	0	27	0	12	55
Tofutti LF Supreme Coffee								
Marshmallow Swirl	100	1	0	0	24	0	14	77
LF Supreme Vanilla Fudge	120	2	1	0	24	0	16	90
Vanilla, No Sugar Added	190	11	2	0	20	0	0	90
LF Supreme Strawberry Banana	100	1	0	0	23	0	17	92
Vanilla Strawberry Sundae, No Sugar	80	0	0	0	19	0	0	95
LF Supreme Choc Fudge	120	2	1	0	25	0	18	98
Premium Choc Cookie Crunch	210	9	2	0	26	1	13	100
Whole Soy Glace' all (avg)	230	13	3	0	23	2	15	6
BARS AND SANDWICHES *(1 BAR OR SANDWICH UNLESS NOTED)*								
Rice Dream Bars (avg)	220	13	10	0	27	0	15	60
Soy Delicious Bars (avg)	260	13	6	0	31	1	15	25
Soy Dream Heavenly Pie (avg)	290	14	5	0	40	2	20	55
Rocket Bar	220	12	4	0	25	2	15	60
Dreamwich	130	6	0	0	16	1	9	65
Tofutti Totally Fudge Pops	95	2	0	0	19	0	14	53
Choc Fudge Treats	30	0	0	0	6	0	0	86
Crumb Cake Bar, Strawberry	220	15	6	0	20	0	15	90
Hip Hip Hooray Bar	150	9	2	0	10	0	0	90
Monkey Bar, Peanut Butter	220	13	8	0	22	1	18	105
Cuties Snack Size Sandwiches (avg)	130	5	1	0	16	0	9	110

Food	Cal	Fat	Sat	Chol	Carb	Fib	Sug	Sod

ICE CREAM CONES & TOPPINGS

CONES

Food	Cal	Fat	Sat	Chol	Carb	Fib	Sug	Sod
Cone, cake or wafer-type, 1	17	0	0	0	3	0	3	6
Sugar cone, 1	40	0	0	0	8	0	8	32
Ice cream cone, waffle, 1 oz cone	121	2	0	0	23	1	-	42

BRANDS ...
Most brands are within the generic range.

TOPPINGS

Food	Cal	Fat	Sat	Chol	Carb	Fib	Sug	Sod
Pineapple or strawberry, 2 tbsp (avg)	109	0	0	0	28	0	27	5
Chocolate, 2 tbsp	100	0	0	0	24	0	21	35
Hot Fudge, 2 tbsp	140	4	1	0	24	1	16	60
Butterscotch or caramel, 2 tbsp	103	0	0	0	27	1	18	143

BRANDS ...

CHOCOLATE AND FRUIT TOPPINGS
Most brands are within the generic range.

BUTTERSCOTCH AND CARAMEL TOPPINGS

Food	Cal	Fat	Sat	Chol	Carb	Fib	Sug	Sod
Wagner Butterscotch, 2 tbsp	150	2	2	5	33	1	21	65

MUFFINS & SCONES

(see Muffins & Scones, pg 29)

PASTRIES & COFFEECAKES

(also see Snack Cakes, Pies & Sweet Snacks, pg 86)

Food	Cal	Fat	Sat	Chol	Carb	Fib	Sug	Sod
Strudel, apple, 1 oz	78	3	1	2	12	1	-	76
Coffeecakes:								
Creme-filled w/choc frosting, 1 oz	94	3	1	20	15	1	-	92
Cheese, 1 oz	96	4	2	24	13	0	-	96
Cinnamon w/crumb topping, 1 oz	119	7	2	9	13	1	-	100
Fruit, 1 oz	88	3	1	2	15	1	-	109
Eclair, custard-filled w/choc glaze, 1 oz	74	5	1	36	7	0	-	96
Cream puff, custard-filled w/choc glaze, 1 oz	73	4	1	38	7	0	-	97
Sweet roll, cheese, 1 oz	102	5	2	22	12	0	-	101
Danish pastries:								
Fruit, 1 oz	105	5	1	32	14	1	-	100
Lemon, 1 oz	105	5	1	11	14	1	-	100
Nut, 1 oz	122	7	2	13	13	1	-	103
Cinnamon, 1 oz	114	6	2	6	13	0	-	105
Cheese, 1 oz	106	6	2	5	11	0	-	128
Sweet roll, cinnamon w/raisins, 1 oz	106	5	1	19	14	1	-	109

DESSERTS & SWEETS
Pies & Cobblers

Food	Cal	Fat	Sat	Chol	Carb	Fib	Sug	Sod
PASTRIES AND COFFEECAKES								
Cinnamon roll, 1	130	2	0	0	21	1	21	200
Refrg dough w/frosting, 1 oz	94	4	1	0	15	0	-	217
Popovers, mix, 1 oz	105	1	0	0	20	0	-	257
BRANDS . . . *(2 OZ UNLESS NOTED)*								
FROZEN/REFRIGERATED								
Athens Baklava Pastry, 1 oz	135	8	1	1	15	1	9	58
Delizza Mini Cream Puffs, 2.7 oz	291	24	14	111	15	1	10	77
Mini Eclairs, 3.6 oz	333	21	13	63	32	1	20	128
Rich's Bavarian Creme Eclair, 2 oz	190	9	8	40	24	0	18	80
New York Hazelnut Eclair, 2 oz	220	12	10	36	26	0	20	85
Robin's Nest Cheese Filled Rolls, FF, 2.7 oz (avg)	43	0	0	0	4	2	0	135
MIX								
Martha's Old Fashioned Buttermilk Coffee Cake, 1.8 oz	127	1	0	0	33	0	14	70
READY-TO-EAT								
Bahlsen Deloba w/Fruit & Filling, 0.9 oz	120	5	2	0	19	1	7	80
Entenmann's								
Pecan Danish Coffee Cake, 1.5 oz	188	11	2	23	19	1	9	120
Lemon Twist Coffee Cake, 1.9 oz	130	0	0	0	31	1	17	130
Raspberry Danish Twist, Light, 1.2 oz	140	0	0	0	32	1	18	180
Cheese Filled Crumb	200	9	4	40	25	1	12	190
Pineapple Topped, NF, 2.9 oz	170	0	0	0	40	1	25	190
Pineapple Cheese, NF, 1.9 oz	120	0	0	0	28	1	16	190
Kings Hawaiian Mini Sweet Rolls, 1	90	2	1	10	15	0	4	85
Svenhard's Cinnamon Rolls, 1.1 oz	140	-	-	-	23	1	11	160
Raisin Snails, 1 pc	250	-	-	-	33	2	17	180
*Toufayan Cinnamon Raisin Ring, 1.6 oz	120	2	0	0	24	1	5	180
*Wolferman's								
Povitica, English Walnut, 1.8 oz	180	10	2	25	20	1	11	80
Rugelach, 1.2 oz	130	8	2	5	14	0	7	85
Povitica, Cream Cheese, 1.8 oz	150	7	3	35	19	0	11	105
Cinnamon Almond Coffee Cake, 2 oz	250	13	2	40	29	1	19	180
Baklava, 1.7 oz	337	19	4	10	44	2	29	187
Blueberry Crumble Coffee Cake, 2 oz	230	13	3	45	27	0	16	190

PIES & COBBLERS

(also see Snack Cakes, Pies & Sweet Snacks, pg 86)

Food	Cal	Fat	Sat	Chol	Carb	Fib	Sug	Sod
Choc creme pie, 1/6	344	22	6	6	38	2	-	154
Lemon meringue pie, 1/6	303	10	2	51	53	1	-	165

Food	Cal	Fat	Sat	Chol	Carb	Fib	Sug	Sod
PIES AND COBBLERS								
Egg custard pie, 1/6	221	12	3	35	22	2	-	252
Cherry pie, 1/6	304	13	3	0	47	1	-	288
Pumpkin pie, 1/6	229	10	2	22	30	3	-	307
Apple pie, 1/6	277	13	4	0	40	2	-	311
Peach pie, 1/6	261	12	2	0	39	1	-	316
Banana creme pie, no-bake mix, prep, 1/6	309	16	9	36	39	1	-	357
Blueberry pie, 1/6	271	12	2	0	41	1	-	380
Pecan pie, 1/6	452	21	4	36	65	4	-	479
Choc mousse pie, no-bake mix, prep, 1/6	329	19	10	44	37	-	-	583
BRANDS ...								
FROZEN/REFRIGERATED								
Amy's Apple Pie, 4 oz	240	8	5	25	37	2	15	135
Marie Callendar Peach Cobbler, 1/4	370	18	3	0	47	0	24	170
Pepperidge Farm Apple Turnover, 1	330	14	3	0	48	6	5	180
Weight Watchers Smart Ones								
Choc Chip Cookie Sundae, 1 serv	190	5	2	5	35	1	15	120
Mississippi Mud, 1 serv	160	5	0	45	24	5	13	120
Choc Mousse, 1 serv	190	5	2	5	31	3	14	150
Brownie A La Mode, 1 serv	190	4	2	30	33	2	15	190
MIX (also see Pie Fillings, pg 9 and Puddings & Gelatins below)								
Chef Hans Apple Crisp, 1/2 cup	280	1	0	0	64	0	45	85

PIES - SNACK

(see Snack Cakes, Pies & Sweet Snacks, pg 86)

PUDDINGS & GELATINS

GELATIN

Food	Cal	Fat	Sat	Chol	Carb	Fib	Sug	Sod
Unflavored gelatin, 1 envl	25	0	0	0	0	0	0	15
Regular gelatin, 1/2 cup	80	0	0	0	19	0	19	80
Sugar free, 1/2 cup	10	0	0	0	0	0	0	60
BRANDS ...								
MIX								
*Calorie Control, all, 1/2 cup	10	0	0	0	1	0	0	0
Hain Dessert Mix, 1/2 cup (avg)	70	0	0	0	20	1	19	10
PUDDING								
Custard, mix for 1/2 cup serv	86	1	0	54	17	0	12	59
Chocolate pudding:								
Regular (cooked), mix for 1/2 cup serv	90	1	0	0	22	0	17	88
Ready-to-eat, 1/2 cup	150	5	1	3	26	1	15	146
FF, 1/2 cup	76	0	0	0	15	0	12	136
Instant, mix for 1/2 cup serv	89	0	0	0	22	1	17	357

DESSERTS & SWEETS
Puddings & Gelatins

Food	Cal	Fat	Sat	Chol	Carb	Fib	Sug	Sod
PUDDING								
Rice pudding:								
Ready-to-eat, 1/2 cup	185	8	1	5	25	0	19	97
Mix for 1/2 cup serv	102	0	0	0	25	0	15	99
Lemon pudding:								
Regular (cooked), mix for 1/2 cup serv	76	0	0	0	19	0	12	106
Ready-to-eat, 1/2 cup	142	4	0	0	28	0	19	159
Instant, mix for 1/2 cup serv	95	0	0	0	24	0	14	333
Tapioca pudding:								
Mix for 1/2 cup serv	85	0	0	0	22	0	15	110
Ready-to-eat, 1/2 cup	134	4	1	5	22	0	20	180
Vanilla pudding:								
Regular (cooked), mix for 1/2 cup serv	81	0	0	0	21	0	16	166
Ready-to-eat, 1/2 cup	147	4	1	8	25	0	18	153
Ready-to-eat, FF, 1/2 cup	74	0	0	0	17	0	12	170
Instant, mix for 1/2 cup serv	92	0	0	0	23	0	19	360
Banana pudding:								
Regular (cooked), mix for 1/2 cup serv	83	0	0	0	20	0	16	173
Ready-to-eat, 1/2 cup	144	1	1	0	24	0	15	157
Instant, mix for 1/2 cup serv	92	0	0	0	23	0	17	375
Plum pudding, mix, 1/3 pkg	460	10	3	0	87	5	58	240
Coconut cream, instant, mix for 1/2 cup serv	97	1	1	0	22	0	17	302
BRANDS . . .								
MIX *(1/2 CUP UNLESS NOTED)*								
Bird's Dessert Mix, 1/4 pkt	25	0	0	0	6	0	0	30
*Calorie Control Mousse, all	50	3	1	0	6	0	0	25
Key Lime Pie Filling & Mousse	60	3	2	0	7	0	0	40
Custard	20	0	0	0	4	0	3	40
Choc Chip Cheesecake	60	2	1	5	7	0	4	80
Choc Mint Instant	70	2	1	0	10	1	8	110
Hain Choc or Vanilla, 1/4 pkg	80	0	0	0	19	1	14	35
Junket Custard, 0.4 oz mix (avg)	44	0	0	0	10	0	10	0
Mori Nu Lemon, 1/4 pkg	120	3	2	0	22	0	19	5
Choc, 1/4 pkg	110	2	2	0	22	1	18	20
Manischewitz Noodle	160	3	1	95	28	1	10	20
Nestle Mousse European Style, 1/4 pkg	90	2	2	0	15	1	14	20
Choc Raspberry Truffle or Milk								
Choc Irish Cream	90	3	2	0	14	2	12	30
Oetker Tiramisu, 1/5 pkg	150	5	3	5	25	0	15	18
Mousse, Choc, 3 tbsp mix	100	4	3	0	15	0	13	45
Mousse, Strawberry, 3 tbsp mix	75	3	2	0	13	0	11	55
Creme Brulee, 1/4 pkg	110	2	1	10	23	0	18	90

Food	Cal	Fat	Sat	Chol	Carb	Fib	Sug	Sod
PUDDING								
*Royal Instant Caramel Custard	70	0	0	0	18	0	17	30
*Sans Sucre Mousse								
Cappuccino, Choc, or Strawberry ...	50	2	1	0	7	0	0	25
French Vanilla, Lemon, or Mocha	50	2	1	0	7	0	0	25
Key Lime	60	3	2	0	7	0	0	40
Cheesecake or Choc Cheesecake ..	60	2	1	5	8	0	4	80
Pumpkin, mix, 1/14 pkg	50	2	1	0	7	1	4	80
White House Choc Fudge, Light	100	1	0	0	20	0	-	120

NOTE: Most of the above pudding mix values listed above do not include milk or other added ingredients.

READY-TO-EAT *(1/2 CUP UNLESS NOTED)*

Food	Cal	Fat	Sat	Chol	Carb	Fib	Sug	Sod
Hunt's Snack Pack Lemon Meringue	130	3	1	0	26	0	21	55
Imagine Natural Lemon, 1 cup	150	3	0	0	31	1	18	35
Banana, 1 cup	140	3	0	0	28	0	17	40
Butterscotch, 1 cup	140	3	0	0	28	1	16	55
Choc, 1 cup	160	3	0	0	34	1	21	85
Jell-O Puddin' Pie								
Caramel Apple, 3.5 oz	170	7	2	0	26	0	20	125
Kozy Shack Creme Caramel Flan	140	4	3	45	23	0	22	105
Real Choc	140	4	2	15	24	1	19	140
Creamy Banana or Vanilla (avg)	130	3	2	15	22	0	18	150

RICE PUDDING & TAPIOCA

MIX *(1/2 CUP PREP UNLESS NOTED)*

Food	Cal	Fat	Sat	Chol	Carb	Fib	Sug	Sod
Bascom Instant Rice, 1 oz mix	100	0	0	0	24	0	11	80
*Lundberg Rice Puddings, all,								
1 serv (avg)	70	1	0	0	15	1	5	0
Minute Tapioca, 1 1/2 tsp	20	0	0	0	5	0	0	0
Uncle Ben's Rice Pudding								
w/Cinnamon & Raisins	160	1	0	0	37	1	16	150

READY-TO-EAT *(3.5 OZ UNLESS NOTED)*

Food	Cal	Fat	Sat	Chol	Carb	Fib	Sug	Sod
Hunt's Snack Pack, Tapioca	130	5	2	0	20	0	14	135
Kraft Handi-Snacks, Tapioca	120	4	1	0	20	0	14	115

SAUCES & TOPPINGS

(also see Whipped Toppings, pg 62 and Ice Cream Cones & Toppings, pg 81)

Food	Cal	Fat	Sat	Chol	Carb	Fib	Sug	Sod
Strawberry, 2 tbsp	107	0	0	0	28	0	-	9
Marshmallow cream, 2 tbsp	91	0	0	0	22	0	-	14
Pineapple, 2 tbsp	106	0	0	0	28	0	-	27
Choc fudge sauce, 2 tbsp	133	3	2	1	24	1	16	131
Butterscotch or caramel sauce, 2 tbsp .	103	0	0	0	27	0	-	143

DESSERTS & SWEETS
Snack Cakes, Pies & Sweet Snacks

Food	Cal	Fat	Sat	Chol	Carb	Fib	Sug	Sod
SAUCES AND TOPPINGS								
BRANDS . . . *(1 TBSP UNLESS NOTED)*								
Steel's Fudge, Amaretto, Caramel, Espresso or Butterscotch (avg)	100	8	4	10	16	0	12	16
Wax Orchards Fudge Sauces, FF, Fruit Sweetened, all	90	0	0	0	20	4	18	40

SNACK CAKES, PIES & SWEET SNACKS

Food	Cal	Fat	Sat	Chol	Carb	Fib	Sug	Sod
Cake, sponge, creme-filled, 1.5 oz	157	5	1	7	27	0	-	157
Cupcake, choc w/frosting, 1.5 oz	131	2	0	0	29	2	-	178
Cupcake, choc w/frosting, creme-filled, 1.8 oz	188	7	1	9	30	0	-	213
Pie, fruit filled, fried, 4.6 oz (avg)	405	21	3	0	55	3	-	479
BRANDS . . .								
Dolly Madison Creme Cakes, 1 oz	105	4	2	12	16	0	11	115
Devil's Food Zinger, 1.5 oz	150	5	3	10	25	0	18	140
Cinnamon Stix, 1.3 oz	170	9	4	15	21	0	14	140
Choc Snack Squares, 1.6 oz	210	10	6	10	28	0	22	150
Ferrara Panettone, 1.8 oz	180	7	3	70	27	0	12	95
Hostess Pecan Spinners, 1	110	5	1	0	15	0	-	65
Brownie Bites, 1.3 oz	170	9	2	30	21	1	17	80
Mini-Muffins, Choc Chip, 1.2 oz	160	9	3	0	17	0	8	100
Mini-Muffins, Banana Walnut, 1.2 oz	160	9	1	25	16	2	8	100
Zingers, Raspberry Cream-Filled, 1.9 oz	160	7	3	5	24	0	20	100
Crumb Cake, LF, 1 oz	90	1	0	0	19	0	16	100
Crumb Coffee Cake, 1 oz	130	5	2	10	19	0	10	110
Lance Fig Cake, LF, 1 oz	110	2	1	0	21	1	14	70
Peanut Bar, 1.6 oz	240	14	3	0	22	2	10	70
Creme-Filled Wafer, 1.5 oz	220	12	3	0	25	1	16	120
Dunking Stick, 1.4 oz	180	9	3	5	22	1	15	130
Little Debbie								
Cookie Wreaths (seasonal), 1 pkg	90	5	1	0	11	0	-	45
Ginger Cookies, 1 pkg	90	3	1	5	14	1	-	55
German Choc Rings	140	8	4	0	18	1	11	65
Marshmallow Supremes, 1 pkg	140	5	1	0	22	1	15	65
Star Crunch, 1.1 oz	150	6	2	0	22	0	12	70
Pecan Pinwheels, 1 oz	100	4	1	0	16	0	7	80
Caramel Cookie Bar, 1.2 oz	160	8	2	0	22	0	16	85
Fudge Rounds, 1.2 oz	150	4	1	0	23	1	14	85
Strawberry Cupcakes, 1.7 oz	210	10	3	0	29	1	22	100
Frosted Fudge Cake, 1.5 oz	200	10	3	5	25	1	18	105

Food	Cal	Fat	Sat	Chol	Carb	Fib	Sug	Sod
SNACK CAKES, PIES AND SWEETS								
Little Debbie (cont'd)								
Nutty Bars, 2 oz (2)	310	18	4	0	32	1	20	110
Banana Marshmallow Pie, 1.5 oz	180	6	2	0	30	0	18	110
Raisin Creme Pie Cookie, 1.2 oz	140	5	1	0	23	0	16	120
Golden Cremes, 1	150	-	-	-	26	0	17	125
Madeleine Choc Chip French, 1.1 oz	130	5	1	20	18	1	10	70
Salerno Scooter Pie, 1.2 oz	140	5	3	0	23	0	14	80
Sara Lee Pound Cake, Strawberry Swirl, 1.5 oz	95	6	2	30	22	0	13	70
***Tastykake** Kreme Bars, 1 oz	120	6	4	3	18	1	12	33
Kandy Kakes, Coconut, 1.4 oz	160	9	7	0	21	1	15	55
Kandy Kakes, Mint, 1.4 oz	160	8	5	0	23	1	16	65
Koffee Kake, Creme-Filled, 1 oz	120	5	1	15	18	0	11	65
Kandy Kakes, Strawberry, 1.4 oz	180	9	5	10	23	0	18	75
Kandy Kakes, Choc, 1.4 oz	170	9	5	0	24	1	16	80
Kandy Kakes, Peanut Butter, 1.4 oz	180	9	5	10	21	1	14	85
Kandy Kakes, Frosty, 1.4 oz	170	8	5	0	23	0	17	85
Koffee Kake, LF Apple-Filled, 1 oz	85	1	0	0	17	1	10	85
Creamies, Witchy Treat, 1.4 oz	150	6	1	30	24	0	16	90
Koffee Kake, LF Raspberry-Filled, 1 oz	85	1	0	0	18	1	8	90
Koffee Kake, LF Lemon-Filled, 1 oz	90	2	0	5	18	0	11	90
Krimpets, Strawberry Kreme Filled, 1.1 oz	130	5	1	28	20	0	14	100
Creamies, Bunny Trail Treats, Cupid, Kringle, or Sparkle, 1.4 oz (avg)	150	5	1	30	25	0	17	105
Tastyklair, 2 oz	195	10	2	45	25	0	13	145
Peach Pie, 2 oz	135	6	1	0	22	1	11	145
Apple or Cherry Pie, 2 oz (avg)	138	6	1	0	22	1	11	150

Food	Cal	Fat	Sat	Chol	Carb	Fib	Sug	Sod

DIET & NUTRITIONAL FOODS

DIET & NUTRITIONAL DRINKS

(also see Sports & Energy Drinks, pg 18)

Food	Cal	Fat	Sat	Chol	Carb	Fib	Sug	Sod
Meal replacement, mix, 3 tbsp	140	2	0	0	14	2	11	170
Diet, ready-to-drink, 8 fl oz	165	2	0	6	32	4	-	188
Nutritional, ready-to-drink, 8 fl oz	240	4	1	5	40	0	-	200
Diet, mix, prep w/skim milk, 8 fl oz	200	1	0	8	38	6	-	280

BRANDS . . .

DIET DRINKS

MIX *(3 TBSP MIX UNLESS NOTED)*

Food	Cal	Fat	Sat	Chol	Carb	Fib	Sug	Sod
*Atkins Shakes								
Choc, 2 scoops	180	9	2	5	3	2	1	80
Cappuccino, Strawberry, or Vanilla,								
2 scoops (avg)	170	8	1	5	2	0	1	12
Slim Fast								
Ultra, all choc mixes (avg)	120	2	1	5	23	5	15	100
Choc, Choc Malt, or Vanilla (avg)	100	1	1	5	20	2	17	115
Ultra, Strawberry or Vanilla (avg)	100	1	1	5	25	5	18	130

READY-TO-DRINK *(8 FL OZ UNLESS NOTED)*

Food	Cal	Fat	Sat	Chol	Carb	Fib	Sug	Sod
*Atkins, Choc, 11 oz	170	9	2	15	5	3	2	140
Strawberry or Vanilla, 11 oz	170	9	2	15	4	2	2	140
Calorie Shed Shake, FF, No								
Sugar, all	140	0	0	10	42	4	6	90
Slim Fast, 11 oz (avg)	220	3	1	5	40	5	35	220

NUTRITIONAL DRINKS

READY-TO-DRINK *(8 FL OZ UNLESS NOTED)*

Food	Cal	Fat	Sat	Chol	Carb	Fib	Sug	Sod
Boost Butter Pecan, Strawberry,								
Choc Malt, or Choc Mocha (avg)	240	4	1	5	40	0	23	130
Ensure Coffee Latte or Butter Pecan	250	6	5	5	40	0	18	200
Grainaissance Amazake most								
(avg)	180	2	0	0	35	4	30	20
Gimme Green Rice Shake	190	3	1	0	37	4	29	35
Rice Nog	190	2	0	0	39	4	34	65
RW Knudsen Mega C	140	0	0	0	33	0	30	15
Morning Blend	140	0	0	0	31	0	25	15
High Antioxident	140	0	0	0	29	0	28	20
Gingko Alert	120	0	0	0	31	0	27	25
Mega Green	120	0	0	0	30	0	25	35

Food	Cal	Fat	Sat	Chol	Carb	Fib	Sug	Sod

DIET, ENERGY & NUTRITIONAL BARS

There are many low-sodium diet, energy and nutritional bars, the following have less than 125mg per serving.

BRANDS . . .

FROZEN/REFRIGERATED *(3.5 OZ UNLESS NOTED)*

Food	Cal	Fat	Sat	Chol	Carb	Fib	Sug	Sod
Cold Fusion Protein & Energy (avg)	80	0	0	0	21	0	21	0

READY-TO-EAT *(1.8 OZ BAR UNLESS NOTED)*

*Atkins

Advantage, 2.1 oz bars:

Food	Cal	Fat	Sat	Chol	Carb	Fib	Sug	Sod
Choc Decadence	220	11	7	2	25	11	0	65
Frosted Cinnamon Swirl	230	11	7	2	21	10	0	95
Choc Coconut	230	11	8	2	21	9	0	100
Creamy Berry Cheesecake	240	11	7	2	20	9	0	100
Almond Brownie	220	8	4	5	21	7	0	105
Pralines 'N Creme	250	13	7	2	18	7	0	105
Choc Mocha Crunch	220	10	6	2	22	10	0	120
Choc Peanut	240	12	6	2	21	10	1	125
Endulge Candy Bars, all, 1.1 oz	150	12	7	5	2	3	0	20
Balance								
Gold:								
Rocky Road	210	7	4	0	22	1	12	80
Triple Choc Chaos	200	6	4	0	22	1	12	85
Caramel Nut Blast	210	7	4	0	22	1	13	110
Choc Peanut Butter	210	7	4	0	22	1	11	125
Almond Brownie	200	6	2	5	23	2	18	115
Yogurt Berry, 1.8 oz	100	6	3	5	22	0	17	120
Carbolite Choc Crisp, 1 oz	140	9	6	5	15	1	0	10
Choc Almond, 1 oz	130	9	5	5	14	1	0	16
Choc Peanut Butter, 1 oz	140	10	4	5	15	1	0	30
Carb Solutions								
Candy Bars, 1.1 oz:								
Choc w/Almonds	140	11	5	5	15	1	0	20
Choc	140	10	6	10	17	1	0	25
High Protein Bars, 2.1 oz:								
Frosted Blueberry	230	8	3	5	15	1	3	115
Choc Toffee Hazelnut, Choc Mint, or Choc Fudge Almond (avg)	245	9	4	0	14	1	0	115
Choice Nutrition Bars, all, 1.3 oz	140	5	3	5	19	3	9	80
Clif Bar Choc Chip, 2.4 oz	250	3	1	0	51	3	15	45
Carrot Cake, 2.4 oz	240	4	1	0	42	5	14	50
Cookies 'n Cream, 2.4 oz	250	5	1	0	42	5	14	80
Apricot, 2.4 oz	220	3	0	0	43	5	21	90

DIET & NUTRITIONAL FOODS
Diet, Energy & Nutritional Bars

Food	Cal	Fat	Sat	Chol	Carb	Fib	Sug	Sod
DIET, DNERGY AND NUTRITIONAL BARS								
Creme De La Creme, all, 1.4 oz (avg)	200	14	2	0	15	5	9	0
Delta Natural Fiber, 1/2 cup	20	0	0	0	2	20	-	20
EAS Advant Edge Carb Control								
Blueberry, 2.1 oz	200	5	3	5	21	3	2	125
Lemon Cheesecake or Apple								
Cinnamon, 2.1 oz	210	5	3	5	19	2	1	125
Ensure Glucerna Lemon Crunch, 1 bar	140	4	1	5	24	4	10	100
Fi-Bar, 1 bar (avg)	130	4	2	0	25	3	16	35
GeniSoy Xtreme Carrot Cake								
Quaker, 1.6 oz	190	7	3	0	24	1	18	90
Glenny's, all, 1 bar	180	7	2	0	28	4	17	20
Go Lean Malted Choc Chip, 2.8 oz	280	5	4	20	51	6	29	85
Cookies 'N Cream, 2.8 oz	290	6	4	0	54	7	35	100
Honey Bars, all, 1.4 oz (avg)	180	9	2	0	21	2	13	20
Luna Lemon Zest, 1.7 oz	180	4	3	0	26	2	14	50
Nutz Over Chocolate, 1.7 oz	180	5	3	0	24	2	12	100
Met Rx								
Protein Plus Bars, 3 oz:								
Choc Roasted Peanut	320	9	5	5	29	1	2	75
Choc Choc Chip	310	6	1	10	32	2	2	80
Food Bars, 3.5 oz:								
Choc Graham Cracker Chip	320	3	2	10	48	1	26	95
Fudge Brownie	320	3	1	10	52	2	29	110
Choc Chip, 3 oz	340	4	2	10	50	0	29	110
Choc Choc Chip, 3 oz	310	6	1	10	32	2	2	80
Nutiva Flax-Choc, 1.4 oz	200	12	2	0	19	5	10	5
Hempseed, 1.4 oz	210	14	2	0	11	5	5	5
Flax-Raisin, 1.4 oz	280	19	2	0	12	6	5	10
Nutritious Creations Snack Bars								
all, 3 oz (avg)	100	0	0	0	32	5	12	45
Omega Smart Cinnamon Apple, 1	220	5	0	0	36	7	22	65
Power Bar Harvest, 2.3 oz (avg)	240	4	1	0	45	4	16	80
Regular, 2.3 oz (avg)	230	3	1	0	45	3	14	90
Slim Fast								
Snack Bars, 1 oz:								
Choc Peanut or Chewy Choc Nougat	120	4	3	5	20	0	16	70
Rich Chewy Caramel	120	4	3	0	22	2	12	75
Peanut Butter Crunch	130	4	2	0	21	1	20	80
Meal Bars, 1.2 oz:								
Breakfast/Lunch, Dutch Choc	140	5	3	5	20	2	12	80
Oatmeal Raisin	220	5	4	5	36	2	22	100
Milk Choc Peanut	220	5	3	5	37	2	24	125

Food	Cal	Fat	Sat	Chol	Carb	Fib	Sug	Sod
DIET, DNERGY AND NUTRITIONAL BARS								
Tigers Milk								
Peanut Butter Crunch, 1.3 oz	160	8	2	0	19	2	16	70
Peanut Butter, 1.3 oz	170	7	2	0	19	0	13	80
Original, 1.3 oz	160	6	1	0	20	0	13	90
Worldwide Pure Protein								
Blueberry or Strawberry								
Cheesecake, 1.8 oz (avg)	190	3	2	5	20	0	3	40
Chewy Choc Chip, 1.8 oz	170	4	3	5	17	1	1	60
S'Mores, 1.8 oz	190	3	3	5	22	1	2	65
Cinnamon Graham, 1 .8 oz	180	4	3	5	17	1	2	75
Lemon Chiffon, 1.8 oz	170	3	3	5	17	0	1	90
Peanut Butter, 1.8 oz	180	5	3	5	16	1	1	100
Zoe Foods Nutri Bar								
Flax/Soy, Choc, 1.9 oz b	190	6	2	0	28	4	11	40
Flax/Soy, Apple Crisp, 1.9 oz	180	6	1	0	28	4	11	50
Flax/Soy, Lemon, 1.9 oz	190	5	1	0	28	5	12	70
Flax/Soy, Peanut Butter, 1.9 oz	210	8	1	0	27	4	11	95
Peanut Butter & Honey, 1.3 oz	150	5	1	0	19	0	13	100

(SEAWEED)

Food	Cal	Fat	Sat	Chol	Carb	Fib	Sug	Sod
Agar, fresh, 1 oz	0	0	0	0	2	-	0	3
Nori, fresh, 1 oz	10	0	0	0	1	-	0	14
Spirulina, fresh, 1 oz	7	0	0	0	1	-	0	28
Spirulina, dried, 1 oz	83	2	1	0	7	-	0	309

BRANDS . . .

Most brands are within the generic range.

(WHEAT GERM)

Food	Cal	Fat	Sat	Chol	Carb	Fib	Sug	Sod
Wheat germ, 2 tbsp	50	1	0	0	6	2	1	0

BRANDS . . .

Most brands are within the generic range.

Food	Cal	Fat	Sat	Chol	Carb	Fib	Sug	Sod

DINNERS, ENTREES & SIDE DISHES

APPETIZERS & SNACKS

Food	Cal	Fat	Sat	Chol	Carb	Fib	Sug	Sod
Mozzarella cheese sticks, 1.5 oz	150	8	3	11	12	1	1	370
Egg roll, 3 oz	190	7	2	15	29	2	2	440
Pizza snacks, cheese & pepperoni, 3 oz	290	14	3	24	30	1	3	650
Buffalo wings, 3.3 oz	100	7	0	35	1	0	0	920

BRANDS . . .

FROZEN/REFRIGERATED

Food	Cal	Fat	Sat	Chol	Carb	Fib	Sug	Sod
Amy's Cheese Pizza Snacks, 3 pcs	90	3	2	5	11	1	2	145
Anchor Golden Crisp Diced Jalapeño & Cheddar Mini Hot Shots, 2 pcs	100	4	3	10	14	1	1	220
Athens Three Cheese Blend Appetizers, 4-5 pcs	540	31	5	5	62	2	34	230
Health is Wealth								
Spinach Munchies, 1 oz	60	3	0	0	9	1	0	105
Mexican Munchies, 1 oz	49	1	0	0	8	1	0	110
Spinach & Feta Munchies, 1 oz	70	3	1	5	9	1	0	115
Broccoli Munchies, 1 oz	60	2	0	0	10	1	0	170
Vegie Munchies, 1 oz	50	1	0	0	9	1	0	170
Veg Potstickers, 1.6 oz	90	3	1	0	11	5	0	190
Spring Rolls, 1.6 oz	70	2	1	0	10	5	0	200
Mozzarella Sticks, 1.3 oz	120	5	3	15	14	0	0	250
Michelina's Yu Sing Egg Rolls								
Sweet & Sour Pork, 3 oz	180	5	2	8	28	2	-	135
Shrimp, 3 oz	180	6	2	10	20	2	-	230
Sweet & Sour Chicken, 3 oz	200	6	2	13	30	2	-	230
TGIF Friday's Mozzarella Sticks, 1.6 oz	100	6	2	10	9	1	1	160
White Wave Spring Rolls, 1.5 oz	70	2	1	0	10	5	0	200

BLINTZES & CREPES

Food	Cal	Fat	Sat	Chol	Carb	Fib	Sug	Sod
Fruit, 2.2 oz	100	3	1	3	13	3	6	130
Cheese, 2.2 oz	100	3	1	10	15	2	4	155
Potato, 2.2 oz	95	3	1	5	16	2	2	265

BRANDS . . .

FROZEN/REFRIGERATED *(2.2 OZ UNLESS NOTED)*

Food	Cal	Fat	Sat	Chol	Carb	Fib	Sug	Sod
Flaum Cheese & Blueberry, 3 oz	135	4	-	-	22	-	-	105
Potato, Potato Spinach, or Cheese, 3 oz (avg)	110	4	-	-	16	-	-	110

Food	Cal	Fat	Sat	Chol	Carb	Fib	Sug	Sod
BLINTZES AND CREPES								
***Empire Kosher** Blintzes*								
Apple	110	3	-	3	18	-	-	130
Cheese	90	2	-	15	13	-	-	135
Cherry	100	2	-	5	19	-	-	140
Blueberry	90	1	-	10	18	-	-	150
Ian's Crepes Apple Cinnamon Filled	120	4	1	40	18	1	11	115
***J & J** Potato Blintz, 2.3 oz	90	5	1	14	13	1	1	130
Cheese Blintz, 2.3 oz	132	4	-	7	10	-	-	132
King Kold Blintzes								
Cherry or Blueberry, 2.5 oz (avg)	90	1	0	25	19	0	6	98
Cheese, 2.5 oz	90	2	1	30	13	0	5	160
Potato, 2.5 oz	80	3	0	25	13	0	0	170
***Ratner's** Blintzes*								
Cheese	90	1	-	20	15	-	-	15
Blueberry or Blueberry Cheese	100	1	-	15	17	-	-	15
Cherry	100	1	-	15	20	-	-	15
Potato	110	3	-	15	17	-	-	130
***Tuv Taam** Apple Cinnamon Crepes, 2.5 oz*	110	2	-	-	21	-	-	90
Diet Cheese/Cherry Blintzes, 2.5 oz	100	3	-	-	15	-	-	90
Cheese Blintzes, Sugar Free, 2.5 oz	70	3	-	-	12	-	-	105
Cheese Blintzes, 2.5 oz	95	3	-	-	13	-	-	110
Potato Blintzes, 2.5 oz	115	4	-	-	18	-	-	110

BREAKFAST MEALS

(also see Pancakes & Waffles, pg 35)

Food	Cal	Fat	Sat	Chol	Carb	Fib	Sug	Sod
Breakfast burrito, ham/cheese, 3.5 oz	212	7	2	192	28	1	-	405
Scrambled eggs & sausage w/hash brown potatoes, 6.3 oz	361	27	7	283	17	1	-	772
Sausage, egg & cheese on a biscuit, 5.5 oz	490	30	12	110	36	3	4	1110
BRANDS ...								
FROZEN/REFRIGERATED								
Health is Wealth Breakfast Munchies, all, 1 oz (avg)	70	4	0	0	9	1	1	190
Hot Pockets								
Sausage, Egg & Cheese, 2.3 oz	180	10	4	35	16	1	6	260
Bacon, Egg & Cheese, 2.3 oz	170	9	4	45	17	1	6	260
State Fair Pancake/Sausage Stick, 1	240	14	5	20	22	1	9	320
Sunny Fresh Bagel French Toast w/Maple Syrup, 1 serv	190	5	1	128	21	0	6	283

DINNERS, ENTREES & SIDE DISHES
Dinners & Entrees - Canned

Food	Cal	Fat	Sat	Chol	Carb	Fib	Sug	Sod
BREAKFAST MEALS								
Swanson Great Starts								
Sticks w/Syrup, 1 pkg	320	10	5	25	50	2	16	260
Cinnamon Roll French Toast & Sausage, 1 pkg	410	20	7	100	47	2	30	450

DINNERS & ENTREES - CANNED

Food	Cal	Fat	Sat	Chol	Carb	Fib	Sug	Sod
Beef stew, 8.3 oz	218	12	5	37	16	3	2	947
Macaroni & cheese, 9 oz	199	6	3	8	29	3	2	1058
Spaghetti & meatballs, 7.5 oz	230	7	4	20	29	2	2	1060

BRANDS . . .

No low-sodium alternatives.

DINNERS & ENTREES - FROZEN

Food	Cal	Fat	Sat	Chol	Carb	Fib	Sug	Sod
ASIAN MEALS								
Chicken chow mein w/egg roll, 9 oz	210	7	4	30	28	3	-	850
Oriental beef, 9 oz	250	7	4	30	31	3	3	960
Chicken teriyaki rice bowl, 10.9 oz	430	6	1	25	77	1	-	1210
BRANDS . . . *(11 OZ UNLESS NOTED)*								
Amy's Organic Thai Stir Fry, 9.5 oz	270	11	7	0	36	2	4	420
Cedarlane LF Rice & Veg Teriyaki Wrap, 8 oz	280	3	0	0	56	2	5	480
Ethnic Gourmet								
Pad Thai w/Tofu Rice Bowl	390	9	2	0	68	4	20	160
Vegetarian Teriyaki Rice Bowl, 12 oz	350	3	1	0	73	4	12	210
Teriyaki Chicken Rice Bowl	360	5	1	30	66	2	9	270
Vegetable Paneer, 8 oz	320	10	2	5	50	4	7	380
Kung Pao Chicken Rice Bowl, 12 oz	340	6	1	30	56	3	9	400
Chicken Biryani Rice Bowl	340	9	1	25	52	3	7	430
Shrimp Fried Rice Bowl	400	10	1	50	64	4	5	430
Thai Chef Veg Chicken w/Lemon & Basil	390	11	6	0	61	7	13	470
Veg Lo Mein w/Organic Tofu	410	10	6	35	58	6	6	490
Weight Watchers Smart Ones								
Chicken Chow Mein, 9 oz	200	2	1	25	34	3	5	490

FISH & SEAFOOD MEALS *(also see Fish & Seafood - Prepared Entrees, pg 118)*

Food	Cal	Fat	Sat	Chol	Carb	Fib	Sug	Sod
Fish 'n chips, 10 oz	490	20	4	45	59	5	18	1030
Tuna noodle casserole, 10 oz	360	16	5	30	36	2	5	1060
BRANDS . . .								
Healthy Choice Lemon Pepper Fish, 10.7 oz	320	7	2	30	50	5	20	480

Food	Cal	Fat	Sat	Chol	Carb	Fib	Sug	Sod
HISPANIC MEALS								
Bean & cheese burrito, 4.9 oz	270	5	2	5	46	7	-	530
Enchiladas w/beans & rice, 11 oz	360	11	5	20	55	9	7	1390
Tamales, beef enchiladas w/beans & rice, 13.4 oz	508	20	7	26	68	8	-	1812
BRANDS . . .								
***Amy's** Organic*								
Black Bean & Veg Enchilada, 9.5 oz	170	5	1	0	26	3	2	390
Cheese Enchilada, 9.5 oz	210	12	6	35	13	2	2	440
***Atkins** Roasted & Shredded Pork*								
Enchilada, 4.8 oz	190	11	4	35	11	8	0	410
Grilled Steak Fajitas, 4.8 oz	300	18	8	40	16	10	2	500
Cedarlane								
LF Garden Veg Enchiladas, 1	140	3	2	10	20	3	4	310
Quesadillas, 3 pcs	250	11	6	25	27	0	4	420
LF Beans & Rice Cheese Style Burritos, 1	260	1	0	0	48	7	2	490
***Delimex** Beef Taquitos, 5 oz*	350	12	2	25	44	7	0	460
Chicken Taquitos, 5 oz	370	14	3	30	47	8	0	480
***El Monterey** Bean & Cheese Burrito,*								
Reduced Fat, 4 oz	210	4	1	0	35	3	1	180
Beef/Bean Burrito, Reduced Fat, 4 oz	260	9	3	15	34	3	1	190
Bean & Cheese Burrito, 5 oz	290	9	3	10	44	4	2	270
Beef & Bean Burrito, 5 oz	420	21	8	30	44	4	2	320
Spicy Red Hot Beef & Bean Burrito, 5 oz	370	17	6	20	43	4	2	330
Beef/Bean Green Chili Burrito, 5 oz	370	17	6	20	42	4	1	340
Beef & Cheese Chimichanga, 5 oz	310	13	5	35	35	1	1	340
Chicken/Cheese Chimichanga, 5 oz	320	13	5	25	38	2	1	350
***Jose Ole** Beef & Cheese Mini*								
Taquitos, 3 oz	160	5	2	10	22	2	1	330
Shredded Beef Taquitos, 3 oz	160	5	1	10	24	2	0	330
Chicken & Cheese Mini Tacos, 3 oz	140	5	2	15	20	2	1	350
Chicken Taquitos, 3 oz	160	5	1	20	21	2	0	380
Beef & Cheese Mini Tacos, 3 oz	200	10	4	15	23	2	1	410
Chicken & Cheese Mini Burritos, 3 oz	180	5	1	10	26	1	1	410
Cheese Mini Burritos, 3 oz	180	7	2	5	26	1	1	460
***Senor Felix's** Sonora Style Burrito, 1*	280	8	2	10	45	3	4	240
Black Bean Soy Burrito, 1	240	7	1	0	36	3	6	360
Whole Foods Market 365								
Chicken Taquitos, 5 oz	260	5	1	35	40	4	0	230

95

DINNERS, ENTREES & SIDE DISHES
Dinners & Entrees - Frozen

Food	Cal	Fat	Sat	Chol	Carb	Fib	Sug	Sod
INTERNATIONAL MEALS								
Cascadian Farm Organic Indian Meal, 10.1 oz	350	6	0	0	61	6	5	330
Organic Moroccan Meal, 10.1 oz	310	4	0	0	59	11	12	440
Organic Aztec Meal, 10.1 oz	290	4	0	0	54	10	1	480
MEAT & POULTRY MEALS								
Sliced beef w/gravy, mashed potatoes & peas, 9.1 oz	270	10	4	71	19	4	12	742
Veal parmigiana w/tomato sauce, mashed potatoes & peas, 9.1 oz	362	19	6	26	35	7	15	964
Turkey w/gravy, stuffing, mashed potatoes & corn, 9.4 oz	280	10	3	52	34	3	7	1061
Salisbury steak w/mashed potatoes & corn, 9.6 oz	398	25	9	51	28	3	-	1140
Fried chicken w/mashed potatoes & corn, 8.1 oz	470	27	9	89	35	2	3	1500
BRANDS . . . *(8 OZ UNLESS NOTED)*								
Atkins Chicken Cacciatore, 5 oz	90	1	0	10	10	4	4	25
Budget Gourmet								
Orange Glazed Chicken, 8.6 oz	300	3	1	20	56	2	13	460
Cascadian Farm Chicken Bowl, Orange Dijon Veggie, 8.5 oz	240	3	1	35	42	3	7	360
Healthy Choice								
Country Breaded Chicken, 10.3 oz	380	8	2	25	57	7	22	450
Meatloaf, 12 oz	330	7	4	35	52	6	17	460
Salisbury Steak, 11.5 oz	330	7	3	50	48	6	24	470
Sweet & Sour Chicken, 11 oz	360	7	2	35	54	3	21	470
Mesquite Beef w/BBQ Sauce, 11 oz	320	9	3	55	38	5	16	490
Stouffer's Lean Cuisine Café Classics, Chicken a L'Orange, 9 oz	230	2	1	40	33	2	9	300
Skillet Sensations, Chicken Primavera	180	3	1	20	28	1	11	430
Skillet Sensations, Roasted Turkey	150	2	1	15	24	3	7	450
Skillet Sensations, Three Cheese Chicken	200	5	2	25	26	2	5	460
Café Classics, Glazed Chicken, 8.5 oz	230	5	1	55	25	0	7	480
Skillet Sensations, Garlic Chicken	200	4	2	25	32	2	4	500
Weight Watchers Smart Ones								
Honey Mustard Chicken, 1 serv	200	2	-	30	33	6	9	340
Lemon Herb Chicken Piccata, 9 oz	190	2	1	25	34	3	8	460

Food	Cal	Fat	Sat	Chol	Carb	Fib	Sug	Sod
VEGETARIAN MEAT DISHES								
Hain Vegetarian Classics, Pepper								
Steak, 10 oz	310	6	-	0	41	-	-	440
PASTA MEALS *(also see Pasta Entrees, pg 100)*								
Spaghetti w/meat sauce, 10 oz	350	12	4	35	46	5	-	570
Fettuccine alfredo, 10 oz	653	39	16	64	58	2	4	902
Macaroni & cheese, 12 oz	370	15	8	38	48	2	-	1070
Lasagne w/meat sauce, 10.5 oz	370	14	7	45	39	-	-	1050
BRANDS . . . *(10 OZ UNLESS NOTED)*								
Amy's Organic								
Cannelloni Whole Meal, 9 oz	330	12	8	35	34	6	10	390
Skillet Meal Pasta & Veg Alfredo	220	8	4	20	27	4	6	460
Skillet Meal Country Cheddar	250	11	3	5	27	3	3	480
*Atkins Baked Ziti, 5 oz	200	8	5	30	10	4	4	300
Meatballs & Pasta, 5 oz	80	6	2	36	10	3	3	430
Bird's Eye Pasta Secrets								
Zesty Garlic, 6 oz	240	10	3	5	31	2	6	310
Primavera, 6.8 oz	230	10	3	10	26	3	4	430
Ranch, 6.8 oz	300	15	6	25	29	2	8	460
Budget Gourmet								
Light & Healthy, Penne Pasta								
w/Chunky Tomatoes & Sausage	270	6	1	10	46	3	4	410
Angel Hair Pasta w/Chunky Tomatoes	240	5	2	10	39	3	6	450
Cedarlane								
LF Garden Veg Lasagna, 5 oz	180	3	2	10	26	2	2	390
Eggplant Parmesan, 5 oz	160	8	3	15	16	3	3	390
Cascadian Farm Organic Indian Meal								
Penne Marinara, 10.1 oz	280	5	3	5	50	4	5	410
Pasta Primavera, 9 oz	280	8	3	10	41	3	4	440
Celentano								
Penne w/Roasted Veg	120	4	1	0	19	3	5	390
Roasted Veg Lasagne	170	9	1	0	21	5	8	430
Eggplant Parmigiana	340	24	4	0	26	5	10	450
Stuffed Shells w/Sauce, 7 oz	320	12	5	70	36	2	4	470
Lasagne Primavera	420	5	2	70	73	6	7	480
Healthy Choice								
Solos, Cheese Ravioli, 9 oz	260	5	3	30	44	4	14	340
Solos, Beef Macaroni, 8.5 oz	220	4	2	20	34	5	9	450
Stuffed Pasta Shells, 11.2 oz	290	6	3	20	40	5	10	470
Michael Angelo's Mini Calzone								
Sausage & Pepperoni, 3 oz	240	8	4	20	32	4	8	360
Manicotti w/Sauce	230	12	6	55	11	5	5	390
Lasagna w/Meat Sauce	294	10	8	50	26	4	5	490

97

DINNERS, ENTREES & SIDE DISHES
Dinners & Entrees - Shelf-Stable

Food	Cal	Fat	Sat	Chol	Carb	Fib	Sug	Sod
PASTA MEALS - FROZEN								
Stouffer's Lean Cuisine								
Everyday Favorites, Penne Pasta								
w/Tomato Basil Sauce	260	4	1	0	50	5	13	390
Tyson Garlic Chicken & Pasta	190	5	2	15	23	0	1	380
Oriental Style Chicken & Pasta	180	5	2	15	19	0	2	380
Weight Watchers Smart Ones								
Pasta w/Tomato Basil Sauce, 1 serv	260	9	4	10	33	5	3	360
Spicy Penne & Ricotta, 1 serv	280	6	2	5	45	5	5	370
QUICHES, PIES & SOUFFLES								
Turkey pot pie, 7 oz	350	18	6	32	35	2	-	695
Beef pot pie, 7 oz	449	24	9	38	44	2	-	737
Chicken pot pie, 7.8 oz	484	29	10	41	43	2	8	857
BRANDS . . .								
Amy's Organic Shepherd's Pie, 8 oz	160	4	0	0	27	5	5	490
***Atkins** 4 Cheese Crustless Quiche, 1	290	24	15	45	2	0	1	270
Smoked Ham & Cheese Crustless								
Quiche, 1	290	24	13	170	2	0	2	490
Spinach, Tomato & Feta Souffle, 1	170	13	7	200	4	2	2	490
Dimitri Delights Pita Cheese &								
Spinach Pie, 5 oz	370	23	-	35	32	-	-	460
Fillo Factory Broccoli/Cheese Pie, 6 oz	350	12	5	20	50	3	1	370
Shelton's Pies								
Organic Chicken, 9.1 oz	260	13	7	65	20	2	2	280
Turkey w/whole wheat flour, 10 oz	220	10	5	50	18	3	0	360
Chicken w/sunbleached flour, 10 oz	230	10	5	55	18	1	0	370
Chicken w/whole wheat flour, 10 oz	230	10	5	55	18	3	3	370

NOTE: Although not listed, Trader Joe's carries many frozen entrees with less than 500mg sodium per serving.

(DINNERS & ENTREES - SHELF-STABLE)

Food	Cal	Fat	Sat	Chol	Carb	Fib	Sug	Sod
Macaroni & cheese, microwave, 7.5 oz	260	10	5	25	35	1	-	840
Spaghetti & meatballs, micro, 7.5 oz	230	6	4	25	35	1	-	900
Cheese tortellini, 10 oz	340	10	3	15	49	6	-	1000
BRANDS . . .								
***Atkins** Menu Classics, 8 oz:								
Beef Teriyaki	211	7	3	65	9	1	0	302
Chicken Teriyaki	160	5	1	69	9	1	0	313
Chicken Marsala	169	6	1	69	9	1	0	366
My Own Meal								
Chicken Mediterranean, 1 pkg	270	9	2	45	28	4	-	320

Food	Cal	Fat	Sat	Chol	Carb	Fib	Sug	Sod

DINNER MIXES & HELPERS

Food	Cal	Fat	Sat	Chol	Carb	Fib	Sug	Sod
Tuna mix/helper, cheese, 1 cup	290	11	-	20	32	1	-	890
Hamburger mix/helper, cheese, 1 cup	310	15	-	60	30	1	-	920
Shrimp stir fry, 9.8 oz	200	2	0	105	28	5	17	1330

BRANDS ...

BOXED/PACKAGED
Bumble Bee Tuna Mixes, all, 1 pkg	75	0	0	0	15	0	-	15

FROZEN/REFRIGERATED
Bird's Eye Easy Recipe Meal Starter Sweet & Sour w/Pineapple, 8.8 oz	200	1	0	0	45	3	41	330
Chef's Choice Shrimp Linguini, 1 1/3 cup	170	1	0	40	30	4	2	450

TOFU MIXES
BRANDS ...
Nasoya Tofu Mate

Food	Cal	Fat	Sat	Chol	Carb	Fib	Sug	Sod
Szechuan Stir Fry, 1/4 pkg	25	0	0	0	4	0	0	280
Eggless Salad, 1/4 pkg	15	0	0	0	4	0	0	310
Mandarin Stir Fry, 1/4 pkg	30	0	0	0	6	0	3	310
Mediterranean Herb, 1/4 pkg	15	0	0	0	3	0	1	330
Breakfast Scramble, 1/4 pkg	15	0	0	0	3	0	0	330
Texas Taco, 1/4 pkg	15	0	0	0	3	0	0	360

FISH & SEAFOOD ENTREES

(see Fish & Seafood - Frozen Prepared Entrees, pg 118)

LUNCH PACKS

(also see Pockets, Sandwiches & Wraps, pg 103)

Food	Cal	Fat	Sat	Chol	Carb	Fib	Sug	Sod
Cheese & salsa nachos, 4.4 oz box	380	21	5	10	39	3	3	1060
Bologna, american cheese & choc chip cookies, 4.2 oz box	470	31	13	80	31	1	9	1340
Lean turkey, cheddar cheese & crackers, 4.5 oz box	360	22	12	70	20	1	4	1740

BRANDS ... *(10 OZ UNLESS NOTED)*
Kosherbles Bagels

Food	Cal	Fat	Sat	Chol	Carb	Fib	Sug	Sod
Cream Cheese & Jelly	450	11	-	30	78	-	-	430
PB&J w/Peanut Butter & Jelly	490	13	-	0	81	-	-	440

MEAT & POULTRY ENTREES

(see Meat, Poultry & Substitutes - Prepared Entrees, pg 125)

DINNERS, ENTREES & SIDE DISHES
Pasta Entrees

Food	Cal	Fat	Sat	Chol	Carb	Fib	Sug	Sod

PASTA ENTREES

(also see Dinners & Entrees - Frozen Pasta Meals, pg 97)

Food	Cal	Fat	Sat	Chol	Carb	Fib	Sug	Sod
Macaroni & cheese, boxed, 1 cup	420	19	5	15	50	2	7	750
Spaghetti, canned, 1 cup	210	2	1	5	41	3	14	940
Macaroni & cheese, canned, 1 cup	197	6	3	8	29	3	-	1047

BRANDS ...

BOXED/PACKAGED *(1 CUP PREP UNLESS NOTED)*

Annie's Homegrown
Mac & Cheese:

Food	Cal	Fat	Sat	Chol	Carb	Fib	Sug	Sod
Mild Cheddar	270	5	2	5	49	2	2	170
Original	270	4	2	10	49	2	7	360
Mild Mexican	280	5	3	10	47	2	2	370
Bunny-Shape	270	4	2	10	47	2	2	370
Alfredo	280	5	3	15	46	2	2	380
Pasta Meal:								
Tomato & Basil	280	3	1	5	49	2	2	390
Garlic & Parmesan	200	3	2	5	34	1	2	430
Cheddar & Broccoli	280	3	2	5	48	2	2	450
Keto Macaroni & Cheese Dinner, 1/3 box	112	0	0	0	5	1	0	120
Near East Basil & Herb Pasta	240	2	1	5	39	3	2	380
Ragu Express!, Sweet Tomato & Garlic, 1 pouch pasta & sauce	200	3	0	0	39	3	8	320

FROZEN/REFRIGERATED *(1 CUP UNLESS NOTED)*

Food	Cal	Fat	Sat	Chol	Carb	Fib	Sug	Sod
A&M Stuffed Shells, 4 oz	240	10	-	100	20	-	-	118
Atkins Chicken Cacciatore, 5 oz	90	1	0	10	10	4	4	25
Baked Ziti, 5 oz	200	8	5	30	10	4	4	300
Bernardi Traditional Stuffed Shells, 2.8 oz	140	6	4	40	12	0	1	260
Contadina Buitoni								
Mushroom/Cheese Tortellini	310	8	3	45	49	2	3	250
Mini Three Cheese Ravioli	260	5	3	30	41	3	3	260
Three Cheese Tortellini	260	6	3	35	41	1	2	290
Light Four Cheese Ravioli	240	5	2	45	38	2	3	300
DiGiorno Lemon Chicken Tortellini	260	5	3	30	40	1	2	310
Good Health Spinach Cheese Ravioli, 5.3 oz	110	1	0	7	23	-	-	21
Putney Pasta Black Bean & Habanero Ravioli	180	0	0	0	38	3	4	250
Rosetto Beef Ravioli, 4.4 oz	250	5	2	20	42	2	3	330
SoyBoy Ravioli, all, 3.6 oz (avg)	180	3	1	0	30	3	2	130

Food	Cal	Fat	Sat	Chol	Carb	Fib	Sug	Sod
PIZZA								
Pepperoni, 12" pizza, 1/4	362	14	4	28	40	-	-	534
Cheese, 12" pizza, 1/4	282	6	4	18	42	4	3	672
Cheese, meat & veg, 12" pizza, 1/4	368	11	3	41	43	-	-	765

BRANDS . . .

FROZEN/REFRIGERATED *(1/4 PIZZA UNLESS NOTED)*

Food	Cal	Fat	Sat	Chol	Carb	Fib	Sug	Sod
A.C. LaRocco Garden Veg, 1/6	216	6	2	9	34	3	2	281
Cheese & Garlic, 1/6	216	6	2	10	34	3	2	284
Greek Sesame, 1/6	224	7	2	11	33	3	2	304
Advantage/10 Roasted Veg, 1/2	263	3	0	0	49	8	13	338
Amy's Pesto, 1/3	310	12	4	10	39	2	3	480
Roasted Vegetable, 1/3	260	8	1	0	43	3	4	490
Spinach or Cheese, 1/3 (avg)	320	11	4	15	39	2	5	490
Bravissimo Roasted Veg Rising Crust	210	3	-	0	38	1	3	470
Connie's								
Thin Crust Cheese, 1/6	200	10	5	25	20	1	3	440
Thin Crust Sausage, Green Pepper, Onion, Mushroom, 1/5	260	13	5	30	21	2	4	490
DiGiorno Rising Crust Veg, 1/2	145	3	2	13	19	2	5	295
*Empire Kosher 4 Cheese	170	7	-	10	25	-	-	332
Cheese	170	4	-	10	27	-	-	370
Farm Foods PizSoy								
Cheese Style, 1/2 pkg	220	0	0	0	46	12	15	410
Jack's								
Pizza Bursts Supercheese, 3 oz	250	12	5	20	25	2	-	460
Naturally Rising, The Works, 9"	280	12	6	30	29	2	-	480
Pizza Bursts, Sausage, 3 oz	250	12	4	20	25	2	-	490
Naturally Rising, Cheese, 12", 1/6	290	10	6	25	35	2	7	500
Pizza Bursts, Combination Sausage & Pepperoni, 3 oz	250	12	4	20	26	2	-	500
Jaclyn's Not Even 1 Gram of Fat, 1/6	200	1	1	0	34	3	6	480
Kid Cuisine Cheese, 8 oz	430	11	3	20	71	5	31	440
Pirate Pizza w/Cheese, 8 oz	430	11	5	30	71	5	34	480
Nature's Hilights Soy Cheese, 1/2	290	2	-	0	52	2	-	430
Small Delivery Organic, 1/3	320	9	5	20	46	1	-	500
Small World Four Cheese, 1	240	6	3	13	83	1	3	350
Tofutti Pan Crust Pizzaz, 1/3	175	5	2	0	24	1	6	320
Tombstone								
Taco Supreme Mexican Style, 1/4	360	17	8	40	37	3	5	360
Light Vegetable, 1/5	240	7	3	10	31	3	5	500
Weight Watchers Smart Ones								
Deluxe Combo, 1	380	11	4	40	47	6	-	500

DINNERS, ENTREES & SIDE DISHES
Pizza Crust & Dough

Food	Cal	Fat	Sat	Chol	Carb	Fib	Sug	Sod
PIZZA								
Wolfgang Puck								
Mushroom Spinach, 5.3 oz	270	8	3	10	36	5	4	380
Grilled Veg Cheeseless, 5.5 oz	200	0	0	0	42	2	3	430
MIX								
***Low Carbolicious** (sauce & crust mix), 1/4 of 12" pizza	177	2	1	0	8	1	1	331
PIZZA BREAD *(also see Pockets, Sandwiches & Wraps, pg 103)*								
Cheese french bread pizza, 6 oz	350	14	5	15	42	3	4	660
BRANDS . . .								
FROZEN/REFRIGERATED *(6 OZ UNLESS NOTED)*								
***Empire Kosher**								
English Muffin, 2.3 oz	120	3	-	5	18	-	-	370
Bagel Cheese, 2.3 oz	140	2	-	5	24	-	-	380
Healthy Choice Cheese French								
Bread	340	5	2	15	51	7	4	480
Stouffer's Lean Cuisine								
Cheese French Bread	320	7	4	20	47	3	7	520

PIZZA CRUST & DOUGH

Food	Cal	Fat	Sat	Chol	Carb	Fib	Sug	Sod
Pizza crust, mix, 1/4	180	3	3	0	33	2	-	264
Refrg, 1/5	150	2	0	0	27	1	-	380
BRANDS . . .								
FROZEN/REFRIGERATED								
***French Meadow** Spelt, 1/4	113	3	0	0	19	3	0	139
Country Sourdough, 1/4	122	2	0	0	20	3	0	148
Giant, 1/6	100	1	0	0	19	4	1	130
House of Pasta, 1/8 of 14"	140	1	0	0	27	1	-	140
Mama Mary's, 1/2 of 7" or 1/6 of 12"	200	5	1	0	32	3	1	135
Tony's Pastry Crust, 1/3	400	21	8	20	0	0	0	0
MIX *(1/8 SLICE UNLESS NOTED)*								
***Carbosense** Garlic & Herb	100	0	0	0	7	4	0	85
***Cause You're Special**	96	0	0	0	21	1	2	156
Eagle Mills	160	2	0	0	29	1	3	170
***Gluten Free Pantry** French Bread &								
Pizza Crust, 1 slice	110	0	0	0	25	1	0	115
***Keto** Pizza Dough	79	1	0	0	5	3	1	95
Martha White Deep Dish, 1 slice	110	1	0	0	23	0	-	110
Regular, 1 slice	100	2	0	0	19	0		125
Sassafras Italian Mix, 1.4 oz	140	0	0	0	30	1	1	135
Watkins, 1.8 oz	180	1	0	0	36	2	5	6

Food	Cal	Fat	Sat	Chol	Carb	Fib	Sug	Sod
POCKETS, SANDWICHES & WRAPS								
Pierogi, potato & cheese, 4 oz	250	8	2	35	38	1	10	430
Pocket sandwich, cheese, 4.5 oz	290	9	4	20	38	3	5	450
Croissant w/chicken, broccoli & cheese, 4.5 oz	300	11	4	35	37	5	5	640
Pocket sandwich, beef & cheese, 4.5 oz	360	18	9	50	36	1	5	830
BRANDS . . .								
FROZEN/REFRIGERATED								
Amy's Pocket Sandwich								
Vegetarian Pizza, 4.5 oz	250	6	3	10	39	4	4	360
Roasted Veg, 4.5 oz	220	8	2	0	35	4	5	480
Veg Pie, 5 oz	300	9	2	0	45	3	5	490
Cedarlane Pesto, Mozzarella & Tomato Bruschetta, 1/8 pc	100	5	2	5	10	1	2	190
Veggie "Pepperoni" Stuffed Focaccia, 1/3	250	6	4	20	34	1	3	430
Mediterranean Stuffed Focaccia, 1/3	296	10	6	22	37	1	4	485
Ethnic Gourmet Kung Pao Tofu Wrap, 8 oz	350	11	2	0	51	4	5	290
Golden Pierogi								
LF Potato Cheese, 4 oz	185	3	1	45	33	1	10	175
LF Potato Onion, 4 oz	182	3	1	36	35	1	9	195
Health is Wealth Whole Wheat Potato & Onion Pierogies, 2.9 oz	140	2	0	0	27	3	1	300
Hot Pockets Toaster Breaks, Double Cheese, 1	170	8	3	10	21	2	2	300
Ian's Natural Foods Stuffed Sandwich, Meatball Parmesan, 4 oz	290	15	3	20	32	2	2	490
Krystal Krystal Sandwich, 1	160	7	3	20	17	1	1	260
Cheese Krystal Sandwich, 1	180	9	4	25	16	2	1	430
Lean Pockets Cheeseburger, 1	290	7	3	25	45	3	9	520
Mrs. T's Potato & Cheese 'Rogies, 7	130	2	1	10	24	0	2	310
Potato & Onion 'Rogies, 3	180	2	0	5	34	2	2	340
Jalapeño & Cheese 'Rogies, 7	130	2	1	5	25	0	2	340
Potato & Cheddar Pierogies, 3	180	3	1	10	34	2	3	430
Old El Paso Pizza Burrito, Cheese, 1	320	9	4	20	27	0	3	430
Pizza Burrito, Sausage, 1	260	9	4	15	32	0	2	420
Tofutti Cheese Pizzaz Pizza Bagel, 1 bagel	175	5	3	0	15	1	2	380
Weight Watchers Smart Ones								
3 Cheese Italian Meatball Sandwich, 4.5 oz	270	7	2	15	39	2	5	520

Food	Cal	Fat	Sat	Chol	Carb	Fib	Sug	Sod

SIDE DISHES

GRAIN SIDES

Tabouli, mix, prep, 2/3 cup	95	0	0	0	22	4	1	340
Couscous w/roasted garlic, mix, prep, 1 cup	200	2	0	0	41	2	1	480
Falafel, mix, 1/4 cup	120	2	0	0	20	4	3	610

BRANDS . . .
No low-sodium alternatives.

KNISHES

Potato, 1 pc	200	4	-	0	38	2	-	530

BRANDS . . .
No low-sodium alternatives.

MISC SIDES *(1/2 CUP UNLESS NOTED)*

*Atkins Savory Sides, Creamy Cheese .	78	3	1	8	9	5	1	159
Original	90	4	2	13	9	5	1	178

POLENTA

Polenta, ready-to-eat, 4 oz	88	0	0	0	20	1	0	376
Mix, prep, 3/8 cup	260	5	2	5	48	4	3	550

BRANDS . . .
Bellino Instant Polenta, 1/4 cup	140	0	0	0	32	4	0	0

POTATOES *(also see Frozen Vegetables - Potatoes, pg 156)*

Mashed potatoes, instant, 1/3 cup mix .	80	0	0	0	18	2	0	20
Hash browns, frozen, 1/2 cup	70	0	0	0	17	2	1	70
Mix, 1 oz mix	100	1	0	0	22	1	1	570
Gnocci, boxed/packaged, 5.2 oz	250	0	0	0	55	1	2	240
Potato pancake, 1 tbsp mix	50	0	0	0	12	1	0	270
Fries, seasoned, frozen, 3 oz	120	4	1	20	20	2	1	360
Potato dumplings, 1 oz mix	90	0	0	0	21	1	0	410
Stuffed potato, cheese, 5 oz	200	9	3	5	24	1	9	550
Scalloped potatoes, 1 oz mix	100	1	0	0	21	1	1	570
Au gratin potatoes, 1 oz mix	100	1	0	0	22	1	1	610

BRANDS . . .

BOXED/PACKAGED *(1/3 CUP MIX UNLESS NOTED)*
Tasty Bite Curried Mashed, 1/2 pkg .	229	6	1	0	23	7	7	121

NOTE: Most instant mashed potato brands are within the generic range, however, flavored potatoes may contain added sodium.

Food	Cal	Fat	Sat	Chol	Carb	Fib	Sug	Sod
POTATOES								
FROZEN/REFRIGERATED (*1/2 CUP UNLESS NOTED*)								
Basic American Redi-Shred Hash								
Browns	134	7	1	0	16	2	0	19
Cascadian Farm Organic								
Oven French Fries, 3 oz	130	4	1	0	24	2	1	10
Hash Browns, 3 oz	70	0	0	0	15	2	1	20
Country Style, 3 oz	60	0	0	0	13	2	2	20
C&W Roasted Parmesan & Garlic								
Potatoes w/Italian Green Beans &								
Sweet Baby Carrots	40	1	0	0	7	1	2	127
Roasted Rosemary & Garlic Potatoes								
w/Sweet Red & Green Peppers	60	1	0	0	10	2	1	213
Dr. Praeger's Homestyle Potato								
Pancakes, 1.5 oz	80	3	1	15	10	1	1	150
Simply Potatoes								
Shredded Hash Browns	70	0	0	0	17	2	1	70
RICE SIDES (*see Rice & Rice Dishes, pg 132*)								
SALADS								
Carrot raisin salad, 1/2 cup	280	11	2	10	20	2	14	125
Cole slaw, 3/4 cup	147	11	2	5	13	-	-	267
Potato salad, 3.4 oz	108	6	1	57	13	-	-	312
Tuna salad, 3 oz	159	8	1	11	8	0	-	342
3 bean salad, 1/2 cup	90	0	0	0	19	6	8	620
Pasta salad, mix, 3/4 cup	240	7	2	5	34	2	5	740
BRANDS ...								
FROZEN/REFRIGERATED								
Hanover 3 Bean, 3.1 oz	100	1	0	0	22	3	14	120
Vegetable, 3.1 oz	80	0	0	0	17	3	15	120
STUFFING & DRESSING								
Cornbread, 1 oz	90	1	0	0	19	1	2	350
Bread, seasoned, 1 oz	90	1	0	0	18	1	3	440
BRANDS ... (*1 OZ UNLESS NOTED*)								
Arnold Unspiced Premium	114	2	0	0	22	0	2	220
Corn	100	2	0	0	18	2	-	280
Herb Seasoned	100	0	0	0	4	2	-	300
Brownberry Herb	100	1	0	0	19	2	-	297
Martin's Potato Bread Stuffing, 1.1 oz	110	1	0	0	19	2	3	150

DINNERS, ENTREES & SIDE DISHES
Side Dishes - Vegetable

Food	Cal	Fat	Sat	Chol	Carb	Fib	Sug	Sod
SIDE DISHES								
Stove Top Chicken, lower sodium	110	1	0	0	21	0	3	270
Wonder Seasoned Stuffing, 1 cup	60	1	0	0	12	0	0	135

Although many of the stuffings listed above exceed sodium guidelines, they are substantially less than the generic.

VEGETABLE SIDE DISHES

Food	Cal	Fat	Sat	Chol	Carb	Fib	Sug	Sod
Succotash, frozen, unprep, 1 cup	145	1	0	0	31	6	-	70
Canned, 1 cup	161	1	0	0	36	7	-	564
Corn grits (hominy), instant, 1 oz	100	0	0	0	22	2	-	320
w/cheese, 1 oz	100	1	0	0	21	1	-	425
Broccoli w/butter sauce, 1/2 cup	50	2	1	5	7	2	-	330
w/cheese sauce, 1/2 cup	110	5	2	5	7	1	-	500
Spinach, creamed, 1/2 cup	169	13	4	16	9	2	-	335

BRANDS . . .

FROZEN/REFRIGERATED

Dr. Praeger's

Food	Cal	Fat	Sat	Chol	Carb	Fib	Sug	Sod
Broccoli Pancakes, 1.3 oz	70	3	1	15	9	1	0	150
Spinach Pancakes, 1.3 oz	70	3	1	15	9	1	0	155
Melrose Zucchini Souffle, 3.6 oz	90	0	0	0	19	3	3	160
*Seneca Succotash, 2/3 cup	100	1	0	0	20	4	2	55

Food	Cal	Fat	Sat	Chol	Carb	Fib	Sug	Sod

ETHNIC FOODS

ASIAN

CONDIMENTS & ADDITIVES

	Cal	Fat	Sat	Chol	Carb	Fib	Sug	Sod
Wasabi:								
Powder, 1 tsp	0	0	0	0	0	0	0	0
Prepared, 1 tsp	15	1	0	0	3	0	0	100
Chinese mustard, 1 tsp	10	0	0	0	1	0	0	70
Miso/soybean paste, 1 tbsp	30	1	0	0	3	1	0	760
BRANDS . . .								
Sun Luck Chinese Mustard, 1 tsp	10	0	0	0	1	0	0	50
Westbrae Natural Mellow Barley								
Miso, 1 tbsp	30	0	0	0	3	0	0	300

EGG ROLLS *(see Appetizers & Snacks, pg 92)*

FORTUNE COOKIES

	Cal	Fat	Sat	Chol	Carb	Fib	Sug	Sod
Fortune cookie, 0.5 oz	56	0	0	0	12	0	5	68
BRANDS . . .								
La Choy, 0.5 oz	55	0	0	0	14	0	7	5
Umeya, 1	28	0	0	0	6	0	3	23

FRIED RICE - MIX

	Cal	Fat	Sat	Chol	Carb	Fib	Sug	Sod
Fried rice seasoning mix, 1 1/3 tbsp	30	0	0	0	6	0	0	490
Fried rice, prep, 1/2 cup	181	6	0	0	29	1	-	900
BRANDS . . .								
No low-sodium alternatives.								

KIM CHEE

	Cal	Fat	Sat	Chol	Carb	Fib	Sug	Sod
Kim chee, 1/4 cup	15	0	0	0	2	1	-	340
BRANDS . . .								
No low-sodium alternatives.								

NOODLES

	Cal	Fat	Sat	Chol	Carb	Fib	Sug	Sod
Chinese, cellophane, or long rice								
noodles, 1 cup	491	0	0	0	121	1	0	14
Chow mein noodles, 1 cup	237	14	2	0	26	2	1	198
Soba noodles, 2 oz	192	0	0	0	43	1	0	451
Udon noodles, 2 oz	190	2	0	0	37	3	5	660
Somen noodles, 2 oz	203	1	0	0	42	3	1	1049
BRANDS . . . *(2 OZ UNLESS NOTED)*								
*Annie Chun's Rice Noodles, all	210	0	0	0	50	0	0	75
Asian Gourmet Wide LoMein	200	0	0	0	45	1	0	1

107

Food	Cal	Fat	Sat	Chol	Carb	Fib	Sug	Sod
NOODLES								
*Eden Organic								
Buckwheat Soba	200	1	0	0	43	3	2	5
Soba	200	2	0	0	38	2	3	70
Organic Somen	200	2	0	0	38	3	1	80
Brown Rice Udon	200	2	0	0	38	3	1	80
Organic Udon	200	2	0	0	38	3	1	115
Sun Luck Saifun Bean Threads	190	0	0	0	47	0	0	10
Tomoshiraga Somen, 3 oz	330	15	2	0	65	2	0	70
Chuka Soba Chow Mein, 3 oz	310	2	0	0	61	0	0	140
SAUCES								
BEAN SAUCE								
Bean sauce, 1 tbsp	30	0	0	0	5	1	4	475
BRANDS . . .								
No low-sodium alternatives.								
CHILI/GARLIC SAUCE								
Chili/garlic sauce, 1 tsp	5	0	0	0	1	0	1	155
BRANDS . . . *(1 TSP UNLESS NOTED)*								
A Taste of Thai Sweet Red or								
Sweet Green Chili	10	0	0	0	2	0	2	40
Dynasty Szechwan Chili	10	0	0	0	1	0	0	80
*Heaven and Earth Dragon Fire								
Chili	8	0	0	0	2	0	2	17
Huy Fong Foods Tuong Ot Toi								
Vietnam Chili	0	0	0	0	1	0	1	70
Robbie's Garlic	0	0	0	0	1	1	0	60
Union International Chili Garlic	5	0	0	0	1	0	1	80
HOISIN SAUCE								
Hoisin sauce, 1 tbsp	35	1	0	0	7	0	7	258
BRANDS . . . *(1 TBSP UNLESS NOTED)*								
*Heaven and Earth Raspberry	20	0	0	0	4	0	4	140
Polynesian	20	0	0	0	5	0	4	80
OYSTER SAUCE								
Oyster sauce, 1 tbsp	130	0	0	0	30	0	21	675
BRANDS . . . *(1 TBSP UNLESS NOTED)*								
Ka-Me	10	0	0	0	3	0	-	260
PEANUT SAUCE								
Peanut sauce, 1 tbsp	45	3	1	0	4	0	3	240
BRANDS . . . *(1 TBSP UNLESS NOTED)*								
*Annie Chun's Thai	60	4	1	0	5	0	4	135
A Taste of Thai Satay	25	2	0	0	3	1	2	30

Food	Cal	Fat	Sat	Chol	Carb	Fib	Sug	Sod
PEANUT SAUCE								
*Heaven and Earth	100	16	0	0	5	0	1	90
*Mr. Spice Thai	15	2	0	0	4	0	4	0
Thai Kitchen Satay	45	3	1	0	4	1	3	70
PLUM SAUCE								
Plum sauce, 1 tbsp	35	0	0	0	8	0	7	140
BRANDS . . . (1 TBSP UNLESS NOTED)								
*Jok 'n' Al	8	0	0	0	2	0	1	42
*Wax Orchards	20	0	0	0	5	1	5	10
SOY SAUCE								
Soy sauce, 1 tbsp	8	0	0	0	1	0	0	914
Lite, 1 tbsp	8	0	0	0	1	0	0	660
BRANDS . . . (1 TBSP UNLESS NOTED)								
Angostura	10	0	0	0	1	0	0	390
House of Tsang LS	10	0	0	0	2	0	0	280
Ginger Flavored, LS	10	0	0	0	2	0	2	280
Rice Road	15	0	0	0	4	0	2	300
Yamasa	10	0	0	0	1	0	0	490

NOTE: Although the soy sauces listed above exceed sodium guidelines, they are substantially less than the generic.

Food	Cal	Fat	Sat	Chol	Carb	Fib	Sug	Sod
STIR-FRY SAUCE								
Stir-fry sauce, 1 tbsp	15	0	0	0	3	0	3	570
BRANDS . . . (1 TBSP UNLESS NOTED)								
*Mr. Spice Ginger	15	0	0	0	4	0	4	0
*New Traditions, mix, 1 tsp	15	0	0	0	2	0	0	0
Rice Road, 1 tbsp	20	0	0	0	4	0	3	310
SWEET AND SOUR SAUCE								
Sweet & sour sauce, 1 tbsp	18	0	0	0	5	0	5	130
BRANDS . . . (1 TBSP UNLESS NOTED)								
Ah-So Chinese-Style Duck	25	0	0	0	7	0	5	8
Asian Gourmet Duck	25	0	0	0	2	0	2	33
Contadina w/Pineapple	20	1	0	0	4	0	3	58
*Heaven and Earth Tangerine	25	0	0	0	6	0	6	5
Ginger Mint	35	0	0	0	9	1	9	10
Four Fruit	20	1	0	0	9	0	9	10
House of Tsang	30	0	0	0	7	0	6	45
Kraft	24	0	0	0	6	0	5	50
La Choy	25	0	0	0	7	0	6	53
*Mr. Spice	18	0	0	0	4	0	4	0
*Robbie's Hawaiian Style	23	0	0	0	6	0	4	6
*Steel's Rocky Mountain	5	0	0	0	1	0	0	78
Sun Luck	31	0	0	0	7	0	6	30

ETHNIC FOODS
Hawaiian

Food	Cal	Fat	Sat	Chol	Carb	Fib	Sug	Sod
SAUCES								
TERIYAKI SAUCE								
Teriyaki sauce, 1 tbsp	15	0	0	0	3	0	3	690
Lite, 1 tbsp	10	0	0	0	2	0	1	260
BRANDS . . . *(1 TBSP UNLESS NOTED)*								
Miko Lite	10	0	0	0	2	-	-	125
World Harbors Maui Mt Hawaiian	35	0	0	0	9	0	8	135

TEMPURA BATTER *(see Batter, Seasoning & Coating Mixes, pg 3)*

VEGETABLES

Food	Cal	Fat	Sat	Chol	Carb	Fib	Sug	Sod
Water chestnuts, 1/4 cup	15	0	0	0	4	1	1	0
Bamboo shoots, 1/2 cup	10	0	0	0	2	1	0	10
Bean sprouts, 1/2 cup	16	0	0	0	2	1	0	20
Chow mein vegetables, 1/2 cup	20	0	0	0	4	1	0	422
BRANDS . . .								
CANNED *(1/2 CUP UNLESS NOTED)*								
Ka-Me Stir Fry Veg	20	0	0	0	4	2	0	10
Sun Luck Mushrooms, Straw	10	0	0	0	8	0	0	0
Mixed Stir Fry Veg	20	0	0	0	4	2	0	10
Baby Corn, all	10	0	0	0	6	4	6	20
Mushrooms, Stir Fry	40	0	0	0	6	4	0	50

FROZEN/REFRIGERATED *(see Frozen Vegetables - Mixed Vegetables, pg 156)*

WRAPPERS

Food	Cal	Fat	Sat	Chol	Carb	Fib	Sug	Sod
Wonton wrapper, 1	23	0	0	1	5	0	0	46
Egg roll wrapper, 1	93	0	0	3	19	1	0	183
BRANDS . . .								
Azumaya Round Wonton, 1	16	0	0	1	3	0	0	37
Egg Roll, 1	57	0	0	3	12	0	0	137
Dynasty Wonton, 1	17	0	0	0	4	0	0	18
Egg Roll, 1	57	0	0	2	12	0	0	60
Melissa's Egg Roll Wraps, 1	65	0	0	0	14	1	1	125

(HAWAIIAN)

Food	Cal	Fat	Sat	Chol	Carb	Fib	Sug	Sod
Poi, 1/3 cup	70	0	0	0	18	2	0	30
Lau lau:								
Vegetable, 1	130	0	0	0	26	6	0	80
Pork, 1	320	21	9	90	5	8	0	980
Chicken, 1	260	21	6	75	5	8	0	1010
Kalua pork, 3 oz	260	18	6	85	0	0	0	200
Kalua chicken or turkey	205	11	3	70	0	0	0	330
Portuguese sausage, 2 oz	180	15	6	35	2	0	1	520

Food	Cal	Fat	Sat	Chol	Carb	Fib	Sug	Sod

HISPANIC

CHILI PEPPERS

Food	Cal	Fat	Sat	Chol	Carb	Fib	Sug	Sod
Whole green chiles, 1.3 oz	15	0	0	0	3	1	1	100
Diced green chiles, 2 tbsp	5	0	0	0	1	1	0	110
Jalapeños, diced, 2 tbsp	10	0	0	0	1	0	0	440

BRANDS . . . *(2 TBSP UNLESS NOTED)*

Food	Cal	Fat	Sat	Chol	Carb	Fib	Sug	Sod
Albertson's Diced Green Chiles	5	0	0	0	1	0	0	75
Casa Fiesta								
Diced Green Chiles	5	0	0	0	1	0	0	75
Whole Green Chiles, 1.1 oz	5	0	0	0	1	0	0	75
Chi-Chi's								
Diced Green Chiles	10	0	0	0	1	0	0	20
Whole Green Chiles	10	0	0	0	1	0	0	20
Diced Jalapeños, 1.1 oz	10	0	0	0	-	0	-	55
LaVictoria Diced Green Chiles	0	0	0	0	1	0	0	70
*Melissa's Fire Roasted Red &								
Green Chiles	10	0	0	0	1	0	0	55
Ortega Diced Jalapeños	10	0	0	0	2	0	1	25

FILLINGS

BRANDS . . .

Food	Cal	Fat	Sat	Chol	Carb	Fib	Sug	Sod
Casa Fiesta Burrito, Bean w/Bacon Flavor, 3 tbsp	60	1	0	0	9	3	2	170

GUACAMOLE *(see Dips, pg 139)*

REFRIED BEANS

Food	Cal	Fat	Sat	Chol	Carb	Fib	Sug	Sod
Refried beans, canned, 1/2 cup	100	1	0	0	17	6	1	530
Mix, prep, 1/2 cup	160	1	0	0	29	11	-	610

BRANDS . . . *(1/2 CUP UNLESS NOTED)*

Food	Cal	Fat	Sat	Chol	Carb	Fib	Sug	Sod
Albertson's, NF	100	0	0	0	19	7	2	290
*Bearitos LF, NSA	140	3	0	0	23	9	2	5
Casa Fiesta All Natural, NF	130	0	0	0	22	7	1	290
All Natural	115	1	0	0	20	3	1	330
Gebhardt Refried Jalapeño	110	2	0	0	19	7	-	320
Old El Paso Refried Black	110	2	0	0	18	7	-	340
ShariAnn's Organic								
Refried Black	110	0	0	0	20	4	0	330
Refried Pintos	110	0	0	0	20	4	0	330
Refried Pintos w/Roasted Garlic	110	0	0	0	20	4	0	330

NOTE: Although many of the beans listed above exceed sodium guidelines, they are substantially less than the generic.

Food	Cal	Fat	Sat	Chol	Carb	Fib	Sug	Sod
SALSA & TACO SAUCE								
Salsa, 2 tbsp	9	0	0	0	2	0	-	139
Salsa, refrg, 2 tbsp	10	0	0	0	2	0	1	250

BRANDS ... *(2 TBSP UNLESS NOTED)*

There are many low-sodium salsas, the following have 90mg or less per serving.

Food	Cal	Fat	Sat	Chol	Carb	Fib	Sug	Sod
American Spoon Mango Habanero	25	0	0	0	8	0	5	70
Cool Coyote Taos Black Bean & Corn	15	0	0	0	4	1	1	80
Del Salsa Fire Roasted (avg)	8	0	0	0	2	0	0	70
Enrico's Chunky Style NSA, Mild	10	0	0	0	3	0	2	55
Chunky Style, Medium	10	0	0	0	2	1	2	70
Chunky Style, Hot	15	0	0	0	3	0	2	75
Chunky Style, Mild	10	0	0	0	3	0	2	80
Floribbean Key Lime	15	0	0	0	3	0	2	0
Mango	15	0	0	0	4	0	3	0
Frontera Tomatillo	10	0	0	0	2	0	1	70
Roasted Corn & Bean	20	0	0	0	4	1	0	90
Chipotle Black Bean	15	0	0	0	3	1	0	90
Frog Ranch Hot	8	0	0	0	3	0	0	23
Garlic Survival Co. Tomatillo Garlic	20	0	0	0	4	1	0	15
Garlic	10	0	0	0	2	0	1	70
Gloria's Santiam Ridge Peach Mango	50	0	0	0	12	0	-	15
Happy Valley Apple	20	0	0	0	4	0	3	45
Goldwater's Cochise Corn & Black Bean	30	2	0	0	4	1	1	80
Mohave Mango	20	0	0	0	5	0	4	85
Papago Peach	15	0	0	0	3	0	3	85
Ruby Raspberry	20	0	0	0	5	0	5	90
Green Mountain Gringo all (avg)	10	0	0	0	2	0	0	85
Hot Cha Cha Medium	5	0	0	0	2	0	0	0
Native South Fiery Peach	15	0	0	0	3	0	3	85
Newman's Own Peach	25	0	0	0	6	1	5	90
Pineapple	15	0	0	0	3	1	3	90
Quinn's Apple Cranberry	15	0	0	0	4	0	3	45
Palmieri, all	10	0	0	0	2	0	2	65
Rainy Day Gourmet Del Sol	10	0	0	0	2	0	0	10
Santa Barbara Roasted Garlic	10	0	0	0	2	0	0	40
Black Bean & Corn, Medium	15	0	0	0	3	0	2	80
Santa Cruz Black Bean & Corn	30	0	0	0	4	1	2	70
Steel's Caribe Mango	24	0	0	0	6	1	4	0
Super G Healthy Ideas	10	0	0	0	2	0	1	55
Tree of Life, all	10	0	0	0	2	0	1	20
Walnut Acres Sweet Southwestern Peach	20	0	0	0	5	0	4	85

Food	Cal	Fat	Sat	Chol	Carb	Fib	Sug	Sod
SAUCES								
CHEESE SAUCE								
Cheese sauce, 2 tbsp	55	4	2	9	2	0	0	261
BRANDS . . . *(2 TBSP UNLESS NOTED)*								
Louise's FF Nacho Queso	15	0	0	0	3	0	1	45
CHILI SAUCE								
Chili sauce, 1 tbsp	20	0	0	0	5	0	4	260
BRANDS . . .								
505 Southwestern Hot Green, 2 tbsp	25	0	0	0	5	1	2	40
ENCHILADA SAUCE								
Enchilada sauce, 1/4 cup	25	1	0	0	2	1	0	310
BRANDS . . . *(1/4 CUP UNLESS NOTED)*								
El Molino Hot	32	2	-	-	4	-	-	200
Old El Paso Mild	20	1	0	0	3	0	1	220
HOT SAUCE								
Hot sauce, 1 tsp	0	0	0	0	0	0	0	120
BRANDS . . .								
No low-sodium alternatives.								
MOLE								
Mole, 2 tbsp	230	15	2	0	12	2	7	460
BRANDS . . .								
Rogelio Bueno, 2 tbsp	150	11	2	0	12	1	4	270
SEASONING MIXES								
Guacamole seasoning mix, 1/8 pkt	15	0	0	0	2	0	0	160
Enchilada sauce mix, 1/6 pkt	20	0	0	0	4	0	1	250
Chili seasoning mix, 1/4 pkt	30	1	0	0	5	2	1	310
Burrito seasoning mix, 1/6 pkt	15	0	0	0	4	0	0	410
Fajita seasoning mix, 1/6 pkt	15	0	0	0	3	0	0	450
Taco seasoning mix, 1/6 pkt	20	0	0	0	5	0	0	550
BRANDS . . . *(1 TSP UNLESS NOTED)*								
Ancho Mama's Chile	0	0	0	0	0	0	0	0
Chipolte Del Sol Southwest	0	0	0	0	0	0	0	0
*Frontier Taco, 1/4 tsp	10	0	0	0	2	0	0	0
Mojave Hot Taco Mix	0	0	0	0	0	0	0	0
*New Traditions Fajita Mix	8	0	0	0	2	0	0	0
Santa Fe Taco Mix	10	0	0	0	2	0	0	0
Old El Paso Taco Mix, 40% Less Salt	8	0	0	0	2	0	0	165
TOMATILLOS								
Tomatillos, raw, diced, 1/2 cup	21	1	0	0	4	1	0	1
Tomatillos, canned, 2.1 oz	15	0	0	0	3	2	1	15

Food	Cal	Fat	Sat	Chol	Carb	Fib	Sug	Sod
TOMATILLOS								
BRANDS . . .								
Most brands are within the generic range.								
TORTILLAS & TACO SHELLS								
Corn tortilla, 6" diam, 1	58	1	0	0	12	1	0	3
Corn tortilla, shelf-stable, 1	50	2	0	0	6	1	0	150
Flour tortilla, 7"-8", 1	159	1	1	0	27	2	0	234
12", 1	380	2	1	0	65	4	0	559
Whole wheat tortilla, 1	120	2	1	0	20	1	0	280
BRANDS . . .								
FROZEN/REFRIGERATED *(1 TORTILLA UNLESS NOTED)*								
***Adios Carbs* Tortillas**								
Flour or Garlic & Herb	87	3	-	-	8	2	0	66
Burrito size	108	4	-	-	10	3	0	82
Garden of Eatin'								
Chapati	120	3	0	0	20	2	1	110
Whole Wheat	140	3	0	0	22	2	1	170
Thin Thin Wraps, Whole Wheat	110	1	0	0	21	0	1	190
Pinata Flour, 8"	100	2	0	0	20	1	1	120
SHELF-STABLE *(1 CORN TACO SHELL UNLESS NOTED)*								
***Casa Fiesta* Jumbo**	160	7	5	5	23	3	0	5
***Diane's* Jumbo**	90	4	1	0	11	1	0	5
La Preferida	55	3	1	0	7	1	0	3
Taco Bell	150	6	3	0	21	2	0	0

Food	Cal	Fat	Sat	Chol	Carb	Fib	Sug	Sod

FISH & SEAFOOD

ANCHOVY PASTE

Food	Cal	Fat	Sat	Chol	Carb	Fib	Sug	Sod
Anchovy paste, 1 tbsp	30	3	1	55	0	0	0	940

BRANDS . . .

No low-sodium alternatives.

CLAM JUICE

Food	Cal	Fat	Sat	Chol	Carb	Fib	Sug	Sod
Clam juice, 1/4 cup	1	0	0	0	0	0	0	280

BRANDS . . . *(1/4 CUP UNLESS NOTED)*

Food	Cal	Fat	Sat	Chol	Carb	Fib	Sug	Sod
Atlantic	0	0	0	0	0	0	0	120
Bookbinder's Restaurant Style	0	0	0	0	0	0	0	135

FISH & SEAFOOD - CANNED

Food	Cal	Fat	Sat	Chol	Carb	Fib	Sug	Sod
Cod, 2 oz	59	0	0	31	0	0	0	123
Oysters, 2 oz	70	3	1	38	3	0	0	145
Smoked, 2 oz	87	3	1	37	7	0	0	267
Mackerel, 2 oz	88	4	1	45	0	0	0	214
Gefilte fish, sweet, 1.5 oz pc	35	1	0	13	3	0	-	220
Tuna, packed in oil, 2 oz	104	4	1	17	0	0	0	221
Packed in water, 2 oz	106	5	1	18	0	0	0	226
Caviar, black or red, 1 tbsp	40	3	1	94	1	0	0	240
Black or golden whitefish, 1 tbsp	25	2	0	45	1	0	0	300
Herring, pickled, 1 oz	74	5	1	4	3	0	-	247
Kippered, boneless, 1 oz	62	4	1	23	0	0	0	260
Mussels, smoked, 2 oz	90	5	2	50	0	0	0	250
Sardines, atlantic, in oil, 2 oz	118	6	0	80	0	0	0	286
Pacific, in tomato sauce, 2 oz	100	7	2	34	0	0	0	232
Salmon, sockeye, 2 oz	87	4	1	25	0	0	0	305
Pink, 2 oz	79	3	1	31	0	0	0	314
Clams, chopped/minced, 2 oz	25	0	0	10	2	0	0	320
Crab, 2 oz	40	1	0	50	20	0	1	400
Anchovies in oil, 1 oz	47	2	1	19	0	0	0	826

BRANDS . . .

ANCHOVIES

No low-sodium alternatives.

CAVIAR

No low-sodium alternatives.

Food	Cal	Fat	Sat	Chol	Carb	Fib	Sug	Sod
FISH AND SEAFOOD - CANNED								
CLAMS *(2 OZ UNLESS NOTED)*								
Geisha Baby Clams	130	9	3	20	0	0	0	60
Pacific Pearl Fancy Smoked Clams	130	9	3	20	4	1	0	60
Baby Clams	45	2	0	30	0	0	0	150
COD								
Most brands are within the generic range.								
CRAB *(2 OZ UNLESS NOTED)*								
Bumble Bee Fancy White	40	1	0	50	0	0	0	300
Crown-Prince Lump Crab	46	0	0	69	1	0	0	276
GEFILTE FISH								
Mother's LS, 1 ball	45	1	0	0	2	0	-	-
HERRING AND KIPPER SNACKS *(1 OZ UNLESS NOTED)*								
Alstertor Herring in Dill-Herb Sauce	55	4	0	7	1	0	1	26
Herring Fillets in Tomato Sauce	55	4	0	7	1	0	1	32
Crown Prince Kipper Snacks	57	4	0	0	0	0	0	119
Season Kipper Snacks, Salmon	54	3	0	20	0	0	0	57
MACKEREL								
Season Fillet of Mackerel, NSA	90	5	-	25	0	0	0	55
MUSSELS *(2 OZ UNLESS NOTED)*								
Pacific Pearl Smoked	120	7	1	13	2	0	1	95
Ty Ling Smoked in Cottonseed Oil	120	7	4	45	2	0	0	118
OYSTERS								
No low-sodium alternatives.								
SALMON *(2 OZ UNLESS NOTED)*								
Crown Prince, Reduced Salt	90	5	1	40	0	0	0	60
Featherweight Pink, NSA	60	1	0	30	0	0	0	40
Gefen Fancy Pink	160	9	-	75	1	0	0	80
Miramonte	70	3	0	30	0	0	0	45
SARDINES *(2 OZ UNLESS NOTED)*								
King Oscar Brisling in Water or Soya Oil	132	5	2	55	0	0	0	35
Reese Skinless/Boneless in Water, LS	60	3	1	15	0	0	0	22
Smoked Brisling in Tomato Sauce & Sherry	110	9	3	40	1	1	1	135
Season Skinless/Boneless in Water, NSA	61	2	-	16	0	0	0	24
Norway Sardines, NSA	77	5	-	58	0	0	0	37
Brisling in Tomato Sauce, NSA	117	9	-	58	1	0	0	61

Food	Cal	Fat	Sat	Chol	Carb	Fib	Sug	Sod
FISH AND SEAFOOD - CANNED								
TUNA (ALBACORE) (2 OZ UNLESS NOTED)								
Bumble Bee Chunk White in Water, LS	70	1	0	30	0	0	0	35
Chicken of the Sea Chunk White								
Very LS, in Spring Water	60	1	0	25	0	0	0	35
LS in Spring Water	60	1	0	30	0	0	0	90
Crown Prince Tongol Light Chunk, NSA	60	0	0	35	0	0	0	50
Albacore in Spring Water, LS	65	0	0	30	0	0	0	80
Featherweight Chunk Light, NSA	60	1	0	30	0	0	0	40
Miramonte NSA	60	0	0	30	0	0	0	5
Natural Sea Chunk, NSA	60	0	0	20	0	0	0	120
Natural Value Albacore, NSA	60	1	0	30	0	0	0	40
Season Chunk Light in Water, NSA	60	1	0	25	0	0	0	100
StarKist Chunk White, LS	60	1	0	25	0	0	0	35
Albacore, LS	60	1	0	25	0	0	0	35
Chunk Light, LS	60	1	0	25	0	0	0	100
Tree of Life NSA	60	0	0	30	0	0	0	5
Lightly Salted	60	0	0	30	0	0	0	140
Whole Foods Market 365 Tongol, NSA	60	0	0	35	0	0	0	50
Albacore, NSA	65	1	0	30	0	0	0	80

FISH & SEAFOOD - FRESH

Food	Cal	Fat	Sat	Chol	Carb	Fib	Sug	Sod
Monkfish, 3 oz	65	1	0	21	0	0	0	15
Trout, rainbow, 3 oz	109	4	1	50	0	0	0	28
Anchovies, 1 oz	37	1	0	17	0	0	0	29
Tuna (albacore), yellowfin, 3 oz	92	1	0	38	0	0	0	31
Pike, northern, 3 oz	75	1	0	33	0	0	0	33
Walleye, 3 oz	79	1	0	73	0	0	0	43
Catfish, wild, 3 oz	81	2	1	49	0	0	0	37
Farmed, 3 oz	115	6	2	40	0	0	0	45
Eel, 3 oz	156	10	2	107	0	0	0	43
Cod, 3 oz	70	1	0	37	0	0	0	46
Halibut, 3 oz	94	2	0	27	0	0	0	46
Sturgeon, 3 oz	89	3	1	51	0	0	0	46
Clams, 3 oz	63	1	0	29	2	0	0	48
Salmon, atlantic, 3 oz	156	9	2	50	0	0	0	50
Chinook, 3 oz	153	9	2	56	0	0	0	40
Pink, 3 oz	99	3	0	44	0	0	0	57
Crayfish, 3 oz	61	1	0	91	0	0	0	53

Food	Cal	Fat	Sat	Chol	Carb	Fib	Sug	Sod
FISH AND SEAFOOD - FRESH								
Perch, 3 oz	77	1	0	77	0	0	0	53
Atlantic, 3 oz	80	1	0	36	0	0	0	64
Snapper, 3 oz	85	1	0	31	0	0	0	54
Orange roughy, 3 oz	59	1	0	17	0	0	0	54
Pompano, 3 oz	139	8	3	43	0	0	0	55
Haddock, 3 oz	74	1	0	48	0	0	0	58
Bass, sea 3 oz	82	2	0	35	0	0	0	58
Freshwater, 3 oz	97	3	1	58	0	0	0	60
Sole (flounder), 3 oz	77	1	0	41	0	0	0	69
Mackerel, pacific, 3 oz	134	7	2	40	0	0	0	73
Atlantic, 3 oz	174	12	3	60	0	0	0	77
King, 3 oz	89	2	0	45	0	0	0	134
Swordfish, 3 oz	103	3	1	33	0	0	0	76
Pollack, 3 oz	75	1	0	60	0	0	0	78
Oysters, pacific, 3 oz	69	2	0	43	4	0	0	90
Eastern, 3 oz	50	1	0	21	5	0	0	151
Shrimp, 3 oz	90	1	0	129	1	0	0	126
Scallops, 3 oz	75	1	0	28	2	0	0	137
Lobster, spiny, 3 oz	95	1	0	60	2	0	0	150
Northern, 3 oz	77	1	0	81	0	0	0	252
Mussels, 3 oz	73	2	0	24	3	0	0	243
Crab, blue or dungeness, 3 oz (avg)	74	1	0	68	0	0	0	250
Alaskan king, 3 oz	71	1	0	36	0	0	0	711
Abalone, raw , 3 oz	89	1	0	72	5	0	0	256
Cuttlefish, 3 oz	67	1	0	95	1	0	0	316

(FISH & SEAFOOD - FROZEN)

NOTE: Frozen fish & seafood have comparable sodium to fresh, however, prepared fish and seafood (i.e. battered or breaded) may contain added sodium.

PREPARED ENTREES

Food	Cal	Fat	Sat	Chol	Carb	Fib	Sug	Sod
Shrimp, breaded, 3 oz	206	10	2	150	10	0	-	292
Fish sticks, breaded, 3.5 oz	290	17	4	30	23	0	-	390
Battered, 3.5 oz	270	18	6	25	20	0	-	540
Fillets, battered or breaded, 3.3 oz	211	11	3	31	15	0	-	484
Crab cakes, 2.1 oz	160	10	2	82	5	0	-	491
Fillets, breaded, seasoned, 3.7 oz	220	11	3	30	21	0	4	600

BRANDS . . . *(4 OZ UNLESS NOTED)*

Dr. Praeger's

Food	Cal	Fat	Sat	Chol	Carb	Fib	Sug	Sod
Minced Fish Sticks, 1.7 oz	90	4	0	18	9	1	0	127
Fish or Salmon Croquettes, 2.2 oz	120	5	1	25	12	1	0	170
Fish Fillet Sticks, 2.9 oz	138	6	1	24	14	1	0	185

Food	Cal	Fat	Sat	Chol	Carb	Fib	Sug	Sod
FISH AND SEAFOOD - FROZEN PREPARED ENTREES								
Dr. Praeger's (cont'd)								
Breaded Fish Fillets, 2.1 oz	113	4	0	24	11	1	0	211
Sandwich Fish Fillets	210	9	1	60	19	1	0	230
Gorton's Grilled Fillets								
Lemon Pepper, 3.8 oz	120	6	1	60	1	0	1	160
Lemon Butter, 3.8 oz	110	5	1	60	0	0	0	270
Kineret Fish Cakes	160	6	1	5	23	1	0	310
Mrs. Pauls Grilled Fillets, Garlic Butter	130	6	1	60	0	0	0	230
SeaPak Coconut Shrimp	250	14	13	70	21	1	3	300
Van de Kamp's								
Fish Sticks, Crunchy, 6	260	14	3	25	21	0	2	250
Fish Fillets, Crispy, 3.5 oz	280	19	3	35	17	0	2	270
Breaded Fillets, 3.5 oz	280	19	3	35	17	0	2	270
Breaded Mini Fish Sticks, 3.3 oz	250	14	2	30	19	0	0	330
Golden Breaded Fish Sticks, 4.1 oz	290	17	3	30	22	0	3	420

FISH BURGERS & PATTIES

BRANDS . . . *(4 OZ PATTY UNLESS NOTED)*

Food	Cal	Fat	Sat	Chol	Carb	Fib	Sug	Sod
*Jeremiah's** Paella Cake w/Shrimp	120	4	1	20	15	1	0	30
Shrimp Scampi Cake, 3 oz	140	4	1	95	15	1	0	100
Pasta Cake, Tuna Noodle	170	4	2	35	22	1	0	130
Salmon & Corn Cake	140	5	2	10	19	0	0	135
Crab Cake, 3 oz	110	3	1	50	11	1	1	160
Scallop & Shrimp Cake, 3 oz	125	4	2	45	12	0	9	270
Omega Wild Pacific Salmon, 3.2 oz	100	2	0	20	3	0	0	150
Ahi Tuna, 3.2 oz	90	1	0	1	3	0	0	182
*Salmolux** Salmon	146	4	-	0	0	0	0	20

FISH & SEAFOOD SUBSTITUTES

Food	Cal	Fat	Sat	Chol	Carb	Fib	Sug	Sod
Shrimp, imitation, 3 oz	86	1	0	0	31	8	-	599
Scallop, imitation, 3 oz	84	0	0	0	18	9	-	676
Crab, imitation, 3 oz	87	1	0	0	17	1	-	715
BRANDS . . .								
Louis Kemp Crab Delights Chunk Style, 3 oz	81	0	0	15	8	-	-	480
Veat Vegetarian Fillet (Salmon), 1.8 oz	170	5	1	0	19	1	1	90

Food	Cal	Fat	Sat	Chol	Carb	Fib	Sug	Sod

FRUITS

FRUIT JUICE

(see Fruit Juice & Fruit-Flavored Drinks, pg 15)

FRUITS - CANNED

The following fruits are listed alphabetically.

Food	Cal	Fat	Sat	Chol	Carb	Fib	Sug	Sod
Applesauce w/salt, 1 cup	194	0	0	0	51	3	42	71
w/o salt, 1 cup	194	0	0	0	51	3	42	8
Apples, sliced, 1 cup	137	1	0	0	34	3	-	6
Apricot, halves, light syrup, 1 cup	159	0	0	0	42	4	-	10
Blackberries, heavy syrup, 1 cup	236	0	0	0	59	9	-	8
Blueberries, heavy syrup, 1 cup	225	1	0	0	56	4	-	8
Boysenberries, heavy syrup, 1 cup	225	0	0	0	57	7	-	8
Cherries, sweet, light syrup, 1 cup	169	0	0	0	44	4	-	8
Cherries, sour, light syrup, 1 cup	189	0	0	0	49	2	-	18
Figs, light syrup, 1 cup	174	0	0	0	45	5	-	3
Fruit cocktail, light syrup, 1 cup	138	0	0	0	36	2	34	15
Fruit salad, light syrup, 1 cup	146	0	0	0	38	3	-	15
Grapefruit sections, light syrup, 1 cup	152	0	0	0	39	1	-	5
Lychees, 5 oz	130	0	0	0	32	0	-	26
Peaches, halves, light syrup, 1 cup	136	0	0	0	37	3	-	13
Pears, halves, light syrup, 1 cup	143	0	0	0	38	4	31	13
Pineapple, light syrup, 1 cup	131	0	0	0	34	2	-	3
Plums, light syrup, 1 cup	159	0	0	0	41	3	-	50
Prunes, heavy syrup, 1 cup	246	0	0	0	65	9	-	7
Raspberries, heavy syrup, 1 cup	233	0	0	0	60	8	-	8
Strawberries, heavy syrup, 1 cup	234	1	0	0	60	4	-	10
Mandarin oranges, light syrup, 1 cup	154	0	0	0	41	2	-	15

BRANDS . . .
Most brands are within the generic range.

FRUITS - DRIED

The following fruits are listed alphabetically.

Food	Cal	Fat	Sat	Chol	Carb	Fib	Sug	Sod
Apple, 1 ring	16	0	0	0	4	1	-	6
Apricot, 1 half	8	0	0	0	2	0	2	0
Currants, 1 cup	408	0	0	0	107	10	-	12
Dates, 1	23	0	0	0	6	1	10	0

Food	Cal	Fat	Sat	Chol	Carb	Fib	Sug	Sod
FRUITS - DRIED								
Fig, 1	48	0	0	0	12	2	-	2
Peach, 1 half	31	0	0	0	8	1	-	1
Pear, 1 half	47	0	0	0	13	1	-	1
Prunes, 1	20	0	0	0	5	1	-	0

BRANDS . . .

Most brands are within the generic range.

FRUITS - FRESH

The following fruits are listed alphabetically.

Food	Cal	Fat	Sat	Chol	Carb	Fib	Sug	Sod
Apple, 1 med	81	0	0	0	21	4	17	0
Apricot, 1	17	0	0	0	4	1	3	0
Banana, 1 med	108	1	0	0	18	8	10	0
Blackberries, 1 cup	75	1	0	0	24	-	11	2
Blueberries, 1 cup	81	1	0	0	20	4	11	9
Cantaloupe, med, 1/4	48	0	0	0	12	1	11	12
Cherries, 1 cup	84	1	0	0	19	3	14	0
Cranberries, 1 cup	47	0	0	0	12	4	-	1
Grapefruit, 1/2	38	0	0	0	9	1	7	0
Grapes, 1 cup	114	1	0	0	28	2	16	3
Guava	46	1	0	0	11	5	5	3
Honeydew, med, 1/4	88	0	0	0	23	2	-	25
Kumquat	12	0	0	0	3	1	-	1
Lemon	22	0	0	0	12	5	1	3
Lime	20	0	0	0	7	2	0	1
Lychee, 1	6	0	0	0	2	0	-	0
Mango, 1 cup	107	0	0	0	28	3	16	3
Nectarine, med	67	1	0	0	16	2	12	0
Orange, med	62	0	0	0	15	3	12	0
Peach, med	42	0	0	0	11	2	8	0
Pear, med	98	1	0	0	25	4	17	0
Pineapple, 1 cup	76	1	0	0	19	2	17	2
Plum	36	0	0	0	9	1	5	0
Pomegranate	105	0	0	0	26	1	19	5
Raspberries, 1 cup	61	0	0	0	14	8	6	0
Strawberries, whole, 1 cup	36	0	0	0	8	3	9	0
Tangerine, med	37	0	0	0	9	2	7	1
Watermelon, 1/16 wedge	92	1	0	0	21	1	20	6

Food	Cal	Fat	Sat	Chol	Carb	Fib	Sug	Sod

FRUITS - FROZEN

The following fruits are listed alphabetically.

Food	Cal	Fat	Sat	Chol	Carb	Fib	Sug	Sod
Apples, unsweetened slices, 1 cup	83	1	0	0	21	3	-	5
Apricots, sweetened, 1 cup	237	0	0	0	61	5	-	10
Blackberries, unsweetened, 1 cup	97	1	0	0	24	8	-	2
Blueberries, unsweetened, 1 cup	79	1	0	0	19	4	-	2
Boysenberries, unsweetened, 1 cup	66	0	0	0	16	5	-	1
Cherries, sour, unsweetened, 1 cup	71	1	0	0	17	2	-	2
Cherries, sweet, sweetened, 1 cup	231	0	0	0	58	5	-	3
Mixed fruit, sweetened, 1 cup	245	0	0	0	61	5	-	8
Loganberries, 1 cup	81	0	0	0	19	7	-	1
Melon balls, 1 cup	57	0	0	0	14	1	-	54
Peaches, sweetened slices, 1 cup	235	0	0	0	60	5	-	15
Raspberries, sweetened, 1 cup	258	0	0	0	65	11	-	3
Rhubarb, 1 cup	29	0	0	0	7	2	-	3
Strawberries, sweetened, 1 cup	199	0	0	0	54	5	-	3
Unsweetened, 1 cup	77	0	0	0	20	5	-	4

JAMS, JELLIES & FRUIT SPREADS

(see Jams, Jellies & Fruit Spreads, pg 38)

Food	Cal	Fat	Sat	Chol	Carb	Fib	Sug	Sod

MEAT, POULTRY & ALTERNATIVES

BREAKFAST MEATS

Food	Cal	Fat	Sat	Chol	Carb	Fib	Sug	Sod
Pork sausage, 1 oz	117	11	4	19	0	0	0	187
Pork bacon, cured, 1 oz	159	16	6	19	0	0	0	208
Canadian-style bacon, 1 oz	43	2	1	14	1	0	0	359
Turkey bacon, 1 oz	60	5	1	20	0	0	0	380

BRANDS . . .

BACON (1 OZ UNLESS NOTED)

Food	Cal	Fat	Sat	Chol	Carb	Fib	Sug	Sod
Armour Turkey Selects	40	3	1	–	0	0	0	100
Bar-S Lower Sodium	75	6	3	15	0	0	0	180
Corn King Less Salt	55	5	2	10	0	0	0	100
Farmland Lower Sodium, 1.3 oz	80	7	3	15	0	0	0	190
Oscar Meyer Lower Sodium	70	5	2	15	1	0	0	170
Smithfield's Less Sodium, Hickory Smoked	35	3	1	5	0	0	0	98

NOTE: Some "lower sodium" bacons may have as much as 230mg sodium per 0.5 oz serving.

SAUSAGE (1 OZ PORK UNLESS NOTED)

Food	Cal	Fat	Sat	Chol	Carb	Fib	Sug	Sod
Farmland Lower Sodium, 0.7 oz	73	7	3	17	0	0	0	140
Healthy Choice Link or Patty, 0.8 oz	25	1	0	8	3	0	1	150
Jones Golden Brown Maple, 0.8 oz	95	9	3	18	0	0	0	130
Brown & Serve Light	110	9	3	18	0	0	0	140
Yorkshire Farms Morning Maple, Turkey, 1 oz	35	2	0	–	–	–	–	140

BREAKFAST MEAT ALTERNATIVES

Food	Cal	Fat	Sat	Chol	Carb	Fib	Sug	Sod
Sausage link, meatless, 1	64	5	1	0	3	1	0	222
Bacon, meatless, 0.5 oz strip	50	5	1	0	1	0	0	234
Sausage patty, meatless, 1.4 oz	97	7	1	0	4	1	0	337

BRANDS . . . (1 OZ UNLESS NOTED)

Food	Cal	Fat	Sat	Chol	Carb	Fib	Sug	Sod
Bocaburger Breakfast Patty, 1	80	4	0	0	5	3	1	260
Lightlife Smart Links, Country Breakfast Style, 1	60	3	1	0	4	0	1	130
Smart Bacon, 0.5 oz	17	1	0	0	1	0	0	135
Smart Links, Sausage Flavor, 1	70	3	0	0	3	1	1	180
Smart Links, Old World Italian, 1	70	3	0	0	3	1	1	180
Heartline Canadian Style NF Vegetarian Bacon, 1 slice	22	0	0	0	1	3	–	135
Morningstar Farms Breakfast Links, 1	30	1	0	0	1	1	0	170
SoyBoy Tofu Breakfast Links	65	3	1	0	6	–	1	130

123

Food	Cal	Fat	Sat	Chol	Carb	Fib	Sug	Sod

BEEF, LAMB & VEAL

CANNED

Food	Cal	Fat	Sat	Chol	Carb	Fib	Sug	Sod
Roast beef w/gravy, canned, 2 oz	75	2	-	38	1	0	0	320
Corned beef hash, canned, 2 oz	120	7	3	50	0	0	0	450
Chopped beef, canned, 2 oz	170	15	-	49	2	0	0	810
Beef stew, 1 cup	220	12	7	30	21	3	0	1250

BRANDS . . .

Food	Cal	Fat	Sat	Chol	Carb	Fib	Sug	Sod
Underwood Roast Beef Light, 2 oz	86	6	2	32	2	0	0	220

DRIED

Food	Cal	Fat	Sat	Chol	Carb	Fib	Sug	Sod
Beef, dried, 1 oz	50	2	1	25	1	0	1	1190

BRANDS . . .

No low-sodium alternatives.

FRESH & FROZEN

Beef:

Food	Cal	Fat	Sat	Chol	Carb	Fib	Sug	Sod
Ribeye steak, lean, 4 oz	150	5	2	65	0	0	0	60
Sirloin tip round, lean, 4 oz	140	5	2	65	0	0	0	65
Porterhouse, lean, 4 oz	177	8	3	63	0	0	0	66
T-bone, lean, 4 oz	164	7	2	54	0	0	0	66
Top sirloin, lean, 4 oz	147	5	2	69	0	0	0	66
Rib roast, lean, 4 oz	181	9	4	67	0	0	0	74
Flank steak, lean, 4 oz	160	7	3	54	0	0	0	75
Ground beef, lean, 4 oz	170	9	5	63	0	0	0	75
Tenderloin, lean, 4 oz	150	6	3	75	0	0	0	75
Tongue, 4 oz	253	18	8	98	4	0	0	78
Top round, lean, 4 oz	140	4	2	65	0	0	0	80
Liver, 4 oz	162	4	2	400	7	0	0	82
Eye of the round, lean, 4 oz	150	5	2	60	0	0	0	85
Strip steak, lean, 4 oz	150	5	2	50	0	0	0	85
Corned beef brisket, 4 oz	224	17	5	61	0	0	0	138

Lamb:

Food	Cal	Fat	Sat	Chol	Carb	Fib	Sug	Sod
Leg, sirloin, lean, 4 oz	210	13	5	76	0	0	0	66
Rib, lean, 4 oz	388	35	15	84	0	0	0	66
Ground, 4 oz	319	26	12	82	0	0	0	67
Loin, lean, 4 oz	316	26	11	82	0	0	0	67
Shoulder, blade, 4 oz	276	21	9	80	0	0	0	71
Cubed, 4 oz	152	6	2	74	0	0	0	74

Veal:

Food	Cal	Fat	Sat	Chol	Carb	Fib	Sug	Sod
Ground, 4 oz	163	7	3	93	0	0	0	93
Shank, lean, 4 oz	122	22	1	85	0	0	0	96
Loin, lean, 4 oz	131	4	1	90	0	0	0	103
Rib, lean, 4 oz	136	4	1	94	0	0	0	108

Food	Cal	Fat	Sat	Chol	Carb	Fib	Sug	Sod
PREPARED ENTREES								
Beef patty w/gravy, 1	200	15	-	45	7	2	-	750
Pot roast, 8 oz	210	6	-	35	25	3	-	780
Beef w/barbecue sauce, 8 oz	296	14	-	56	45	5	-	985

BRANDS . . .

No low-sodium alternatives.

CHICKEN & TURKEY

Food	Cal	Fat	Sat	Chol	Carb	Fib	Sug	Sod
Capon, 4 oz	262	19	5	84	0	0	0	50
Chicken:								
Breast, meat only, 4 oz	123	1	1	65	0	0	0	73
Liver, 4 oz	140	4	1	492	0	0	0	88
Wing, meat only, 4 oz	141	4	1	64	0	0	0	91
Thigh, meat only, 4 oz	133	4	1	93	0	0	0	96
Drumstick, meat only, 4 oz	133	4	1	86	0	0	0	99
Turkey:								
Light meat, w/o skin, roasted, 3 oz	137	3	1	61	0	0	0	56
Dark meat, w/o skin, roasted, 3 oz	170	7	2	78	0	0	0	72
Turkey, ground, lean, 3 oz	128	7	2	68	0	0	0	79
Cornish game hen, 1/2	336	24	7	170	0	0	0	102

BRANDS . . .

CANNED

Food	Cal	Fat	Sat	Chol	Carb	Fib	Sug	Sod
Hormel Turkey, NSA, 2 oz	69	3	2	0	0	0	0	20

FRESH

Foster Farms Chicken Breast

Food	Cal	Fat	Sat	Chol	Carb	Fib	Sug	Sod
Tenders, 3.6 oz	100	1	0	50	0	0	0	60

NOTE: The amount of sodium in packaged poultry varies within brands and cuts of meat. Some may have as much as 190mg sodium per 4-oz serving.

PREPARED ENTREES

Food	Cal	Fat	Sat	Chol	Carb	Fib	Sug	Sod
Chicken:								
Roll, light meat, 2 oz	88	4	1	29	1	0	0	333
Breast, mesquite flavor, 1.5 oz	34	0	0	15	1	0	0	437
Breast, oven-roasted, 1.5 oz	33	0	0	15	1	0	0	457
Nuggets, 5	240	14	4	40	16	0	0	480
Cordon bleu, 6 oz	380	23	8	60	20	4	5	650
Fillets, lightly breaded, 5 oz	270	12	2	50	17	1	1	820
Breast stuffed w/broccoli & cheese, 6 oz	340	19	6	40	20	0	2	870
Strips, buffalo style, 2	230	10	2	45	21	1	1	1250
Turkey:								
Roll, light meat, 2 oz	84	4	1	25	0	0	0	229
Patty, breaded & fried, 2.3 oz	181	12	3	40	10	0	0	512
Ham, 2 oz	73	3	1	32	0	0	0	568

MEAT, POULTRY & ALTERNATIVES
Game Meat

Food	Cal	Fat	Sat	Chol	Carb	Fib	Sug	Sod
PREPARED ENTREES - TURKEY								
Breast, oven-roasted, 2 oz	47	1	0	18	0	0	0	615
Smoked, 2 oz	53	0	0	27	1	0	0	649
BRANDS . . .								
FROZEN/REFRIGERATED *(3 OZ UNLESS NOTED)*								
Dietz & Watson Turkey Breast, NS .	75	3	0	45	0	0	0	84
Turkey Breast, Gourmet Lite, NS	90	3	0	45	3	0	0	84
Health Is Wealth								
Chicken Nuggets	150	6	2	40	9	0	0	180
Chicken Patties	150	6	2	40	9	0	0	180
Shelton's Turkey Burgers, 4 oz	170	10	3	90	0	0	0	110
Steak-umm Sliced Steaks, 1.3 oz	110	7	3	30	0	0	0	30
Tyson Time Trimmers Breast, Diced								
or Strips	90	1	0	45	0	0	0	240
Boneless Skinless Chicken Breast,								
7.1 oz	170	4	1	85	0	0	0	290

GAME MEAT

Rabbit, 3 oz	97	2	1	69	0	0	0	42
Buffalo (bison), top round, 3 oz	93	1	1	56	0	0	0	43
Ground, 3 oz	187	13	6	59	0	0	0	55
Deer, 3 oz	102	2	1	72	0	0	0	43
Elk, 3 oz	93	1	0	47	0	0	0	49
Duck, meat only, 3 oz	111	5	2	65	0	0	0	62
Goose, meat only, 3 oz	135	6	2	71	0	0	0	73

BRANDS . . .
Most brands are within the generic range.

HAM & PORK

Pork loin roast, boneless, lean, 3 oz	120	6	3	48	0	0	0	39
Pork, whole leg (ham), 3 oz	210	15	6	63	0	0	0	39
Pork, ground, 3 oz	225	18	6	60	0	0	0	48
Pork ribs, lean, 3 oz	135	6	3	54	0	0	0	57
Pork shoulder, boneless, lean, 3 oz	120	6	3	54	0	0	0	69
Pork, cured ham, canned, 3 oz.............	162	12	3	33	0	0	0	1056
25% less sodium, 3 oz	255	24	9	60	0	0	0	840
Ham steak, boneless, extra lean, 3 oz .	105	3	0	39	0	0	0	1080
Chopped ham, canned, 1 oz	204	15	6	42	0	0	0	1161

BRANDS . . .
No low-sodium alternatives.

126

Food	Cal	Fat	Sat	Chol	Carb	Fib	Sug	Sod

HOT DOGS, FRANKFURTERS & SAUSAGES

HOT DOGS & FRANKFURTERS

Food	Cal	Fat	Sat	Chol	Carb	Fib	Sug	Sod
Beef, 1.6 oz	142	13	5	27	1	0	0	462
Corn dog, 2.7 oz	180	10	3	35	15	1	1	490
Beef & pork, 1.6 oz	144	13	5	22	1	0	0	504
Chicken, 1.6 oz	116	9	3	45	3	0	0	617
Turkey, 1.6 oz	102	8	3	48	1	0	0	642

BRANDS ... *(1 HOT DOG OR FRANK UNLESS NOTED)*

BEEF AND/OR PORK

Food	Cal	Fat	Sat	Chol	Carb	Fib	Sug	Sod
A & H Beef, Reduced Fat & Sodium	100	8	-	25	0	0	0	195
Boar's Head Lite Beef	90	6	3	25	0	0	0	270
Hatfield Reduced Sodium	170	15	5	35	1	0	1	300
Healthy Choice LF	60	2	1	15	5	0	2	350
Hebrew National Beef, Reduced Fat	120	10	4	25	1	0	0	350
Jordan's Healthy Trim, LF	70	3	1	25	3	0	-	350
Shofer Beef, Reduced Fat	120	10	4	25	0	0	0	360

CHICKEN OR TURKEY

Food	Cal	Fat	Sat	Chol	Carb	Fib	Sug	Sod
*Empire Kosher Turkey Frank	50	2	1	-	-	-	-	320
Shelton's Uncured Chicken	90	8	3	45	0	0	0	340
Uncured Turkey	70	6	2	35	0	0	0	360

NOTE: Although many of the hot dogs & frankfurters listed above exceed sodium guidelines, they are substantially less than the generic.

SAUSAGES

Food	Cal	Fat	Sat	Chol	Carb	Fib	Sug	Sod
Bratwurst, 1 oz	85	7	3	17	1	0	0	158
Italian sausage, 1 oz	98	9	3	20	0	0	0	207
Kishka, 1 oz	80	6	-	8	5	1	-	215
Polish sausage, 1 oz	92	8	3	20	1	0	0	248
Vienna sausage, 1 oz	101	7	3	15	1	0	0	269
Knockwurst, 1 oz	87	8	3	16	1	0	0	286
Kielbasa, 1 oz	88	8	3	19	1	0	0	305
Turkey kielbasa, 1 oz	50	3	-	20	1	0	0	258
Braunschweiger, 1 oz	102	9	3	44	1	0	0	324
Chorizo, 1 oz	129	11	4	25	1	0	0	350

BRANDS ...

No low-sodium alternatives.

LUNCHEON, DELI & SANDWICH MEATS

Food	Cal	Fat	Sat	Chol	Carb	Fib	Sug	Sod
Pastrami, 1 oz	40	2	0	15	0	0	0	255
Turkey pastrami, 1 oz	40	2	1	15	0	0	0	296
Bologna, 1 oz	89	8	3	16	1	0	0	289
Turkey bologna, 1 oz	50	4	1	20	1	0	0	270

MEAT, POULTRY & ALTERNATIVES
Luncheon, Deli & Sandwich Meats

Food	Cal	Fat	Sat	Chol	Carb	Fib	Sug	Sod
LUNCHEON, DELI AND SANDWICH MEATS								
Salami, 1 oz	71	6	2	18	1	0	0	302
Turkey salami, 1 oz	56	4	1	23	0	0	0	285
Chicken, 1 oz	30	1	0	15	1	0	0	330
Turkey, oven-roasted, FF, 1 oz	24	0	0	9	1	0	0	334
Smoked, FF, 1 oz	26	0	0	11	1	0	0	360
Ham, extra lean, 1 oz	37	1	1	13	0	0	0	405
Turkey ham, 1 oz	36	1	1	16	0	0	0	282
Beef, 1 oz	50	1	1	12	2	0	0	408
BRANDS . . . *(1 OZ UNLESS NOTED)*								
BEEF								
Best's Kosher Cooked Corned Beef	40	2	1	15	0	0	0	180
Boar's Head Beef, NSA	45	2	1	15	0	0	0	20
Deluxe Top Round, NSA (avg)	45	2	1	15	0	0	0	40
Pepper Seasoned Eye Round	45	2	1	20	0	0	0	65
Sara Lee Roast Beef, 1 slice, 0.8 oz	30	2	1	13	0	0	0	130
BOLOGNA								
Best's Kosher Beef Bologna	80	7	3	15	2	0	0	180
Boar's Head Bologna, lower sodium	75	7	3	15	0	0	0	205
Dietz & Watson Gourmet Lite Bologna	30	1	0	8	2	0	2	19
Hillshire FF Bologna, 1 slice	30	2	-	-	0	0	0	190
Russer Light Bologna	60	4	2	15	2	0	0	200
HAM								
Boar's Head Branded Deluxe Ham, LS	30	1	0	13	1	0	1	230
PASTRAMI								
Hillshire Flavor Pack Pastrami, 90-99% FF Light, 1 slice	30	2	-	-	1	0	0	185
SALAMI								
Best's Kosher Beef Salami	85	7	3	18	2	0	0	180
Jordan's Genoa Salami	92	8	3	21	1	0	1	125
Russer Light Salami	45	3	2	20	2	0	0	200
TURKEY AND CHICKEN								
Boar's Head Premium Turkey								
Breast, skinless, Lower Sodium	30	0	0	13	0	0	0	170
Oven Roasted Turkey Breast, Skinless	30	1	0	0	0	0	0	175
Smoked Turkey	30	0	0	13	0	0	0	180
Jordan's Healthy Trim Turkey (avg)	30	1	1	15	2	0	0	180
Healthy Trim Chicken (avg)	30	1	1	15	2	0	0	180
Weight Watchers Deli Thin Smoked Turkey Breast, 5 slices	10	0	0	5	0	0	0	80

Food	Cal	Fat	Sat	Chol	Carb	Fib	Sug	Sod

LUNCHEON, DELI AND SANDWICH MEATS

OTHER MEATS
Boar's Head Lite Braunschweiger

Liverwurst	60	4	3	25	1	0	0	225

NON-MEAT SUBSTITUTES

BURGERS & PATTIES

Veg burger, garden-style, 2.5 oz	120	3	2	10	15	3	2	390

BRANDS . . .

FROZEN/REFRIGERATED *(1 BURGER OR PATTY UNLESS NOTED)*

Boca Burgers Grilled Veg	80	1	0	0	6	5	1	300
Dr. Praeger's California Veggie	100	3	0	0	10	4	0	190
Bombay	100	3	0	0	10	4	0	190
Salmon Veggie	100	3	0	7	11	3	0	200
Veggie Royale w/Cheese	120	4	1	5	12	2	2	258
Gardenburger								
Gourmet Style Santa Fe	130	3	1	20	20	4	1	280
Gourmet Style Veggie Medley	90	0	0	0	18	3	2	280
Flame Grilled Hamburger Style	120	4	0	0	7	4	0	300
Harvest Farms Soy Burgers	280	1	0	0	32	18	-	15
***Jeremiah's** Patties, 4 oz*								
Mushroom Walnut Cake	150	7	2	5	16	1	0	105
Roasted Veg Cake	130	5	2	5	19	1	0	110
Red Pepper & Jack Cheese Cake	140	5	3	10	19	1	0	150
Pasta Cake, Macaroni & Cheese	280	15	9	70	25	1	1	255
Lightline Barbecue Grilles	120	4	2	0	11	0	3	180
Morningstar Farms Grillers	140	7	2	0	5	3	1	260
Trader Joe's French Village Burger	190	3	1	10	29	6	0	120

MIX *(1/4 CUP UNLESS NOTED)*

***Authentic Foods** Falafel	100	1	0	0	17	3	2	240
Fantastic Nature's Burger	170	3	0	0	30	5	2	320

ENTREE SUBSTITUTES

Textured veg protein (TVP), 1/4 cup	80	0	0	0	7	4	3	594

BRANDS . . .

CANNED

Worthington LF Vegetarian, 1/4 cup	60	2	0	0	2	1	0	270

FROZEN/REFRIGERATED *(4 OZ UNLESS NOTED)*

Bocaburger Ground Burger	70	1	0	0	7	4	0	220
Field Roast Wild Mushroom, 2 oz	87	1	0	0	11	1	0	174
Lentil Sage, 2 oz	90	0	0	0	8	1	0	240
Smoked Tomato, 2 oz	90	0	0	0	8	1	1	260

MEAT, POULTRY & ALTERNATIVES
Non-Meat Substitutes

Food	Cal	Fat	Sat	Chol	Carb	Fib	Sug	Sod
NON-MEAT SUBSTITUTES - FROZEN/REFRIGERATED ENTREES								
Harvest Direct TVP Poultry, Chunks								
or Ground, 1 cup	280	1	0	0	32	18	-	15
Lightlife								
Smart Ground Taco & Burrito, 2 oz	70	0	0	0	7	4	0	170
Smart Ground Original, 2 oz	70	0	0	0	5	3	0	210
Smart Menu Crumbles, 2 oz	80	1	0	0	7	3	1	280
Loma Linda Fried Chick'N w/Gravy	80	5	1	0	7	3	0	260
Morningstar Farms Harvest Burgers								
Recipe Crumbles	70	0	0	0	5	3	0	200
Sovex Better Than Burger	165	2	1	0	25	9	2	52
Veat Gourmet-Bites, 1.8 oz	90	3	1	0	24	2	1	280
White Wave Chicken Style, 3 oz	130	0	0	0	7	3	0	170
Whole Foods Market 365 Garlic, 2.5 oz	80	1	0	5	7	4	0	240
Gourmet, 2.5 oz	100	2	1	5	9	4	0	290
Yves Veggie Cuisine Veggie or Italian								
Ground Round, 1/3 cup	60	0	0	0	4	3	0	270

HOT DOGS & FRANKFURTERS

Food	Cal	Fat	Sat	Chol	Carb	Fib	Sug	Sod
Hot dog, 1.5 oz	90	2	0	0	3	2	1	350
BRANDS . . . *(1 HOT DOG OR FRANK UNLESS NOTED)*								
Lightlife Tofu Pups, Original	60	3	1	0	2	0	2	240
Loma Linda Big Franks, LF, 1.8 oz	80	3	1	0	3	2	0	220
Big Franks, 1.8 oz	110	4	1	0	2	2	0	240
NewMenu VegiDog, 1.5 oz	45	0	0	0	1	0	0	170
SoyBoy Tofu Hot Dogs	95	3	1	0	10	-	1	200
Zoglo's Vegetarian Franks, 2.6 oz	125	5	1	0	5	2	1	240

LUNCHEON & SANDWICH MEATS

Food	Cal	Fat	Sat	Chol	Carb	Fib	Sug	Sod
BRANDS . . . *(1 OZ UNLESS NOTED)*								
Lightlife Veggie Salami	50	0	0	0	1	0	0	180
Foney Baloney, 3 slices	60	0	0	0	2	0	0	240
Smart Deli Pepperoni	45	0	0	0	3	1	1	290
Smart Deli Roast Turkey Style, 3 slices	40	0	0	0	1	0	2	290
Smart Deli Country Ham Style, 3 slices	60	0	0	0	3	0	1	300
Smart Deli Old World Bologna, 3 slices	50	0	0	0	2	0	0	300
Smart Deli Pastrami, 3 slices	45	0	0	0	1	0	0	300

TEMPEH

Food	Cal	Fat	Sat	Chol	Carb	Fib	Sug	Sod
Tempeh, 4 oz	160	9	2	0	8	4	1	8

BRANDS . . .
Most brands are within the generic range.

Food	Cal	Fat	Sat	Chol	Carb	Fib	Sug	Sod
TOFU								
Tofu, 1/2 cup	183	11	2	0	5	3	-	18

BRANDS ...

Most brands are within the generic range.

(PATE)

(see Pates & Spreads, pg 41)

(SANDWICH SPREADS)

(also see Pates & Spreads, pg 41)

Chicken, 1 oz	55	3	1	15	2	0	0	205
Roast beef, 1 oz	65	5	2	20	1	0	0	205
Deviled ham, 1 oz	75	6	2	18	0	0	0	230
Ham salad, 1 oz	61	4	1	11	3	0	0	259
Pork & beef, 1 oz	67	5	2	11	3	0	0	287
Ham & cheese, 1 oz	70	5	2	17	1	0	0	339

BRANDS ...

No low-sodium alternatives.

(SAUSAGE)

(see Breakfast Meats, pg 123)

Food	Cal	Fat	Sat	Chol	Carb	Fib	Sug	Sod

PASTA, NOODLES, RICE & GRAINS

GRAINS

(also see Flour, pg 6)

Food	Cal	Fat	Sat	Chol	Carb	Fib	Sug	Sod
Bran:								
Wheat, 1/2 cup	63	1	0	0	19	12	0	1
Oat, 1/2 cup	116	3	1	0	31	7	0	2
Corn, 1/2 cup	95	0	0	0	33	33	0	3
Rice, 1/2 cup	191	12	2	0	29	12	0	3
Couscous, dry, 1 cup	650	1	0	0	134	9	-	17
Barley, pearl, 1 cup	704	2	0	0	155	31	-	18
Buckwheat groats, roasted, 1 cup	567	4	1	0	123	17	-	18
Bulgur, 1 cup	479	2	0	0	106	26	-	24
Quinoa, 1 cup	636	10	1	0	117	10	0	36

BRANDS . . .
Most brands are within the generic range.

GRAIN DISHES *(see Grain Side Dishes, pg 104)*

PASTA & NOODLES

Food	Cal	Fat	Sat	Chol	Carb	Fib	Sug	Sod
Lasagne, dry, 2 oz	210	1	0	0	40	2	0	0
Farfel, matzo, 1 oz	105	0	0	0	21	-	-	0
Macaroni & spaghetti, dry, 2 oz	212	1	0	0	43	1	0	4
Macaroni & spaghetti, whole wheat, dry, 2 oz	198	1	0	0	43	9	0	5
Spaghetti, brown rice, dry, 2 oz	210	2	1	0	44	3	3	5
Noodles, egg, dry, 2 oz	217	2	1	54	41	2	0	12

BRANDS . . .
Most brands are within the generic range.

PASTA & NOODLE DISHES *(see Pasta Entrees, pg 100)*

RICE & RICE DISHES

RICE

Food	Cal	Fat	Sat	Chol	Carb	Fib	Sug	Sod
Brown rice, uncooked, 1/4 cup	150	1	0	0	33	1	0	0
Wild rice, uncooked, 1/4 cup	143	0	0	0	30	2	0	3
Instant rice, 1/2 cup	190	1	0	0	43	1	0	15

BRANDS . . .
Most brands are within the generic range.

Food	Cal	Fat	Sat	Chol	Carb	Fib	Sug	Sod
RICE DISHES *(also see Fried Rice - Mix, pg 107)*								
Risotto, mix, 1/4 cup	150	0	0	0	34	0	0	420
Rice w/vegetables, frozen, 1 cup	180	4	2	10	31	2	2	480
Rice & beans, mix, 1/4 cup	160	0	0	0	35	3	1	490
Rice pilaf, mix, prep, 1 cup	210	5	1	0	41	1	0	710
Long grain & wild rice, mix, prep, 1 cup	220	5	1	0	42	2	0	800
Flavored rice, mix, prep, 1 cup	320	2	0	0	51	2	2	1070
1/3 less salt, prep, 1 cup	280	1	0	0	53	1	2	640
Spanish rice, mix, prep, 1 cup	300	2	1	0	65	2	2	1000
Fried rice, mix, prep, 1 cup	260	1	0	0	47	1	3	1095
BRANDS . . .								
MIX *(1 CUP PREP UNLESS NOTED)*								
Atkins Savory Sides								
Mexican Fiesta, 1/2 cup	57	1	0	0	9	5	0	10
Broccoli Au Gratin, 1/2 cup	79	3	1	8	9	5	0	170
Creamy Mushroom, 1/2 cup	75	2	1	3	9	5	0	188
Country Veg or Stir Fry, 1/2 cup	61	1	0	13	9	5	0	194
Grey Owl Pilafs								
Amerimati Garden, 1/4 pkg	160	1	0	0	32	-	0	0
Country Kitchen Wild Rice, 1/4 pkg	150	1	0	0	31	-	0	10
Garden, 1/4 pkg	160	2	0	0	32	-	0	10
Country Garden Wild Rice, 1/4 pkg	160	2	0	0	32	-	0	10
Chef's Favorite Micro-Wild Rice, 1/4 pkg	190	1	0	0	31	-	0	25
Neera's Northern Indian Biryani	132	1	0	0	29	-	0	4
Indian Dal w/Chaunk	140	1	0	0	23	-	0	4
Indian Urad & Channa Dal	104	1	0	0	18	-	0	4
Jamaican-Style Dirty Rice	175	6	-	0	28	-	0	5
Indian Shahi Pilau	286	8	-	0	48	-	0	6
Zatarain's New Orleans Spanish	100	0	0	0	21	3	0	280

Food	Cal	Fat	Sat	Chol	Carb	Fib	Sug	Sod

SNACKS FOODS

CHIPS & NIBBLERS

CORN & TORTILLA CHIPS

Food	Cal	Fat	Sat	Chol	Carb	Fib	Sug	Sod
Tortilla chips, regular, 1 oz	142	7	1	0	18	2	0	150
Ranch, 1 oz	139	7	1	0	18	1	0	174
Nacho, 1 oz	141	7	1	1	18	2	0	201
Nacho, light, 1 oz	126	4	1	1	20	1	0	284
Corn chips, regular, 1 oz	153	10	1	0	16	1	0	179
Barbecue, 1 oz	148	9	1	0	16	2	0	216
Nacho, 1 oz	152	9	8	1	16	1	0	270
Onion, 1 oz	142	6	1	0	19	1	0	278

BRANDS . . . *(1 OZ UNLESS NOTED)*

Food	Cal	Fat	Sat	Chol	Carb	Fib	Sug	Sod
Barbara's Bakery Blue Corn, NSA	140	7	1	0	16	1	1	0
Blue Corn	140	7	1	0	16	1	1	40
Bearito's Little Bear Corn Chips	150	10	2	0	15	1	0	0
Blue Chips, NSA	140	7	1	0	18	2	0	10
Blue Chips	140	7	1	0	18	2	0	60
Little Soy or Sunny Blues	140	7	1	0	18	2	0	70
Red, White, or Yellow Chips	140	7	1	0	18	2	0	70
Black Bean or Garden Grains (avg)	140	7	1	0	18	2	0	70
Blue Farm Blue Corn, NSA	150	1	0	0	17	1	0	0
El Ranchero Natural	140	6	0	0	19	0	0	0
Garden of Eatin'								
Mini Yellow Rounds	140	7	1	0	18	2	0	60
Mini White Rounds or Strips	140	6	1	0	19	2	0	60
Guiltless Gourmet Unsalted Yellow Corn	110	1	0	0	22	2	0	26
Naturally Preferred Yellow Corn	140	6	1	0	19	1	0	40
Que Pasa, all	135	6	1	0	19	2	0	42
Snyder's of Hanover Organic White Corn-Tillas w/3 Bean & Garlic	140	7	1	0	18	-	-	90
Tostitos Restaurant Style	130	6	1	0	19	1	0	80
Santa Fe Gold	140	6	1	0	19	1	0	80
Trader Joe's Unsalted	140	4	1	0	22	4	0	0

FRUIT AND VEGETABLE CHIPS *(also see Potato Chips, pg 136)*

Food	Cal	Fat	Sat	Chol	Carb	Fib	Sug	Sod
Banana chips, 1 oz	147	10	8	0	17	2	-	2
Taro chips, 1 oz	141	7	2	0	19	2	-	97
Potato sticks, 1 oz	148	10	3	0	15	1	-	71

Food	Cal	Fat	Sat	Chol	Carb	Fib	Sug	Sod
FRUIT AND VEGETABLE CHIPS								
BRANDS . . . *(1 OZ UNLESS NOTED)*								
Roberts American Gourmet								
American Buds, Apple & Potato	130	6	1	0	21	2	7	85
Sweet Potato w/Soy	140	7	1	0	17	2	8	90
Original Veggie	130	5	5	0	19	2	2	130
Seneca Apple, 12 chips	140	7	1	0	20	2	11	15
Terra Sweet Potato, NS	140	7	1	0	18	1	2	10
Mesquite BBQ or Jalapeño Sweet Potato	140	7	2	0	18	1	4	65
Weight Watchers Apple Chips or								
Apple Cinnamon, 0.8 oz	70	0	0	0	18	3	13	125
Peach & Strawberry, 0.8 oz	50	0	0	0	13	2	11	125
NIBBLERS AND CRUNCHIES								
Oriental mix, rice based, 1 oz	156	7	1	0	15	4	-	117
Corn nuts, regular, 1 oz	125	4	1	0	21	2	-	157
Nacho, 1 oz	124	4	1	0	20	2	-	180
Barbecue, 1 oz	124	4	1	0	20	2	-	277
Chex mix, 1 oz	121	5	2	0	19	2	-	288
Cheese puffs, 1 oz	157	10	2	1	151	-	-	298
Pork skins, plain, 1 oz	155	9	3	27	0	0	0	521
Barbecue, 1 oz	159	9	3	33	1	0	-	756
BRANDS . . . *(1 OZ UNLESS NOTED)*								
Burns & Ricker Garlic Bagel Chips	110	0	0	0	22	1	2	30
Party Mix	107	0	0	0	23	1	2	38
Fall River Wild Rice Chips	140	7	1	0	17	1	0	65
Nejaimes Pita Bites, all, 0.5 oz (avg)	40	0	0	0	9	1	1	58
New York Style Plain Bagel Chips	130	5	1	0	19	1	1	70
Cinnamon Raisin Bagel Chips	130	5	1	0	20	1	7	105
Nu-World Foods Amaranth Snackers								
Chili Lime, 1 cup	117	2	0	0	20	3	1	10
BBQ Sweet & Sassy, 1 cup	118	3	0	0	20	3	1	36
BBQ Hot & Spicy, 1 cup	113	2	0	0	20	3	1	47
French Onion, 1 cup	115	2	0	0	20	3	1	56
Garden Burst, 1 cup	114	2	0	0	20	3	1	69
Old London Cinnamon Raisin Bagel								
Snacks, 0.5 oz	60	1	0	0	12	1	2	65
Organic Garden Soynutty Crunchies								
Unsalted, 1/4 cup	113	5	1	0	8	6	0	4
Roberts American Gourmet								
Fruit Booty w/Orange & Cherry	125	5	0	0	18	2	5	20
Power Puffs	110	0	0	0	29	4	4	29
Veggie Booty w/Spinach & Kale	125	5	0	0	18	2	0	70

Food	Cal	Fat	Sat	Chol	Carb	Fib	Sug	Sod
NIBBLERS AND CRUNCHIES								
Roberts American Gourmet (cont'd)								
Pirate's Booty w/Caramel	120	2	0	0	23	1	15	70
Past Life	130	6	1	0	15	3	1	125
Snyder's of Hanover Bread Nibblers, NS	120	0	0	0	25	-	-	50
Weight Watchers Cheese Curls, 0.5 oz	70	3	1	0	10	0	0	85
Zambetti's Wheat Star Chips	0	0	0	0	0	0	0	0
POTATO CHIPS								
Potato chips, regular, 1 oz	152	10	3	0	15	1	1	168
Reduced fat, 1 oz	134	6	1	0	19	2	-	140
Sour cream & onion, 1 oz	151	10	3	2	15	2	-	177
Barbecue, 1 oz	139	9	2	0	15	1	-	213
Cheese, 1 oz	141	8	2	1	16	2	-	225
BRANDS . . . (*1 OZ UNLESS NOTED*)								
Jays NSA	150	10	2	0	14	1	0	0
Kettle Chips NS	150	9	1	0	15	1	0	10
Lightly Salted	150	9	1	0	15	1	0	110
Michael Seasons LF, Unsalted	130	6	1	0	17	0	1	5
Lightly Salted, Reduced Fat	140	7	1	0	17	0	1	130
Snyder's of Hanover Unsalted	140	6	2	0	19	-	-	0
***Terra** Yukon Gold Onion & Garlic	130	5	1	0	19	1	1	65
Red Bliss Olive Oil & Fine Herbs	140	7	1	0	18	3	1	70
Terra Chips	140	7	1	0	18	3	1	70
Trader Joe's Hawaiian Style, NS	150	9	1	0	16	1	0	10
Utz NS	150	9	2	0	14	1	1	5
Regular, Kettle Classics, or Wavy	150	9	2	0	14	1	1	95
Ripple	150	10	3	0	14	1	0	95

CRACKERS

Food	Cal	Fat	Sat	Chol	Carb	Fib	Sug	Sod
Whole wheat, 0.5 oz	63	2	1	0	10	2	3	94
Wheat, 0.5 oz	67	3	1	0	9	1	-	113
Cheese, 0.5 oz	71	4	1	2	8	0	1	141
BRANDS . . . (*0.5 OZ UNLESS NOTED*)								

There are many low-sodium crackers, the following have less than 100mg per serving.

Food	Cal	Fat	Sat	Chol	Carb	Fib	Sug	Sod
***Breton** Thin Wheat, LS	70	3	2	0	8	0	1	30
Thin Wheat, Reduced Fat/Sodium	60	2	0	0	9	0	1	75
***Ener-G** Sesame	79	5	1	-	8	-	0	41
Seattle Crackers	32	1	0	0	5	-	1	54
Garlic	73	4	1	-	9	-	0	91
Health Valley Rice Bran	110	30	-	70	3	4	3	19
Original Amaranth	120	30	-	80	3	4	3	22

Food	Cal	Fat	Sat	Chol	Carb	Fib	Sug	Sod
CRACKERS								
Health Valley (cont'd)								
Original Oat Bran	120	30	-	80	3	4	3	22
Bruschetta Vegetable, NSA	60	2	-	0	15	1	1	40
Heavenly Desserts Gourmet, 0.8 oz .	32	1	0	0	5	0	0	38
Hol-Grain Whole Wheat, Unsalted, 8 .	50	0	0	0	11	0	0	0
Brown Rice or Sesame, Unsalted, 7 .	60	0	0	0	13	0	0	0
Brown Rice, 7	60	0	0	0	13	0	0	45
Onion & Garlic, 7	60	0	0	0	13	0	0	45
Whole Wheat, LS, 8	44	0	0	0	11	0	0	50
Kavli Thin Crisp Bread	60	0	0	0	13	2	0	40
Keebler Town House, LS	80	5	1	0	10	1	1	75
Club, Reduced Sodium	70	3	1	0	9	0	1	80
Kemach Snackers, Unsalted, 9	160	8	-	0	19	-	-	80
Nabisco Ritz Crackers, LS, 1 oz	80	4	1	0	10	0	1	35
Triscuits, LS, 1 oz	140	5	1	0	22	4	0	75
Wheat Thins, LS, 1 oz	140	6	1	0	20	1	3	75
Osem Sunny Wheat, NSA	120	4	-	0	21	-	-	95
Partners, all (avg)	65	3	2	3	8	1	2	60
Pepperidge Farm Goldfish, Cheddar								
Cheese Baked, LS	75	3	1	5	9	1	0	88
Distinctive Butter Thins	70	3	1	10	10	0	1	95
Cracker Quartet	70	3	1	5	10	1	1	95
Sesmark Sesame Wheat Thins, NSA,								
1 oz	120	2	0	0	25	1	0	1
Trader Joe's Water, all (avg)	60	2	0	0	11	0	1	70
Tree of Life FF, all (avg)	55	0	0	0	12	0	1	80
Upper Crust Sesame Pepper Crostini, 1	35	2	0	0	5	0	1	5
Blue Cheese & Walnut, 1	45	3	1	0	4	0	0	35
Venus Cracked Pepper or Garden								
Veg (avg)	60	0	0	0	12	0	1	80
Garlic & Herb	60	0	0	0	12	0	1	90
CRISPBREAD AND FLATBREAD								
Crispbread, rye, 0.5 oz	52	0	0	0	12	2	0	90
BRANDS . . . *(1 OZ UNLESS NOTED)*								
Bran-a-Crisp, 0.5 oz	20	0	0	0	6	2	0	0
Gold'N Krackle Garlic, 0.5 oz	58	1	0	0	11	0	0	15
Grillé French Crisp Toast, NS, 0.6 oz.	68	1	0	0	13	0	1	6
Orgran, 1 oz	72	0	0	0	17	1	0	60
GRAHAM CRACKERS								
Graham crackers, 1 oz	120	3	0	0	22	1	9	172
Chocolate, 1 oz	137	7	4	0	19	1	9	83

SNACK FOODS
Crackers

Food	Cal	Fat	Sat	Chol	Carb	Fib	Sug	Sod
GRAHAM CRACKERS								
BRANDS . . . *(1 OZ UNLESS NOTED)*								
Albertson's Cinnamon	130	5	1	0	19	1	11	85
Honey	120	4	1	0	21	1	6	95
Keebler, LF Honey	120	2	0	0	25	1	9	130
LF Cinnamon Crisp	110	2	0	0	23	1	10	135
Cinnamon Crisp	130	3	1	0	23	1	9	140
New Morning Choc	120	3	0	0	21	1	6	120
Cinnamon	100	2	0	0	20	1	5	125
MATZOS AND TAM TAMS								
Matzo, plain, 1 oz	112	0	0	0	24	0	-	1
Whole wheat, 1 oz	100	0	0	0	22	3	-	1
Egg & onion, 1 oz	111	1	0	13	22	1	-	81
BRANDS . . . *(1 OZ UNLESS NOTED)*								
Manischewitz Matzo, Unsalted	110	1	0	0	24	0	1	0
Tams, Unsalted	138	7	-	0	18	0	-	10
***Streit's** Matzo, Unsalted	100	1	0	0	23	1	0	0
MELBA TOAST								
Melba toast, plain, 0.5 oz	55	1	0	0	11	1	1	118
Whole wheat, 0.5 oz	53	0	0	0	11	1	0	119
Rye, 0.5 oz	55	1	0	0	11	1	0	127
BRANDS . . . *(0.5 OZ UNLESS NOTED)*								
Devonsheer Unsalted, all	50	1	0	0	10	2	0	0
Old London Unsalted, most (avg)	50	0	0	0	11	2	0	0
Salted, most (avg)	50	0	0	0	11	1	0	85
RICE CRACKERS								
Rice crackers, salted, 0.5 oz	50	0	0	0	11	0	0	65
Unsalted, 0.5 oz	50	0	0	0	11	0	0	0
BRANDS . . .								
Most brands are within the generic range.								
SALTINES								
Saltines, 0.5 oz	62	2	0	0	10	0	0	185
BRANDS . . . *(0.5 OZ UNLESS NOTED)*								
Keebler Zesta Saltines								
Unsalted Tops	60	2	1	0	11	0	0	60
Reduced Sodium	60	2	1	0	11	0	0	75
Nabisco Premium LS Saltines	60	2	0	0	10	0	0	35
***Liebers** Saltines, Unsalted Tops	60	2	0	0	10	0	0	115
***Rokeach** Saltines, Unsalted Tops	70	2	-	0	11	-	-	110

Food	Cal	Fat	Sat	Chol	Carb	Fib	Sug	Sod
SANDWICH CRACKERS *(1 PKG UNLESS NOTED)*								
Wheat w/cheese filling, 1 pkg	200	11	3	5	22	2	4	320
Cheese w/peanut butter filling, 1 pkg	200	11	2	0	21	1	4	420
BRANDS . . . *(1 PKG UNLESS NOTED)*								
Lance S'mores on Nekot Poppers	220	11	3	5	28	1	14	125
Malt	190	10	2	0	18	1	2	130
Peanut Butter on Captain's	210	13	3	0	19	1	3	170
Toasty	190	11	2	0	17	1	3	220
Reduced Fat Toastchee	180	7	2	0	23	2	2	230

(DIPS)

(also see Salad Dressings - Mix, pg 44 and Hispanic - Salsa & Taco Sauce, pg 112)

Food	Cal	Fat	Sat	Chol	Carb	Fib	Sug	Sod
Guacamole, 2 tbsp	60	5	1	0	3	0	2	140
Creamy herbal, refrigerated, 2 tbsp	100	9	2	5	2	1	1	190
BRANDS . . .								
FROZEN/REFRIGERATED *(1 OZ UNLESS NOTED)*								
Cedarlane Reg Hummus	45	2	0	0	5	0	0	90
Roasted Garlic Hummus	45	2	0	0	5	0	0	90
Roasted Eggplant & Red Pepper Dip	30	2	0	0	2	2	0	90
Cedar's Hommus Tahini, NSA	50	2	0	0	5	3	0	70
Baba Ghannouj	50	2	0	0	5	3	0	80
Garden of Atlantis Spinach &								
Artichoke or Spinach & Cheese	40	2	1	5	3	1	0	80
Spinach & Parmesan	37	2	1	0	2	0	0	106
Two Shieks Hummus, all (avg)	50	3	0	0	4	1	0	105
MIX								
Sheila's Select, all, 1/8 tsp (avg)	5	0	0	0	1	0	0	10
To Market To Market Spice Up Your								
Life Dip & Spread, all, 2 tsp	0	0	0	0	0	0	0	0
SHELF-STABLE *(1 OZ UNLESS NOTED)*								
Classic	80	7	1	0	3	1	0	5
Classy Delight Balsamic Black Bean	30	0	0	0	5	1	1	75
El Paso Chili Co. Cajun Red Bean	25	0	0	0	5	2	1	20
Esparrago Mild or Zesty Asparagus	10	0	0	0	2	0	1	95
Garden of Eatin' Baja Black Bean	25	0	0	0	5	1	1	80
Spicy Chipotle Red Bean	25	0	0	0	5	2	1	90
Guiltless Gourmet Bean, Spicy or Mild								
Spicy or Mild	30	0	0	0	5	1	1	100
Jardine's 7J Ranch Black Bean	30	0	0	0	5	0	1	80
Oasis FF Black Bean Dip	11	0	0	0	2	1	0	38
Santa Cruz FF Spicy Black Bean	30	0	0	0	5	1	0	50

SNACK FOODS
Jerky & Meat Snacks

Food	Cal	Fat	Sat	Chol	Carb	Fib	Sug	Sod

GRANOLA & CEREAL BARS

(see Cereal, Granola & Breakfast Bars, pg 31)

JERKY & MEAT SNACKS

Food	Cal	Fat	Sat	Chol	Carb	Fib	Sug	Sod
Beef sticks, smoked, 1 oz	156	14	6	38	2	0	0	420
Beef jerky, chopped & formed, 1 oz	116	7	3	14	3	1	0	627

BRANDS . . .

Food	Cal	Fat	Sat	Chol	Carb	Fib	Sug	Sod
Rustlers Roundup, 5 pc	20	2	1	5	1	1	0	115
Shelton's Turkey, 1 oz	100	2	0	50	2	0	0	250
Tofurky Jurky, 1 oz	70	2	0	0	14	1	0	190

NUTS & SEEDS

Food	Cal	Fat	Sat	Chol	Carb	Fib	Sug	Sod
Nuts, unsalted:								
Almonds, 1 oz	164	14	1	0	6	3	0	0
Hazelnuts, 1 oz	178	17	1	0	5	3	0	0
Pecans, 1 oz	196	20	2	0	4	3	0	0
Pistachios, 1 oz	156	12	2	0	8	3	0	0
Macadamia nuts, 1 oz	203	22	3	0	4	2	0	1
Pine Nuts, 1 oz	161	14	2	0	4	1	0	1
Walnuts, 1 oz	185	19	2	0	4	2	0	1
Cashews, 1 oz	163	13	3	0	9	1	0	4
Nuts, dry roasted w/salt:								
Macadamia nuts, 1 oz	203	22	3	0	4	2	0	75
Almonds, 1 oz	169	15	1	0	6	3	0	96
Pecans, 1 oz	201	21	2	0	4	3	0	109
Pistachios, 1 oz	161	13	2	0	8	3	0	121
Cashews, 1 oz	163	13	3	0	9	1	0	181
Mixed nuts, 1 oz	168	15	2	0	7	3	0	190
Seeds:								
Sunflower seeds, 1 oz	162	14	7	0	5	-	0	1
Sesame seeds, 1 oz	104	10	2	0	4	-	0	2
Nuts & Seed Snacks:								
Trail mix, regular, 1 oz	131	8	2	0	13	-	-	65
Tropical mix, 1 oz	115	5	2	0	19	-	-	3
Mix w/choc chips, 1 oz	137	9	2	1	13	-	-	34
Sesame sticks, 1 oz	153	10	2	0	13	1	-	422

BRANDS . . .
Most brands are within the generic range. NOTE: Nuts that are smoked and/or with added spices (barbecue, chili, etc.) may contain as much as 245mg sodium per 1 oz serving.

140

Food	Cal	Fat	Sat	Chol	Carb	Fib	Sug	Sod
PEANUT BARS								
Peanut bar, 1 oz	148	10	1	0	13	2	12	44
BRANDS . . .								
Lance, 1.6 oz	240	14	3	0	22	2	10	70
Planters, 1.6 oz	230	14	2	0	22	2	13	20

POPCORN

Food	Cal	Fat	Sat	Chol	Carb	Fib	Sug	Sod
Air-popped, 1 oz (2 1/2 cups)	108	1	0	0	22	4	0	1
Caramel-coated w/o peanuts, 1 oz	122	4	1	1	22	2	-	58
w/peanuts, 1 oz	113	2	0	0	23	1	-	84
Oil-popped, 1 oz (2 1/2 cups)	142	8	1	0	16	3	-	251
Cheese-flavor, 1 oz (2 1/2 cups)	149	9	2	3	15	3	-	252
BRANDS . . .								
MICROWAVE *(3 CUPS UNLESS NOTED)*								
Bearitos Organic, NS	110	2	0	0	23	5	0	0
Newman's Own Light Butter Flavor	94	3	1	0	26	3	0	77
Orville Redenbacher's								
Gourmet SF or SF Butter	100	6	1	0	11	3	-	0
Gourmet Light or Light Butter	70	3	1	0	8	3	-	115
Weight Watchers, 1 oz	100	1	0	0	20	7	0	0
READY-TO-EAT *(1 OZ UNLESS NOTED)*								
Bearitos Organic, Lite, NS, 4 cups	120	2	0	0	24	1	0	0
Cracker Jack	120	2	0	0	23	1	15	70
Estee Caramel, no sugar, 1 cup	120	2	0	0	26	1	1	90
Jiffy Pop Bag Lite, 3 cups	70	3	0	0	11	2	-	110
Glazed Popcorn Clusters	120	2	0	5	25	1	-	120
Roberts American Gourmet								
Nude Food	92	0	0	0	18	0	0	0
Organic Bubble Tea	130	4	1	0	20	3	0	70
Nude Food, Hot n' Spicy	120	3	1	0	20	2	0	125
Utz All Natural, 3 cups	120	1	0	0	25	5	0	0
Walden Farms Caramel Light	90	0	0	0	24	1	15	80
Weight Watchers								
Butter Toffee, less fat, 0.9 oz	110	3	1	0	21	1	11	90
Butter Flavored, less fat, 0.7 oz	90	3	0	0	14	3	0	100
White Cheddar Cheese, less fat, 0.7 oz	90	4	1	0	12	2	0	125
Ya Ya's, 2.5 cups	160	10	1	0	15	2	0	110

PRETZELS

Food	Cal	Fat	Sat	Chol	Carb	Fib	Sug	Sod
Pretzel, plain, 1 oz	110	2	1	0	22	1	1	370
Choc coated, 1 oz	130	5	2	0	20	-	-	161
Sourdough, 1 oz	109	0	0	0	22	1	1	400

Food	Cal	Fat	Sat	Chol	Carb	Fib	Sug	Sod

PRETZELS

BRANDS . . .

FROZEN/REFRIGERATED

New York Soft Pretzel, 3.5 oz 270	1	0	0	57	0	2	75
SuperPretzel Soft, 2.2 oz 170	0	0	0	37	2	2	140

READY-TO-EAT *(1 OZ UNLESS NOTED)*

Anderson Unsalted Bavarian Baldies 111	1	0	0	21	1	1	34
Estee Unsalted 120	1	0	0	25	1	0	30
Dutch Unsalted 118	1	0	0	24	1	1	36
Newman's Own Unsalted Round 110	1	0	0	24	1	1	105
*Roberts American Gourmet w/Soy 102	1	0	0	21	3	2	110
Snyder's of Hanover Unsalted Mini. 110	0	0	0	25	0	0	75
Organic Unsalted Pretzels 120	1	0	0	24	0	0	75
Nibblers, Sourdough Honey							
Mustard & Onion, 1 oz 118	3	0	0	21	1	1	86
Unsalted Hard Pretzels, 1 oz 100	0	0	0	22	0	0	90

(RICE & POPCORN SNACKS)

Rice cakes, 1 cake (avg) 35	0	0	0	7	0	-	20
Popcorn cakes, 0.5 oz 70	0	0	0	16	0	0	55

BRANDS . . . *(0.5 OZ UNLESS NOTED)*

Energy Food Factory Poprice							
Original Rice, NS 45	0	0	0	11	0	0	1
Gift of Nature Plain, NS...................... -	0	0	0	11	0	0	0
Hain, most (avg) 50	0	0	0	12	1	4	15
Innovative Foods Roasted Sweet							
Corn, 1 pkg.. 76	0	0	0	17	2	2	5
*Lundberg Brown Rice Cake, SF, 1 .. 70	0	0	0	16	0	0	0
Buttery Caramel, Apple Cinnamon, or							
Honey Nut Rice, 1 80	1	0	0	18	1	2	0
Mother's Butter Flavor or Unsalted							
Popcorn 70	0	0	0	14	0	0	0
Quaker SF Rice 56	0	0	0	11	0	0	0
Apple Cinnamon 50	0	0	0	11	0	4	0
Lightly Salted Rice 35	0	0	0	7	0	0	15
Caramel Corn 50	0	0	0	11	0	4	25
*Tree of Life Mini Rice, all (avg) 60	0	0	0	13	0	1	5

(RICE BARS & SNACKS)

Crisped rice bar, choc chip, 1 oz 115	4	2	0	21	1	-	79

BRANDS . . .
Most brands are within the generic range.

Food	Cal	Fat	Sat	Chol	Carb	Fib	Sug	Sod

SOUPS, STEWS & CHILI

BOUILLON, BROTHS & BASES

Food	Cal	Fat	Sat	Chol	Carb	Fib	Sug	Sod
Chicken broth, 1 cup	38	1	0	0	1	0	0	763
Reduced sodium, 1 cup	10	0	0	0	0	0	0	450
Beef broth, 1 cup	17	1	0	0	0	0	0	782
Beef bouillon, prep, 1 cup	6	0	0	0	1	0	0	864
Vegetable bouillon, prep, 1 cup	5	0	0	0	1	0	0	980
Chicken bouillon, prep, 1 cup	10	0	0	1	1	0	0	1152
BRANDS . . .								
CANNED (1 CUP UNLESS NOTED)								
Campbell's Chicken Broth, LS	30	2	1	4	2	0	1	107
*Hain Chicken Broth, Home-Style								
Natural, FF	10	0	0	25	0	0	0	60
Chicken Broth, NSA	40	2	1	25	0	0	0	150
Healthy Veg Broth, FF, NSA	25	0	0	0	6	1	2	170
Health Valley Beef Broth, FF, NSA	15	0	0	0	0	0	3	150
Chicken Broth, FF, NSA	40	2	1	25	0	0	0	150
Veg Broth, FF, NSA	20	0	0	0	5	0	1	210
Pacific Natural Chicken Broth	40	0	0	0	4	0	0	110
Shelton's Chicken Broth, FF, LS	10	0	0	0	0	0	0	60
Chicken Broth, Organic, FF, LS	20	0	0	0	0	0	0	135
CONCENTRATED, CUBED AND POWDERED (1 CUP PREP UNLESS NOTED)								
*Bernard Soup & Gravy Base, Cream								
of Chicken or Cream of Mushroom	30	1	0	0	5	0	1	5
Croyden House LS Instant Soup Mix	15	0	0	0	3	0	0	5
Diamond Crystal Beef Bouillon, LS	10	0	0	0	2	0	0	10
Chicken Bouillon, LS	15	0	0	0	2	0	0	20
Emes Beef or Chicken Base	18	0	0	0	2	0	0	10
Featherweight Chicken Bouillon	10	0	0	0	1	0	1	5
Beef Bouillon	20	0	0	0	3	0	2	20
*Gourmet Award Beef or Chicken								
Base, SF	25	1	0	0	3	0	0	0
Herb-Ox Beef or Chicken Bouillon, LS	10	0	0	0	2	0	1	5
Home Again SF Beef or Chicken Base	25	1	0	0	4	-	-	0
L.B. Jamison's Beef Flavored								
Bouillon, LS	25	1	0	0	3	0	2	48
RC Beef or Chicken Bouillon, LS	10	0	0	0	1	0	0	35
Redi-Base Beef or Chicken Bouillon, LS	10	0	0	0	1	0	0	35
Wyler's Chicken Bouillon SF	10	0	0	0	2	0	0	5

SOUPS, STEWS & CHILIS
Chili

Food	Cal	Fat	Sat	Chol	Carb	Fib	Sug	Sod
BOULLON, BROTHS AND BASES								
FROZEN/REFRIGERATED (*1 CUP UNLESS NOTED*)								
Perfect Addition Veg Stock, NSA	40	1	0	0	6	2	4	50
Fish Stock, NSA	32	0	0	0	2	0	0	100
Chicken or Veal Stock, NSA	40	0	0	0	4	0	0	110
Beef Stock, NSA	30	0	0	0	4	0	0	130

CHILI

Food	Cal	Fat	Sat	Chol	Carb	Fib	Sug	Sod
Chili mix, prep, 1 cup	150	1	0	0	29	9	5	460
Chili w/o beans, 1 cup	430	28	8	35	18	2	3	1150
Chili w/beans, 1 cup (avg)	287	14	6	44	31	11	5	1337
Less sodium, 1 cup	340	17	7	60	30	9	3	710
BRANDS . . .								
CANNED (*1 CUP UNLESS NOTED*)								
Ginny's Roasted Pepper	130	1	0	0	24	7	4	220
Savory Soy	150	1	9	9	24	6	5	299
Health Valley Mild Vegetarian, NSA ..	160	1	0	0	30	11	9	65
Spicy Vegetarian, NSA	160	1	0	0	30	11	9	65
Mild Vegetarian Lentil, NSA	160	1	0	0	28	11	9	65
Chili in a Cup:								
Mild Black Bean, 3/4 cup	120	1	0	0	21	6	3	290
Spicy Texas Style, 3/4 cup	120	1	0	0	21	6	3	290
99% FF Chilis:								
Mild Black Bean	160	1	0	0	28	12	7	320
Spicy Black Bean	160	1	0	0	28	12	7	320
Mild 3 Bean	160	1	0	0	28	12	7	320
Pritikin, all (avg)	230	1	0	5	37	13	4	140
MIX (*1 CUP PREP UNLESS NOTED*)								
Ass Kickin' Chili Fixin's	180	1	0	0	33	0	0	75
Green Chili & Corn Stew	80	1	0	0	18	0	0	110
Hurst HamBeens Chili Beans, 1 serv	130	1	0	0	22	10	1	170
Just Delicious Black Bean Chili	85	0	0	0	16	0	0	10

Although some of the soups listed above exceed sodium guidelines, they are substantially less than the generic.

CHILI SEASONING MIX
BRANDS . . .

Food	Cal	Fat	Sat	Chol	Carb	Fib	Sug	Sod
New Traditions Chili Mix, 1 tsp mix .	15	0	0	0	3	0	0	0
WhoopAss Chili Mix, 1 oz mix	60	1	0	0	12	0	0	40
Williams Original Chili Seasoning, NSA, 1/8 pkt	10	0	0	0	2	1	1	0

Food	Cal	Fat	Sat	Chol	Carb	Fib	Sug	Sod

SOUPS & STEWS

Food	Cal	Fat	Sat	Chol	Carb	Fib	Sug	Sod
Clam chowder, manhattan, 1 cup	78	2	0	2	12	2	3	578
New england, 1 cup	164	7	3	22	17	2	6	992
Gazpacho, 1 cup	46	0	0	0	4	1	0	739
Tomato, 1 cup	161	6	3	17	22	3	7	744
Chicken w/rice, 1 cup	60	2	0	7	7	1	-	815
Minestrone, 1 cup	127	3	1	5	21	6	-	864
Cream of mushroom, 1 cup	203	14	5	20	15	1	0	918
Cream of celery, 1 cup	90	6	1	15	9	1	-	949
Chicken gumbo, 1 cup	56	1	0	5	8	2	-	954
Split pea w/ham, 1 cup	185	4	2	7	27	4	1	965
Bean w/ham, 1 cup	231	9	3	22	27	11	2	972
Cream of chicken, 1 cup	117	7	2	10	9	0	-	986
Vegetable, 1 cup	78	2	1	5	10	0	-	791
Onion, 1 cup	58	2	0	0	8	1	0	1053
Cream of potato, 1 cup	73	2	1	5	11	0	-	1000
Oyster stew, 1 cup	135	8	5	32	10	0	-	1041
Chicken noodle, 1 cup	75	2	1	7	9	1	-	1160
Mix, prep, 1 cup	60	2	1	10	10	0	1	960
Black bean, 1 cup	116	2	0	0	20	4	-	1198
Beef stew, 1 cup	220	12	7	30	21	3	0	1250

BRANDS . . .

CANNED *(1 CUP UNLESS NOTED)*

Food	Cal	Fat	Sat	Chol	Carb	Fib	Sug	Sod
Campbell's Split Pea, LS, 1 can	240	4	3	5	38	5	6	50
Tomato w/Tomato Pieces, Ready-to-Serve, LS, 1 can	180	6	3	0	27	2	17	50
Cream Of Mushroom, LS, 1 can	200	14	4	20	18	3	5	65
Chicken w/Noodles, LS, 1 can	170	5	2	50	18	2	3	120
Hain Chicken Noodle, NSA	100	3	-	15	14	-	-	65
*Health Valley Organic Lentil, NSA	100	1	0	0	21	8	5	25
Organic Mushroom Barley, NSA	70	0	0	0	17	3	4	25
Organic Black Bean, NSA	130	1	0	0	25	5	7	25
Organic Potato Leek, NSA	70	0	0	0	15	3	5	35
Organic Tomato, NSA	80	0	1	0	18	1	14	35
Organic Veg, NSA	80	0	0	0	18	4	5	40
Organic Minestrone, NSA	70	0	0	0	17	3	5	45
Organic Split Pea, NSA	110	0	0	0	23	8	5	115
Country Corn & Veg, FF	70	0	0	0	17	7	8	135
Manischewitz Borscht, Unsalted	80	0	0	0	20	0	20	35
Borscht, Reduced Sodium	80	0	0	0	21	0	20	350
*Pritikin Cup of Soup, 1 pkg (avg)	110	0	0	0	22	4	4	140
Ready-to-eat (avg)	90	0	0	0	18	3	2	290

145

SOUPS, STEWS & CHILIS
Soups & Stews

Food	Cal	Fat	Sat	Chol	Carb	Fib	Sug	Sod
SOUPS AND STEWS								
***Rokeach** Borscht, Unsalted*	80	0	0	0	20	0	20	35
ShariAnn's Organic								
Indian Black Bean	150	1	0	0	30	4	0	320
French Green Lentil	130	0	0	0	22	1	0	320
True Foods Split Mong Bean	35	1	0	0	5	1	2	40
FROZEN/REFRIGERATED (7.5 OZ UNLESS NOTED)								
***Tabachinack** Mushroom Barley, NSA	70	0	0	0	13	3	0	98
Cabbage	60	0	0	0	14	2	9	160
Woodstock Organic Creamy Potato								
or Tomato Rice	110	0	0	0	23	3	7	340
MIX (1 CUP PREP UNLESS NOTED)								
Arrowhead Mills								
Bean & Barley, 1/4 cup mix	170	0	0	0	35	7	0	0
Ass Kickin' Tortilla & Bean	150	4	0	0	23	-	-	290
***Aunt Patsy's** Navy Bean	120	0	0	0	21	2	1	160
Bean Cuisine, most (avg)	100	0	0	0	18	6	2	10
Bob's Red Mill								
13 Bean, 1/2 cup mix	322	2	0	0	56	6	2	19
Vegi Soup Mix, 1/2 cup mix	330	2	0	0	60	8	0	28
Canterbury Cuisine Uptown Black								
Bean Soup, 1/4 cup mix	130	1	0	0	25	4	2	5
Cook in the Kitchen Welsh Potato,								
1.4 oz	130	0	0	5	24	1	7	50
***Goodman's** Alphabet Noodle	210	1	0	0	42	-	-	0
Noodleman LS	50	1	0	10	9	1	2	95
Onion LS	30	1	0	0	6	1	3	115
Hurst's HamBeens								
Cajun 15 Bean, 6 oz serv	120	1	0	0	20	9	1	100
Chili 15 Bean, 6 oz serv	120	1	0	0	20	9	1	170
Vegetarian 15 Bean, 6 oz serv	120	1	0	0	20	9	1	250
***Just Delicious**								
Champagne Red Lentil Soup	84	0	0	0	15	0	0	14
Corn Chowder	116	0	0	0	22	-	-	19
Minestrone	116	0	0	0	22	-	-	19
Seafood Chowder	116	0	0	0	22	-	-	19
Gourmet Winter Sunshine, 1/4 cup mix	160	0	0	0	30	6	3	20
Manischewitz Veg w/Mushrooms	120	0	0	0	22	3	1	70
Rainy Day Mushroom Chowder,								
1 tbsp mix	60	0	0	0	14	0	14	0
***Streit's** Variety Veg	100	0	0	0	21	4	0	10
Barley Mushroom	110	0	0	0	22	5	1	70

Food	Cal	Fat	Sat	Chol	Carb	Fib	Sug	Sod

VEGETABLES, BEANS & LEGUMES

BEANS & LEGUMES - CANNED

ADUKI (ADZUKI) BEANS

Aduki beans, 1/2 cup	351	0	0	0	82	0	0	323

BRANDS . . . *(1/2 CUP UNLESS NOTED)*

Eden Organic Aduki	110	0	0	0	19	5	0	10

BAKED BEANS - PORK & BEANS

Baked beans, 1/2 cup	118	1	0	0	26	7	10	504
Pork & beans, 1/2 cup	124	2	0	9	25	6	16	557

BRANDS . . . *(1/2 CUP UNLESS NOTED)*

Eden Baked w/Sorghum & Mustard	150	0	0	0	27	7	6	130
McIlhenny Spicy	28	0	0	0	4	4	1	76

BLACK BEANS (TURTLE BEANS)

Black beans, 1/2 cup	70	0	0	0	17	6	1	480

BRANDS . . . *(1/2 CUP UNLESS NOTED)*

American Prairie Organic	110	0	0	0	20	5	4	35
Eden Organic	100	0	0	0	18	6	0	15
w/Ginger & Lemon	150	0	0	0	21	7	1	200
Nature's Choice Black Turtle	150	1	0	0	28	9	0	10
S&W 50% Less Salt	70	0	0	0	17	6	1	260
Westbrae Natural Organic	100	0	0	0	19	5	4	140

BROAD BEANS *(see Fava Beans)*

BUTTER BEANS *(see Lima Beans)*

CANNELLINI BEANS (WHITE BEANS)

Cannellini beans, 1/2 cup	100	1	0	0	18	5	0	270

BRANDS . . . *(1/2 CUP UNLESS NOTED)*

American Prairie Organic	110	0	0	0	20	7	0	35
Eden Organic	100	1	0	0	17	5	1	40

CHICKPEAS *(see Garbanzo Beans)*

CHILI BEANS

BRANDS . . . *(1/2 CUP UNLESS NOTED)*

Westbrae Natural	100	0	0	0	19	5	2	150

FAVA BEANS (BROAD BEANS)

Fava beans, 1/2 cup	110	1	0	0	20	5	0	250

BRANDS . . .
No low-sodium alternatives.

Food	Cal	Fat	Sat	Chol	Carb	Fib	Sug	Sod
GARBANZO BEANS (CHICKPEAS)								
Garbanzo beans, 1/2 cup	143	2	0	0	27	6	0	359
BRANDS . . . *(1/2 CUP UNLESS NOTED)*								
American Prairie Organic	120	2	0	0	20	6	3	35
*Eden Organic	120	2	0	0	19	5	0	10
S&W 50% Less Salt	110	1	0	0	19	4	1	220
*Westbrae Natural Organic	110	2	0	0	18	5	3	140
GREAT NORTHERN BEANS								
Great northern beans, 1/2 cup	100	1	0	0	19	7	0	300
BRANDS . . . *(1/2 CUP UNLESS NOTED)*								
American Prairie Organic	110	0	0	0	20	8	2	35
*Eden Organic	110	1	0	0	20	8	1	65
*Westbrae Natural Organic	100	0	0	0	19	6	2	140
GREEN BEANS *(see Green Beans, pg 151)*								
KIDNEY BEANS (RED BEANS)								
Kidney beans, 1/2 cup	104	0	0	0	19	5	0	444
BRANDS . . . *(1/2 CUP UNLESS NOTED)*								
American Prairie Organic	110	0	0	0	20	5	2	35
Organic Small Red	110	0	0	0	20	8	2	35
*Eden Organic	100	0	0	0	18	10	0	15
Organic Small Red	100	1	0	0	17	5	1	65
Finest Light Red	120	1	0	0	21	7	1	210
Natural Value Red	100	0	0	0	18	6	0	95
S&W 50% Less Salt	120	1	0	0	21	6	4	220
*Westbrae Natural Organic Kidney	100	0	0	0	18	5	2	140
Red	100	0	0	0	19	7	2	140
LENTILS								
Lentils, 1/2 cup	115	0	0	0	20	8	0	236
BRANDS . . . *(1/2 CUP UNLESS NOTED)*								
*Westbrae Natural								
Organic Black Beluga	100	0	0	0	16	4	0	120
Organic	100	0	0	0	19	7	2	150
LIMA BEANS (BUTTER BEANS)								
Lima beans, 1/2 cup	95	0	0	0	18	6	0	405
BRANDS . . . *(1/2 CUP UNLESS NOTED)*								
American Prairie Organic Baby	110	0	0	0	20	7	3	35
C&W Baby	90	1	0	0	15	5	1	80
*Eden Organic Baby	100	1	0	0	17	4	0	35
*Seneca Lima Beans, NSA	80	0	0	0	18	5	2	25
Stokely No Salt or Sugar Added	80	0	0	0	16	0	0	5

Food	Cal	Fat	Sat	Chol	Carb	Fib	Sug	Sod
MISCELLANEOUS BEANS								
BRANDS . . . *(1/2 CUP UNLESS NOTED)*								
*Westbrae Natural Jackson Wonder	100	0	0	0	19	5	0	135
European Soldier	90	0	0	0	16	5	0	140
Scarlet Runner	100	0	0	0	20	7	1	140
Trout	100	0	0	0	18	6	0	140
MIXED BEANS								
BRANDS . . . *(1/2 CUP UNLESS NOTED)*								
American Prairie Organic 3 Beans	110	0	0	0	20	6	3	35
*Westbrae Natural Soup Beans	100	0	0	0	19	6	2	140
Salad Beans	100	1	0	0	19	5	2	150
NAVY BEANS								
Navy beans, 1/2 cup	148	1	0	0	27	7	0	587
BRANDS . . . *(1/2 CUP UNLESS NOTED)*								
American Prairie Organic	110	0	0	0	20	8	2	35
*Eden Organic	110	1	0	0	20	7	0	15
PINTO BEANS								
Pinto beans, 1/2 cup	103	1	0	0	18	6	0	353
BRANDS . . . *(1/2 CUP UNLESS NOTED)*								
American Prairie Organic	110	1	0	0	20	8	2	35
*Eden Organic	100	0	0	0	18	6	0	15
Spicy w/Jalapeño & Red Pepper	125	0	0	0	24	7	2	195
*Westbrae Natural Organic	100	0	0	0	19	7	2	140
PORK & BEANS *(see Baked Beans - Pork & Beans, pg 147)*								
SOYBEANS								
Soybeans, 1/2 cup	149	8	1	0	9	5	0	204
BRANDS . . . *(1/2 CUP UNLESS NOTED)*								
American Prairie Black	130	6	1	0	10	3	2	35
*Eden Organic Black	120	6	1	0	8	7	1	30
*Westbrae Natural Organic	150	7	1	0	11	3	3	140
WAX BEANS *(see Wax Beans, pg 154)*								
WHITE BEANS *(see Cannellini Beans, pg 147)*								

BEANS & LEGUMES - DRIED/RAW

Food	Cal	Fat	Sat	Chol	Carb	Fib	Sug	Sod
Soybeans, 1/2 cup	387	19	3	0	28	9	9	2
Aduki (adzuki) beans, 1/2 cup	324	1	0	0	62	13	-	5
Black beans, 1/2 cup	331	1	0	0	61	15	-	5
Fava beans (broad beans), 1/2 cup	102	1	0	0	44	19	4	10
Lentils, 1/2 cup	325	1	0	0	55	29	5	10

VEGETABLES, BEANS & LEGUMES
Beans & Legumes - Frozen

Food	Cal	Fat	Sat	Chol	Carb	Fib	Sug	Sod
BEANS AND LEGUMES - DRIED/RAW								
Pinto beans, 1/2 cup	328	1	0	0	61	24	-	10
Great northern beans, 1/2 cup	310	1	0	0	57	19	-	13
Navy beans, 1/2 cup	349	1	0	0	63	26	-	15
Lima beans (butter beans), 1/2 cup	301	1	0	0	57	17	8	16
Kidney beans (red beans), 1/2 cup	307	1	0	0	55	23	-	22
Garbanzo beans (chickpeas), 1/2 cup	364	6	1	0	61	18	1	24

BRANDS . . .
Most brands are within the generic range.

(BEANS & LEGUMES - FROZEN)

LIMA BEANS

Food	Cal	Fat	Sat	Chol	Carb	Fib	Sug	Sod
Baby, 1/2 cup	108	0	0	0	21	5	-	43
Fordhook, 1/2 cup	85	0	0	0	16	4	-	46
Speckled, 1/2 cup	100	0	0	0	20	4	1	130
w/butter sauce, 1/2 cup	133	3	2	5	18	6	1	330

NOTE: Lima beans are often frozen in brine and may contain as much as 213mg sodium per serving.

BRANDS . . . *(1/2 CUP UNLESS NOTED)*

Food	Cal	Fat	Sat	Chol	Carb	Fib	Sug	Sod
Birds Eye Fordhook	100	0	0	0	19	5	3	10
Freshlike Fordhook	90	0	0	0	17	5	-	10
Seabrook Speckled	145	0	0	0	28	2	-	23
Southern Speckled	135	0	0	0	25	0	-	30

(VEGETABLES - CANNED)

ARTICHOKE

Food	Cal	Fat	Sat	Chol	Carb	Fib	Sug	Sod
Artichoke hearts, marinated, 1/2 cup	80	8	0	0	8	4	0	320
Artichoke hearts, 1/2 cup	20	0	0	0	4	2	1	420

BRANDS . . .

Food	Cal	Fat	Sat	Chol	Carb	Fib	Sug	Sod
Reese Hearts, Quartered, 1/2 cup	30	0	0	0	6	1	0	240

ASPARAGUS

Food	Cal	Fat	Sat	Chol	Carb	Fib	Sug	Sod
Asparagus, 1/2 cup	20	0	0	0	3	1	0	346

BRANDS . . . *(1/2 CUP UNLESS NOTED)*

Food	Cal	Fat	Sat	Chol	Carb	Fib	Sug	Sod
Hogue Farms Pickled, 3 spears	10	0	0	0	1	0	0	75
*Seneca Cuts, NSA	20	0	0	0	3	2	1	20
Stokely Cuts, NSA	20	0	0	0	3	0	-	5

BEETS

Food	Cal	Fat	Sat	Chol	Carb	Fib	Sug	Sod
Beets, 1/2 cup	35	0	0	0	8	1	5	310

BRANDS . . . *(1/2 CUP UNLESS NOTED)*

Food	Cal	Fat	Sat	Chol	Carb	Fib	Sug	Sod
*Seneca, NSA	20	0	0	0	8	2	5	25

Food	Cal	Fat	Sat	Chol	Carb	Fib	Sug	Sod
BEETS - CANNED								
Stokely NS, No Sugar	40	0	0	0	8	0	-	40
Harvard	70	0	0	0	18	0	-	135
BLACK-EYED PEAS								
Black-eyed peas, 1/2 cup	90	1	0	0	18	4	0	300
BRANDS . . . *(1/2 CUP UNLESS NOTED)*								
American Prairie Organic	110	0	0	0	19	3	2	35
***Eden** Organic	90	1	0	0	16	4	1	25
CARROTS								
Carrots, 1/2 cup	35	0	0	0	8	3	5	300
BRANDS . . . *(1/2 CUP UNLESS NOTED)*								
Hogue Farms Pickled, 2 oz	30	0	0	0	7	1	6	5
***Seneca**, NSA	25	0	0	0	6	2	3	30
CORN								
Whole kernel corn, 1/2 cup	82	1	0	0	20	2	6	273
50% less sodium, 1/2 cup	85	1	0	0	19	2	5	176
Creamed corn, 1/2 cup	72	1	0	0	23	2	7	365
BRANDS . . . *(1/2 CUP UNLESS NOTED)*								
Del Monte Whole Kernel Sweet, NSA	60	1	0	0	11	3	7	10
Golden Cream Style Sweet, NSA	90	1	0	0	20	2	5	10
Freshlike Whole Kernel	90	0	0	0	20	3	5	0
Cream Style	90	1	0	0	20	2	5	10
Green Giant Niblets, NS	90	0	0	0	20	3	5	0
***Seneca** Whole Kernel, NSA	80	1	0	0	16	1	3	40
Sun Luck Baby Corn, all	10	0	0	0	6	4	6	20
GARLIC								
Garlic, crushed or chopped, 1 tsp	10	0	0	0	1	0	0	0
BRANDS . . .								
Most brands are within the generic range.								
GREEN BEANS								
Green beans, 1/2 cup	18	0	0	0	4	2	2	311
50% less sodium, 1/2 cup	20	0	0	0	4	1	2	200
BRANDS . . . *(1/2 CUP UNLESS NOTED)*								
Del Monte Cut Green Beans, NSA	20	0	0	0	4	2	2	10
French Style Beans, NSA	20	0	0	0	4	2	2	10
Freshlike Cut, NSA	20	0	0	0	4	0	1	5
***Seneca**, NSA	25	0	0	0	5	2	2	10
Stokely NSA	20	0	0	0	4	0	-	5
Tender Sweet French Cut, NSA	20	0	0	0	4	0	2	5

VEGETABLES, BEANS & LEGUMES

Canned Vegetables

Food	Cal	Fat	Sat	Chol	Carb	Fib	Sug	Sod
MIXED VEGETABLES								
Peas & carrots, 1/2 cup	49	0	0	0	11	3	3	332
BRANDS . . . *(1/2 CUP UNLESS NOTED)*								
Del Monte Peas & Carrots, NSA	40	0	0	0	8	0	3	25
*Seneca Mixed Vegetables, NSA	45	0	0	0	9	2	1	10
Succotash (corn/lima beans), 2/3 cup	100	1	0	0	20	4	2	55
Veg-All NSA	40	0	0	0	8	2	2	25
MUSHROOMS								
Mushrooms, 1/2 cup	19	0	0	0	4	2	1	400
BRANDS . . . *(1/2 CUP UNLESS NOTED)*								
Giorgio Pieces and Stems, NSA	20	0	0	0	3	1	0	20
*Seneca NSA	25	0	0	0	5	3	2	15
Sun Luck Straw	10	0	0	0	8	0	0	0
Stir Fry	40	0	0	0	6	4	0	50
PEAS								
Peas, 1/2 cup	66	0	0	0	12	4	4	310
BRANDS . . . *(1/2 CUP UNLESS NOTED)*								
Del Monte Sweet, NSA	20	0	0	0	11	4	5	10
Freshlike Tender Garden, NSA	50	0	0	0	10	2	4	10
LeSueur 50% Less Sodium	60	0	0	0	11	4	3	190
*Seneca NSA	70	0	0	0	12	4	5	15
Stokely NSA	50	0	0	0	9	0	-	5
Tender Sweet NSA	50	0	0	0	10	2	-	10
POTATOES								
Potatoes, 2/3 cup	54	0	0	0	12	2	0	450
BRANDS . . .								
*Seneca, NSA, 2/3 cup	80	0	0	0	17	2	1	30
PUMPKIN								
Pumpkin, 1/2 cup	42	0	0	0	10	4	4	6
BRANDS . . .								
Most brands are within the generic range.								
SAUERKRAUT								
Sauerkraut, 1/2 cup	10	0	0	0	2	1	0	661
BRANDS . . . *(1/2 CUP UNLESS NOTED)*								
*Cascadian Farms Organic LS	20	0	0	0	4	0	0	480
SPINACH								
Spinach, 1/2 cup	22	0	0	0	3	2	0	373
BRANDS . . . *(1/2 CUP UNLESS NOTED)*								
Del Monte, NSA	30	0	0	0	4	2	0	85
Popeye, LS	35	1	0	0	4	3	0	35
*Seneca, NSA	25	0	0	0	3	2	0	20

Food	Cal	Fat	Sat	Chol	Carb	Fib	Sug	Sod
SWEET POTATOES & YAMS								
Yam, 1/2 cup	130	1	0	0	29	2	23	30
Sweet potato, 1/2 cup	91	0	0	0	21	2	15	53
BRANDS ...								
Most brands are within the generic range.								
TOMATOES								
Tomato puree, 1/4 cup	25	0	0	0	6	1	2	249
Tomato paste, 2 tbsp	27	0	0	0	6	1	3	259
Whole tomatoes, 1/2 cup	25	0	0	0	5	1	3	270
Stewed tomatoes, 1/2 cup	36	0	0	0	9	2	6	282
Diced & chopped tomatoes, 1/2 cup	25	0	0	0	4	1	4	290
Crushed tomatoes, 1/2 cup	74	0	0	0	16	4	6	304
Tomato sauce, 1/4 cup	18	0	0	0	4	1	3	371
Diced & chopped w/spices, 1/2 cup	25	0	0	0	4	1	4	600
BRANDS ...								
TOMATO PASTE (2 TBSP UNLESS NOTED)								
Contadina	30	0	0	0	6	1	3	20
Del Monte	30	0	0	0	7	2	3	25
Hunt's, NSA	30	0	0	0	6	2	3	7
*Muir Glen	30	0	0	0	6	1	3	20
Whole Foods Market 365	33	0	0	0	6	1	3	20
TOMATO PUREE (1/4 CUP UNLESS NOTED)								
Contadina	20	0	0	0	4	1	1	15
*Muir Glen	20	0	0	0	5	1	3	20
TOMATO SAUCE (1/4 CUP UNLESS NOTED)								
America's Choice	20	0	0	0	4	1	-	15
Del Monte, NSA	20	0	0	0	4	1	4	20
Hunt's, NSA	16	0	0	0	3	1	2	15
*Muir Glen, NSA	20	0	0	0	5	1	3	30
*Rokeach w/Mushrooms, NSA	40	1	0	0	7	-	-	25
*Tree of Life	20	0	0	0	4	1	-	9
TOMATOES - CHOPPED/DICED (1/2 CUP UNLESS NOTED)								
Del Monte Diced	25	0	0	0	6	2	4	50
*Eden Diced	30	0	0	0	6	2	4	5
Diced w/Green Chilies	30	0	0	0	5	2	3	35
*Muir Glen Diced, NSA	25	0	0	0	4	1	4	45
Pomi Chopped	20	0	0	0	4	3	4	10
S&W Diced, NSA	25	0	0	0	4	1	3	30
Ready Cut Peeled	25	0	0	0	4	1	3	30
TOMATOES - CRUSHED (1/2 CUP UNLESS NOTED)								
Cento	70	0	0	0	-	-	-	40
*Eden	40	0	0	0	6	2	4	0

VEGETABLES, BEANS & LEGUMES
Vegetables - Dried

Food	Cal	Fat	Sat	Chol	Carb	Fib	Sug	Sod
CANNED VEGETABLES - CRUSHED TOMATOES								
Muir Glen Ground Peeled	20	0	0	0	4	2	4	200
S&W Crushed, Italian Style	40	0	0	0	8	2	4	190
TOMATOES - SLICED *(1/2 CUP UNLESS NOTED)*								
Del Monte	35	0	0	0	9	2	7	50
Hunt's	35	0	0	0	7	2	6	30
S&W, NSA	35	0	0	0	7	2	5	15
TOMATOES - WHOLE *(1/2 CUP UNLESS NOTED)*								
Hunt's	33	0	0	0	7	2	3	31
S&W, Peeled	20	0	0	0	4	1	3	20
WAX BEANS								
Wax beans, 1/2 cup	23	0	0	0	5	2	2	360
BRANDS . . . *(1/2 CUP UNLESS NOTED)*								
Seneca NSA	25	0	0	0	4	2	2	10
Stokely No Salt or Sugar	20	0	0	0	4	0	0	5
YAM *(see Sweet Potatoes & Yams, pg 153)*								
ZUCCHINI								
Zucchini, italian style, 1/2 cup	33	0	0	0	8	0	1	427

BRANDS . . .
No low-sodium alternatives.

VEGETABLES - DRIED

Food	Cal	Fat	Sat	Chol	Carb	Fib	Sug	Sod
Mushrooms, shiitake, 4	44	0	0	0	11	2	0	2
Peppers, sweet, red or green, 1/4 cup	5	0	0	0	1	0	0	3
Tomato halves, 2-3	15	0	0	0	3	1	0	5
Seasoned, 2-3	15	0	0	0	3	1	0	25

BRANDS . . .
Most brands are within the generic range.

VEGETABLES - FRESH

The following vegetables are listed alphabetically.

Food	Cal	Fat	Sat	Chol	Carb	Fib	Sug	Sod
Artichoke, globe or french, med, 4.6 oz	60	0	0	0	13	7	-	120
Asparagus, 5 spears	18	0	0	0	2	2	-	0
Avocado, 1/2	162	15	2	0	7	5	1	10
Beets, 1/2 cup	30	0	0	0	7	2	-	53
Brussel sprouts, 1/2 cup	190	0	0	0	4	2	-	11
Broccoli, 1/2 cup	12	0	0	0	2	1	-	12
Cabbage, green or red, 1/2 cup	9	0	0	0	2	0	-	6
Carrot, 1 med	40	1	0	0	8	1	-	40

Food	Cal	Fat	Sat	Chol	Carb	Fib	Sug	Sod
VEGETABLES - FRESH								
Cauliflower, 1/2 cup	13	0	0	0	3	1	-	15
Celery, 1 med stalk	6	0	0	0	1	1	-	35
Corn, 1/2 cup	66	1	0	0	15	-	-	12
Cucumber, 1/2 cup	7	0	0	0	1	1	-	1
Eggplant, 1/2 cup	11	0	0	0	2	1	-	1
Jerusalem artichoke, sliced, 1 cup	114	0	0	0	26	2	-	6
Kale, 1/2 cup	21	0	0	0	3	1	-	15
Leeks, 1/2 cup	16	0	0	0	4	1	-	5
Lettuce, chopped or shredded, 1 cup	8	0	0	0	1	1	-	4
Mushrooms, 1/2 cup	9	0	0	0	1	0	-	1
Mustard greens, 1/2 cup	7	0	0	0	1	0	-	7
Onion, 1/2 cup chopped	30	0	0	0	7	1	-	2
Peas, green, 1/2 cup	59	0	0	0	10	4	-	4
Peppers, sweet, green or red, 1/2 cup	20	0	0	0	5	1	-	2
Potato w/skin, med, 7.6 oz	149	0	0	0	33	5	2	13
Radish, 1/2 cup	12	0	0	0	2	1	-	14
Rutabaga, 1/2 cup cubed	25	0	0	0	6	2	-	14
Shallots, 1 tbsp	7	0	0	0	2	-	-	1
Spinach, 1 cup	7	0	0	0	1	1	0	24
Squash, winter, all, 1/2 cup cubed	16	0	0	0	5	1	-	2
Summer, crookneck, 1/2 cup cubed	12	0	0	0	3	1	-	1
Spaghetti, 1/2 cup cubed	10	0	0	0	2	1	-	15
Sweet potato, 1/2 cup cubed	70	0	0	0	16	2	-	9
Tomato, 1/2 cup chopped	19	0	0	0	4	1	-	8
Turnips, 1/2 cup cubed	25	0	0	0	6	-	-	14
Zucchini, 1/2 cup cubed	9	0	0	0	2	1	-	2

BRANDS . . .

SALAD KITS *(2 CUPS PREP UNLESS NOTED)*

Many packaged salad kits include salad dressing which may have as much as 420mg sodium per serving. The following have less than 200mg per serving.

Dole Triple Cheese Kit	80	5	3	2	4	1	2	120
Mediterranean Kit	90	8	1	0	5	1	3	180

SPINACH

Most brands are within the generic range. NOTE: Fresh Express packaged spinach has 53mg more sodium per serving than Dole's.

VEGETABLES - FROZEN

Most frozen vegetables have minimal sodium. Those packaged with sauces or for convenience may have added sodium.

ARTICHOKES

Artichoke hearts, 1/2 cup	25	0	0	0	4	5	0	55

155

VEGETABLES, BEANS & LEGUMES
Vegetables - Frozen

Food	Cal	Fat	Sat	Chol	Carb	Fib	Sug	Sod

FROZEN VEGETABLES - ARTICHOKES

BRANDS . . .

Birds Eye Deluxe Hearts, 1/2 cup	40	0	0	0	8	6	1	45

MIXED VEGETABLES *(also see Vegetable Side Dishes, pg 106)*

Stir-fry vegetables w/o sauce, 1 cup....	40	0	0	0	7	2	4	20
Peas & carrots, 1/2 cup	37	0	0	0	8	2	-	55

BRANDS . . . *(1/2 CUP UNLESS NOTED)*
Most brands are within the generic range. NOTE: Mixed vegetables frozen with butter or sauces often contain added sodium.

PEAS

Peas, 1/2 cup	80	0	0	0	13	3	4	140

BRANDS . . . *(1/2 CUP UNLESS NOTED)*

C&W Organic Petite, NSA	47	0	0	0	8	3	4	6
Petite Peas, NSA	53	1	0	0	9	3	5	8
Baby Pea Pods	30	0	0	0	5	2	2	34
Flav-R-Pac NSA	47	0	0	0	8	3	-	10
Southern Petite	73	1	0	0	13	0	0	57

POTATOES *(also see Potato Side Dishes, pg 104)*

French fried potatoes, 10 strips..............	101	4	1	0	16	2	-	15
Whole potatoes, 1/2 cup	71	0	0	0	23	1	-	16
Hash brown potatoes, 1/2 cup	86	1	0	0	19	2	-	23
w/butter sauce, 3 oz.............................	115	6	2	0	16	3	-	65

BRANDS . . .
Most brands are within the generic range.

SPINACH

Spinach, chopped or leaf, 1 cup	37	1	0	0	6	5	-	115

BRANDS . . .
Most brands are within the generic range.

WAX BEANS

BRANDS . . .

Seabrook Cut, 1/2 cup	32	0	0	0	6	1	-	1

ZUCCHINI

Summer squash, zucchini, 5 oz	24	0	0	0	5	2	-	3
Winter squash, butternut, 6 oz..............	97	0	0	0	25	2	-	4

BRANDS . . .
Most brands are within the generic range.

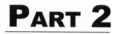

PART 2

QUICK-SERVE
RESTAURANT
CHAINS

Quick-Serve Restaurants:

RESTAURANT	PAGE
Arby's	159
Au Bon Pain	160
Auntie Annes	161
Baja Fresh Mexican Grill	162
Big Apple Bagels	162
Blimpie	163
Bojangles	163
Boston Market	164
Bruegger's Bagels	164
Burger King	165
Carl's Jr.	166
Chick-Fil-A	167
Church's Chicken	168
Cousins Subs	168
Dairy Queen / Brazier	169
D'Angelo	169
Del Taco	170
Denny's	171
Domino's Pizza	172
Donato's Pizza	173
Dunkin' Donuts	173
El Pollo Loco	174
Fazoli's	175
Godfather's Pizza	176
Häagen-Daz	176
Hardee's	177
Hungry Howies Pizza	178
In-N-Out Burger	178
Jack in the Box	178
KFC	180
Koo-Koo-Roo	180

RESTAURANT	PAGE
Krispy Kreme Doughnuts	181
Krystal	182
La Salsa Fresh Mexican Grill	183
Little Caesar's	184
Long John Silver's	184
Manhattan Bagel	185
McDonald's	185
Mrs. Field's Cookies	187
My Favorite Muffin	187
Panda Express	187
Papa John's Pizza	188
Papa Murphy's	188
Pizza Hut	188
Rax	189
Round Table Pizza	190
Rubios Fresh Mexican Grill	191
Schlotzsky's Deli	192
Skipper's	193
Sonic Drive-in	193
Souplantation / Sweet Tomatoes	194
Steak Escape	196
Subway	197
Taco Bell	199
Taco Del Mar	200
Taco John's	200
Taco Time	201
TCBY	202
Wendy's	202
Whataburger	203
White Castle	204

Menu Item	Cal	Fat	Sat	Chol	Carb	Fib	Sug	Sod

ARBY'S

Contact Arby's or their website (www.arbys.com) for nutritional info.

BREAKFAST ITEMS
250MG SODIUM OR LESS
Plain Croissant
500MG SODIUM OR LESS
Croissant w/Bacon • French Toastix w/Syrup or w/o Syrup

SANDWICHES & SUBS
750MG SODIUM OR LESS
Junior Roast Beef

SUBS
EXCEED 1500MG SODIUM
French Dip Sub

SALADS *(W/O DRESSING)*
150MG SODIUM OR LESS
Garden Side Salad • Garden Salad
250MG SODIUM OR LESS
Caesar Salad
750MG SODIUM OR LESS
Roast Chicken Salad

SALAD DRESSINGS AND TOPPINGS
150MG SODIUM OR LESS
Seasoned Croutons
500MG SODIUM OR LESS
Honey French Dressing • Light Buttermilk Ranch Dressing

SIDE ITEMS
150MG SODIUM OR LESS
Plain Baked Potato
250MG SODIUM OR LESS
Baked Potato w/Butter and Sour Cream

CONDIMENTS
150MG SODIUM OR LESS
Bronco Berry Sauce • German Mustard • Ketchup • Mayonnaise •
Light, Cholesterol-Free Mayonnaise • Horsey Sauce
250MG SODIUM OR LESS
Honey Mustard Sauce • Arby's Sauce

DESSERTS AND SHAKES
250MG SODIUM OR LESS
Apple Turnover, Iced • Cherry Turnover, Iced
500MG SODIUM OR LESS
Strawberry, Vanilla, or Choc Shake, 14 oz

AU BON PAIN

Menu Item	Cal	Fat	Sat	Chol	Carb	Fib	Sug	Sod

(AU BON PAIN)

BAKED GOODS

BAGELS AND CROISSANTS (*1 BAGEL OR CROISSANT*)

Menu Item	Cal	Fat	Sat	Chol	Carb	Fib	Sug	Sod
Apple Croissant	220	3	2	20	45	2	17	220
Choc Croissant	380	15	7	20	61	3	26	300
Plain Croissant	250	6	3	25	44	2	6	340
Cinnamon Raisin Croissant	340	5	3	20	69	3	15	350
Cinnamon Crisp Bagel	430	6	1	0	96	3	25	430
French Toast Bagel	420	7	2	0	76	3	14	440

MUFFINS, ROLLS AND SCONES (*1 MUFFIN, ROLL, OR SCONE*)

Menu Item	Cal	Fat	Sat	Chol	Carb	Fib	Sug	Sod
Cinnamon Roll	310	4	2	20	66	2	27	310
LF Triple Berry Muffin	290	2	1	25	61	2	31	310
Cinnamon Scone	480	18	8	125	88	2	23	320
Orange Scone w/Icing	410	14	8	125	62	2	12	340

BREAKFAST

Menu Item	Cal	Fat	Sat	Chol	Carb	Fib	Sug	Sod
Oatmeal Bar	150	3	1	0	27	4	1	0
Chol and FF Eggs	25	0	0	0	1	0	0	70
Egg on a Bagel	400	4	1	120	63	3	5	730

SANDWICHES

Menu Item	Cal	Fat	Sat	Chol	Carb	Fib	Sug	Sod
Mozzarella, Tomato and Pesto	820	43	21	100	67	4	4	1230
Arizona Chicken	580	19	7	95	58	4	3	1590

To reduce fat and sodium, omit cheese.

CREATE-A-SANDWICH

BREADS

Menu Item	Cal	Fat	Sat	Chol	Carb	Fib	Sug	Sod
Lavash	250	0	0	0	55	4	0	280
Country White Sandwich, 1 slice	110	0	0	0	23	1	0	290
Parisienne or Baguette, 1 slice	120	0	0	0	25	1	0	330
Tomato Herb Loaf, 1 slice	140	1	0	0	26	1	0	350

FILLINGS AND TOPPINGS

Menu Item	Cal	Fat	Sat	Chol	Carb	Fib	Sug	Sod
Tomatoes, Lettuce, Onions, Roasted Red Peppers, Sprouts & Honey Mustard (avg)	1-10	0	0	0	1-5	0	0	1-10
Swiss Cheese, 1 portion	160	12	9	30	0	0	0	105
Brie Cheese, 1 portion	150	14	6	30	0	0	0	180
Hummus	100	6	0	0	8	2	0	210
Tuna Salad Mix	170	8	1	0	3	0	1	450
Roast Beef	150	5	2	70	1	0	0	460

WRAPS

Menu Item	Cal	Fat	Sat	Chol	Carb	Fib	Sug	Sod
Fields and Feta	570	17	4	10	91	13	6	850
Chicken Caesar	600	25	8	80	63	5	3	930
Mediterranean	560	23	3	5	77	8	5	960

160

AUNTIE ANNE'S

Menu Item	Cal	Fat	Sat	Chol	Carb	Fib	Sug	Sod
SALADS (W/O DRESSING)								
Charbroiled Salmon Fillet	210	7	1	50	9	2	5	135
Side Garden	90	2	1	0	14	3	3	160
Tomato, Mozzarella w/Basil Pesto	280	19	11	60	11	3	7	180
Mozzarella and Red Pepper	360	25	16	90	10	2	6	380
Garden	160	4	1	0	26	5	6	400
To reduce sodium and fat, omit croutons.								
SALAD DRESSINGS (2 TBSP)								
FF Raspberry	35	0	0	0	8	0	7	80
Caesar	160	16	3	15	3	0	2	220
Lite Olive Oil Vinaigrette	60	6	1	0	3	0	2	230
Lite Honey Mustard	100	6	1	15	11	0	8	240
SOUPS (1 CUP)								
Southwest Vegetable	150	3	1	0	23	4	3	250
Southern Black-Eyed Pea	190	1	0	5	34	12	2	400
Mediterranean Pepper	190	4	0	0	30	7	3	450
CREAM CHEESE (2 OZ)								
Honey Walnut	140	9	6	30	12	0	12	150
Plain	120	11	7	35	4	0	4	180
To reduce sodium and fat, use half the cream cheese.								
DESSERTS								
Fruit Cup, small, 6 oz	70	0	0	0	16	1	15	10
Fruit Cup, large, 12 oz	140	1	0	0	32	2	30	20
Plain Yogurt, LF, 7 oz	190	2	2	10	36	0	31	95
Double Choc Cookie	340	19	10	40	42	2	24	120
Yogurt w/Granola and Fruit, all	310	6	2	10	56	2	36	130
White/Choc Dipped Shortbread Cookie	380	21	15	40	46	2	26	135
Cherry Strudel	390	19	0	0	49	1	5	135
Apple Strudel	410	18	0	0	56	1	19	140
English Toffee Cookie	200	6	4	30	33	0	19	170
Choc Dipped Cranberry Macaroon	320	16	8	0	42	3	33	190
Pecan Brownie	510	31	7	80	55	3	40	200
SPECIALTY DRINKS								
Apple Cider, 16 oz	250	0	0	0	62	0	62	125
Frozen Mocha Blast, 16 oz	270	6	4	25	43	0	41	150

AUNTIE ANNE'S®

	Cal	Fat	Sat	Chol	Carb	Fib	Sug	Sod
PRETZELS (1 PRETZEL)								
Almond w/o Butter	360	2	1	0	72	2	15	390
Almond w/Butter	400	8	5	20	72	2	15	400
Cinnamon Sugar w/o Butter	350	2	0	0	74	2	16	410
Cinnamon Sugar w/Butter	450	9	5	25	83	3	26	430

161

BAJA FRESH MEXICAN GRILL

Menu Item	Cal	Fat	Sat	Chol	Carb	Fib	Sug	Sod

BAJA FRESH MEXICAN GRILL

Contact Baja Fresh or their website (www.bajafresh.com) for nutritional info.

TACOS
500MG SODIUM OR LESS
Baja Style, Charbroiled Steak • Baja Style, Chicken • Baja Style, Wild Gulf Shrimp

SPECIALTIES

QUESADILLAS AND TACQUITOS
EXCEED 1000MG SODIUM
Cheese Mini Quesa-Dita • Chargroiled Chicken Tacquito w/Rice

ENCHILADAS
EXCEED 2000MG SODIUM
Cheese Enchilada • Charbroiled Chicken Enchilada

BURRITOS
EXCEED 1500MG SODIUM
Bean & Cheese Burrito • Grilled Vegetarian Burrito

SALADS *(W/O DRESSING)*
250MG SODIUM OR LESS
Side Salad

MAIN DISH SALADS
EXCEED 1000MG SODIUM
Baja Ensalada, Charbroiled Fish

SALAD DRESSINGS
250MG SODIUM OR LESS
Olive Oil Vinaigrette

SIDE ITEMS
150MG SODIUM OR LESS
Sour Cream • Pico de Gallo Fresh Salsa • Baja Fresh Salsa •
250MG SODIUM OR LESS
Cebollitas • Guacamole, small

BIG APPLE BAGELS

Contact Big Apple Bagels or their website (www.bigapplebagels.com) for nutritional info.

BAGELS *(1/2 BAGEL)*
500MG SODIUM OR LESS
Cinnamon Raisin • Vegetable • Plain • Eight Grain • Whole Wheat

CREAM CHEESE
150MG SODIUM OR LESS
Honey Cinnamon • Very Berry • Soft (plain) • Plain Lite • Onion Chive •
Salsa Ole

Menu Item	Cal	Fat	Sat	Chol	Carb	Fib	Sug	Sod

BLIMPIE

Contact Blimpie or their website (www.blimpie.com) for nutritional info.

SUBS (ON WHITE SUB ROLL)

1000MG SODIUM OR LESS

6" Hot Grilled Chicken • 6" Tuna • 6" Seafood • 6" Hot VegiMax

To reduce sodium, substitute mediterranean flatbread for the sub roll.

WRAPS

EXCEED 1500MG SODIUM

Chicken Caesar

TOPPINGS & SAUCES

150MG SODIUM OR LESS

Oil and Vinegar (for 6" Subs) • Honey Mustard • Swiss Cheese •
GourMayo Wasabi Horseradish, Sun-Dried Tomato, or Chipotle Chili

SALADS (W/O DRESSING)

500MG SODIUM OR LESS

Tuna • Seafood

SALAD DRESSINGS - *nutritional info unavailable*

SOUPS

750MG SODIUM OR LESS

Garden Vegetable

SIDE ITEMS

250MG SODIUM OR LESS

Regular Potato Chips • Cheddar and Sour Cream Potato Chips •
Romano and Garlic Potato Chips • Cole Slaw

COOKIES

150MG SODIUM OR LESS

Macadamia White Chunk

250MG SODIUM OR LESS

Oatmeal Raisin

BOJANGLES

BREAKFAST

Menu Item	Cal	Fat	Sat	Chol	Carb	Fib	Sug	Sod
Egg Biscuit Sandwich	400	30	6	120	26	1	-	630
CHICKEN (1 PIECE UNLESS NOTED)								
Leg, Southern Style	254	15	-	94	11	1	-	448
Thigh, Cajun Spiced	310	23	-	67	11	1	-	465
Breast, Cajun Spiced	278	17	-	75	12	1	-	565
SANDWICHES								
Cajun Filet w/Mayo	437	22	7	55	41	3	-	506
w/o Mayo	337	11	5	45	41	3	-	401
Grilled Filet w/o Mayo	235	5	3	51	25	2	-	540

163

BOSTON MARKET

Menu Item	Cal	Fat	Sat	Chol	Carb	Fib	Sug	Sod
SIDE ITEMS								
Corn on the Cob, 1	140	2	0	0	34	2	–	20
DESSERTS								
Bo Berry Sweet Biscuit	220	10	3	1	29	1	–	410

(BOSTON MARKET)

Contact Boston Market or their website (www.bostonmarket.com) for nutritional info.

ENTREES

250MG SODIUM OR LESS

Marinated Grilled Chicken Breast

500MG SODIUM OR LESS

1/4 Dark Chicken, No Skin • 1/4 White Chicken, No Skin or Wing

SIDE ITEMS

150MG SODIUM OR LESS

Cranberry Walnut Relish • Fruit Salad • Hot Cinnamon Apples •
Steamed Vegetables • Jumpin Juice Squares • New Potatoes

250MG SODIUM OR LESS

Whole Kernel Corn • Sweet Potato Casserole • Green Beans

SALADS *(W/O DRESSING)*

500MG SODIUM OR LESS

Oriental Grill Chicken w/o Noodles • SW Grill Chicken w/o Chips

SOUPS

500MG SODIUM OR LESS

Chicken Noodle

SANDWICHES

750MG SODIUM OR LESS

Marinated Grilled Chicken w/o Mayo

DESSERTS

250MG SODIUM OR LESS

Pecan Pie • Cherry Struesel Pie

(BRUEGGER'S BAGELS)

Contact Bruegger's Bagels or their website (www.brueggers.com) for nutritional info.

BAGELS

500MG SODIUM OR LESS

Honey Grain

750MG SODIUM OR LESS

Plain Garlic • Poppy • Sesame • Onion • Cinnamon Sugar • Jalapeño

CREAM CHEESE

150MG SODIUM OR LESS

Garden Veggie Light • Strawberry Light • Herb and Garlic Light • Plain Light

Menu Item	Cal	Fat	Sat	Chol	Carb	Fib	Sug	Sod

BREAKFAST SANDWICHES

1000MG SODIUM OR LESS
Egg and Cheese

SANDWICHES

BAGEL SANDWICHES

750MG SODIUM OR LESS
Garden Veggie · Atlantic Smoked Salmon

DELI SANDWICHES

1000MG SODIUM OR LESS
Chicken Salad w/Mayo

DESSERTS

150MG SODIUM OR LESS
Mint Brownie · Cappuccino Bar · Raspberry Sammies · Choc Chunk Brownie

---

(BURGER KING)

Contact Burger King or their website (www.burgerking.com) for nutritional info.

BREAKFAST ITEMS

500MG SODIUM OR LESS
French Toast Sticks, 5 sticks · Hash Brown Rounds, small

SANDWICHES

750MG SODIUM OR LESS
Croissan'wich w/Egg and Cheese

BURGERS AND SANDWICHES

750MG SODIUM OR LESS
Original Whopper Jr. w/o Mayo · Original Whopper Jr. · Hamburger

CHICKEN, FISH AND VEGETARIAN SANDWICHES

750MG SODIUM OR LESS
BK Veggie Burger w/o Mayo

1000MG SODIUM OR LESS
BK Veggie Burger w/LF Mayo · Chicken Whopper Jr. w/o Mayo ·
BK Fish Filet Sandwich

CHICKEN

500MG SODIUM OR LESS
Chicken Tenders, 4 pc

SALADS *(W/O DRESSING)*

150MG SODIUM OR LESS
Side Garden Salad

750MG SODIUM OR LESS
Chicken Caesar w/o Croutons

SALAD DRESSINGS - *nutritional info unavailable*

CARL'S JR

Menu Item	Cal	Fat	Sat	Chol	Carb	Fib	Sug	Sod

SIDE ITEMS
250MG SODIUM OR LESS
French Fries, NSA, small
500MG SODIUM OR LESS
Onion Rings, small

DESSERTS AND SHAKES
250MG SODIUM OR LESS
Hershey's Sundae Pie • Vanilla or Strawberry Shake, small

(CARL'S JR.)

Contact Carl's Jr. or their website (www.carlsjr.com) for nutritional info.

BREAKFAST
150MG SODIUM OR LESS
Scrambled Eggs
500MG SODIUM OR LESS
Sourdough Breakfast w/o Ham and American Cheese •
Sunrise Sandwich w/o Meat & Cheese • French Toast Dips w/Syrup or Jam •
Sunrise Sandwich w/o Meat

BREAKFAST SIDES
150MG SODIUM OR LESS
Bacon, 2 strips
250MG SODIUM OR LESS
English Muffin w/o Margarine
500MG SODIUM OR LESS
English Muffin w/Margarine • Blueberry Muffin

BURGERS AND SANDWICHES
500MG SODIUM OR LESS
Hamburger w/o Mustard and Pickle • Hamburger

CHICKEN SANDWICHES
1000MG SODIUM OR LESS
Charbroiled BBQ Chicken

SALADS *(W/O DRESSING)*
150MG SODIUM OR LESS
Garden Salad-to-Go
500MG SODIUM OR LESS
Charbroiled Chicken Salad-to-Go

SALAD DRESSINGS
500MG SODIUM OR LESS
Blue Cheese

BAKED POTATOES
250MG SODIUM OR LESS
Plain Baked Potato • Potato w/Margarine • Potato w/Sour Cream and Chives

Menu Item	Cal	Fat	Sat	Chol	Carb	Fib	Sug	Sod

SIDE ITEMS

150MG SODIUM OR LESS
Breadsticks • Croutons • French Fries, kids
250MG SODIUM OR LESS
French Fries, small

CONDIMENTS

150MG SODIUM OR LESS
Honey Sauce • Table Syrup • Grape or Strawberry Jam •
Sweet n' Sour Sauce
250MG SODIUM OR LESS
Salsa

DESSERTS & SHAKES

250MG SODIUM OR LESS
Strawberry Swirl Cheesecake
500MG SODIUM OR LESS
Strawberry, Vanilla, or Chocolate Shake, small

(CHICK-FIL-A)

Menu Item	Cal	Fat	Sat	Chol	Carb	Fib	Sug	Sod
BREAKFAST								
Danish	430	17	5	25	63	2	16	160
Hashbrowns	170	9	5	10	20	2	1	350
Plain Biscuit	260	11	3	0	38	1	5	670
CHICKEN								
Chick-n-Strips, 4 pc	260	11	3	70	12	0	2	570
SANDWICHES								
Chicken Salad Sandwich	350	15	3	65	32	5	6	880
WRAPS								
Chargrilled Chicken Cool Wrap	390	7	4	70	52	4	6	1030
Spicy Cool Wrap	390	7	4	60	50	3	5	1060
SALADS *(W/O DRESSING)*								
Side Salad	60	3	2	10	5	2	3	75
Chargrilled Chicken Garden Salad	180	6	3	70	9	3	5	660
Chick-n-Strips Salad	350	16	5	85	20	3	6	700
SALAD DRESSINGS *(1.25 OZ)*								
Basil Vinaigrette	210	21	4	0	4	0	4	160
Spicy	165	17	3	8	3	0	2	160
FF Dijon Honey Mustard	60	0	0	0	14	0	11	200
SOUPS								
Hearty Breast of Chicken, 1 cup	140	4	1	25	18	1	2	900
SIDE ITEMS *(1 CUP UNLESS NOTED)*								
Carrot and Raisin Salad	130	5	1	0	22	2	15	90
Waffle Potato Fries, small	280	14	5	15	37	5	0	105
Cole Slaw	210	17	3	20	14	2	9	180

167

CHURCH'S CHICKEN

Menu Item	Cal	Fat	Sat	Chol	Carb	Fib	Sug	Sod
DIPPINGS SAUCES *(1 oz)*								
Dijon Honey Mustard Sauce, 0.4 oz	50	5	1	5	2	0	2	65
Honey Mustard Sauce	45	0	0	0	10	0	10	150
Barbeque Sauce	45	0	0	0	11	0	9	180

CHURCH'S CHICKEN

Contact Church's Chicken or their website (www.churchs.com) for nutritional info.

CHICKEN
150MG SODIUM OR LESS
Leg w/o Batter, Skin Removed
250MG SODIUM OR LESS
Leg w/Batter and Skin
500MG SODIUM OR LESS
Krispy Tender Strips, 1 pc • Thigh w/o Batter, Skin Removed • Breast w/o Batter, Skin Removed
750MG SODIUM OR LESS
Breast

DIPPING SAUCES
150MG SODIUM OR LESS
Purple Pepper • Sweet and Sour • Honey Mustard • Creamy Jalapeño

SIDE ITEMS
150MG SODIUM OR LESS
Corn on the Cob • French Fries, regular
250MG SODIUM OR LESS
Collard Greens • Cole Slaw

DESSERTS
150MG SODIUM OR LESS
Strawberry Cream Pie
250MG SODIUM OR LESS
Double Lemon Pie

COUSINS SUBS

Contact Cousins Subs or their website (www.cousinssubs.com) for nutritional info.

SUBS *(ON ITALIAN BREAD)*
750MG SODIUM OR LESS
Seafood w/Crab, 4" • Tuna, 4" • Provolone (Cheese), 4" • Chicken Salad, 4" • Cold Veggie, 7 1/2"

SOUPS
1000MG SODIUM OR LESS
Cream of Potato, regular

D'ANGELO

Menu Item	Cal	Fat	Sat	Chol	Carb	Fib	Sug	Sod

SALADS *(W/O DRESSING)*

150MG SODIUM OR LESS
Side Salad

500MG SODIUM OR LESS
Garden Salad • Tuna Salad

SALAD DRESSINGS - *nutritional info unavailable*

SIDE ITEMS

250MG SODIUM OR LESS
French Fries, small

DESSERTS

150MG SODIUM OR LESS
Choc Chip Cookie

DAIRY QUEEN / BRAZIER

Contact Dairy Queen or their website (www.dairyqueen.com) for nutritional info.

BURGERS & SANDWICHES

500MG SODIUM OR LESS
DQ Homestyle Hamburger w/o Ketchup and Pickles

750MG SODIUM OR LESS
BBQ Beef Sandwich • DQ Homestyle Hamburger

CHICKEN SANDWICHES

EXCEED 1000MG SODIUM
Grilled Chicken Sandwich

SALADS

EXCEED 1000MG SODIUM
Grilled Chicken w/Honey Mustard • Crispy Chicken w/Honey Mustard •
Grilled Chicken w/FF Italian

SIDE ITEMS

250MG SODIUM OR LESS
Onion Rings

DESSERTS

150MG SODIUM OR LESS
StarKiss • Lemon DQ Freez'r • DQ Vanilla Orange Bar, No Sugar Added •
DQ Fudge Bar, No Sugar Added • DQ Soft Serve, Vanilla or Choc •
Choc Dilly Bar • Vanilla or Choc Cone, small • DQ Sandwich

D'ANGELO

Contact D'Angleo's or their website (www.dangelos.com) for nutritional info.

SUBS *(SMALL SUB ON HONEY WHEAT)*

500MG SODIUM OR LESS
Steak • Hamburger • Salad • Turkey

DEL TACO

Menu Item	Cal	Fat	Sat	Chol	Carb	Fib	Sug	Sod

SANDWICHES *(SMALL SUB ON WHITE ROLL)*
750MG SODIUM OR LESS
Turkey • Turkey Cranberry • Fresh Veggie
POKKET SANDWICHES *(HONEY WHEAT POKKET)*
500MG SODIUM OR LESS
Steak • Classic Veggie No Cheese • Hamburger • Salad • Turkey
WRAPS *(WHITE WRAP)*
500MG SODIUM OR LESS
Steak • Salad • Hamburger • Turkey
KIDZ MEALS
500MG SODIUM OR LESS
Turkey D'Lite • Cheeseburger Sub
SOUPS
750MG SODIUM OR LESS
New England Clam Chowder
SALADS *(W/O DRESSING)*
150MG SODIUM OR LESS
Tossed • Turkey
250MG SODIUM OR LESS
Roast Beef
750MG SODIUM OR LESS
Chicken Stir Fry • Asian Chicken • Lobster
SALAD DRESSINGS
250MG SODIUM OR LESS
Honey Mustard

(DEL TACO)

Contact Del Taco or their website (www.deltaco.com) for nutritional info.

BREAKFAST
750MG SODIUM OR LESS
Breakfast Burrito
TACOS
150MG SODIUM OR LESS
Taco
500MG SODIUM OR LESS
Soft Taco • Ultimate Taco
750MG SODIUM OR LESS
Chicken Soft Taco
BURRITOS
EXCEED 1000MG SODIUM
Bean & Cheese Burrito, Red or Green

Menu Item	Cal	Fat	Sat	Chol	Carb	Fib	Sug	Sod

QUESADILLAS
1000MG SODIUM OR LESS
   Cheddar Quesadilla

BURGERS
750MG SODIUM OR LESS
   Hamburger

SALADS
500MG SODIUM OR LESS
   Taco Salad

SIDE ITEMS
250MG SODIUM OR LESS
   Fries, small

SHAKES
250MG SODIUM OR LESS
   Strawberry or Vanilla Shake, small

(DENNY'S)

Contact Denny's or their website (www.dennys.com) for nutritional info.

BREAKFAST
250MG SODIUM OR LESS
   Belgian Waffle
750MG SODIUM OR LESS
   Vegie-Cheese Omelette

BREAKFAST SIDES
150MG SODIUM OR LESS
   1/2 Grapefruit or Grapes • Banana • Applesauce • Fruit Mix •
   1/4 Cantaloupe or Honeydew • One Egg • Egg Substitute
250MG SODIUM OR LESS
   Toast (dry), 1 slice • English Muffin (dry)

CEREALS
150MG SODIUM OR LESS
   Oatmeal N'Fixins
250MG SODIUM OR LESS
   Quaker Oatmeal

ENTREES
500MG SODIUM OR LESS
   Sirloin Steak Dinner
750MG SODIUM OR LESS
   Grilled Chicken Dinner
NOTE: Values do not include side dishes and bread.

DOMINO'S PIZZA

Menu Item	Cal	Fat	Sat	Chol	Carb	Fib	Sug	Sod

SANDWICHES
1000MG SODIUM OR LESS
Boca Burger • Bacon Lettuce and Tomato

SOUPS
750MG SODIUM OR LESS
Chicken Noodle

SALADS *(W/O DRESSING)*
150MG SODIUM OR LESS
Side Salad
750MG SODIUM OR LESS
Garden Deluxe w/Chicken Breast

SALAD DRESSINGS
150MG SODIUM OR LESS
Honey Mustard
250MG SODIUM OR LESS
Thousand Island • Ranch • Blue Cheese

SIDE ITEMS
150MG SODIUM OR LESS
Sliced Tomatoes, 3 slices • Plain Baked Potato
250MG SODIUM OR LESS
Carrots in Honey Glaze • French Fries

CONDIMENTS & TOPPINGS
150MG SODIUM OR LESS
Whipped Cream • Cherry Topping • Sour Cream • Blueberry Topping •
Strawberry Topping • Maple-Flavored Syrup, Regular and Sugar-Free •
Choc or Fudge Topping • Cream Cheese • Country Gravy •
Whipped Margarine • Chicken Gravy

DESSERTS & SHAKES
150MG SODIUM OR LESS
Single or Double Scoop Sundae • Choc Layer Cake
250MG SODIUM OR LESS
Hot Fudge Cake Sundae • Banana Split

SHAKES
500MG SODIUM OR LESS
Milk Shake or Malted, Vanilla or Choc

(**DOMINO'S PIZZA**)

PIZZAS *(1/8 SLICE UNLESS NOTED)*
Hand Tossed:

Menu Item	Cal	Fat	Sat	Chol	Carb	Fib	Sug	Sod
Cheese, 12" Medium	187	6	5	12	28	2	3	388
14" Large	258	8	7	16	38	2	3	541

172

Menu Item	Cal	Fat	Sat	Chol	Carb	Fib	Sug	Sod
TOPPINGS								
Onions, Mushrooms, Bell Peppers and Pineapple (avg)	3	0	0	0	3	0	1	1
BUFFALO WINGS *(1 PIECE)*								
Barbeque	50	2	1	26	2	0	1	175
Hot Wings	45	2	1	26	1	0	0	354
SIDE ITEMS								
Breadstick, 1	116	4	1	0	18	1	1	152
DESSERTS								
CinnaStix, 1	111	5	1	0	15	1	3	105

DONATOS PIZZERIA

Contact Donato's or their website (www.donatos.com) for nutritional info.

PIZZAS *(7" INDIVIDUAL OR 1/4 OF 14" PIZZA)*
EXCEED 1500MG SODIUM
Serious Cheese, Original Crust • Vegy, Original Crust

SUBS *(WHOLE SUB)*
1000MG SODIUM OR LESS
Steak and Cheese

SALADS *(W/O DRESSING)*
500MG SODIUM OR LESS
Side Salad

SALAD DRESSINGS
500MG SODIUM OR LESS
Italian

SIDE ITEMS
500MG SODIUM OR LESS
Breadstick

DESSERTS
1000MG SODIUM OR LESS
Fruit Dessert Pizza, 1/4 of 14"

DUNKIN' DONUTS

Contact Dunkin' Donuts or their website (www.dunkindonuts.com) for nutritional info.

BREAKFAST SANDWICHES
1000MG SODIUM OR LESS
Egg, Ham and Cheese Croissant
DONUTS
150MG SODIUM OR LESS
Lemon Glazed Cake
250MG SODIUM OR LESS
Sugar Raised • Glazed • Vanilla Kreme Filled

173

EL POLLO LOCO

Menu Item	Cal	Fat	Sat	Chol	Carb	Fib	Sug	Sod

Donuts (cont'd)

500MG SODIUM OR LESS

Strawberry Frosted • Choc Frosted • Marble Frosted • Choc Kreme Filled • Strawberry Kreme Filled • Blueberry Crumb • Jelly Filled • Boston Kreme

MUNCHKINS

250MG SODIUM OR LESS

Lemon Filled • Glazed Cake • Glazed • Powdered • Cinnamon Cake

CRULLERS, DANISHES & FRITTERS

150MG SODIUM OR LESS

French Cruller

250MG SODIUM OR LESS

Strawberry Cheese Danish • Cheese Danish • Apple Danish

FRITTERS

500MG SODIUM OR LESS

Glazed Fritter

MUFFINS , SCONES & OTHER BAKERY ITEMS

500MG SODIUM OR LESS

Cake Stick, all • Blueberry Scone • Maple Walnut Scone • Coffee Roll, all • Carrot Walnut Spice Muffin

BAGELS & CROISSANTS

500MG SODIUM OR LESS

Croissant

750MG SODIUM OR LESS

Berry Berry Bagel • Cinnamon Raisin Bagel

CREAM CHEESE

150MG SODIUM OR LESS

Shedd's Buttermatch Blend • Strawberry

250MG SODIUM OR LESS

Salmon • Plain • Lite

COOKIES

150MG SODIUM OR LESS

Oatmeal Raisin Pecan • Choc Chunk w/Nuts • Choc-White Choc Chunk

SPECIALTY DRINKS

150MG SODIUM OR LESS

Coolatta, all fruit varieties, 16 oz • Vanilla Chai, 10 oz

EL POLLO LOCO

Contact El Pollo Loco or their website (www.elpolloloco.com) for nutritional info.

TACOS

150MG SODIUM OR LESS

Taco Al Carbon

750MG SODIUM OR LESS

Chicken Soft Taco

Menu Item	Cal	Fat	Sat	Chol	Carb	Fib	Sug	Sod

FLAME-BROILED CHICKEN
150MG SODIUM OR LESS
Leg
250MG SODIUM OR LESS
Wing • Thigh
500MG SODIUM OR LESS
Breast

SPECIALTIES
500MG SODIUM OR LESS
Chicken Tamale

BURRITOS
EXCEED 1000MG SODIUM
Mexican Chicken Caesar Burrito • Ultimate Burrito

SALADS *(W/O DRESSING)*
150MG SODIUM OR LESS
Garden Salad

BOWLS
EXCEED 1000MG SODIUM
Flame Broiled Chicken Bowl

SALAD DRESSINGS
250MG SODIUM OR LESS
Hidden Valley Ranch

SIDE ITEMS
150MG SODIUM OR LESS
3" Corn Cobbette • Tortilla Chips, Unsalted • Corn Tortilla, 4 1/2" or 6" •
Fresh Vegetables

SAUCES & TOPPINGS
150MG SODIUM OR LESS
Sour Cream • House Salsa • Jalapeño Hot Sauce • Pico de Gallo
250MG SODIUM OR LESS
Guacamole

DESSERTS
150MG SODIUM OR LESS
Foster's Freeze, w/o Cone • Berry Banana Smoothie, 11 oz •
Kiwi Strawberry Smoothie, 9.5 oz
250MG SODIUM OR LESS
Churros

(**FAZOLI'S**)

PASTAS

Menu Item	Cal	Fat	Sat	Chol	Carb	Fib	Sug	Sod
Spaghetti w/Marinara	420	6	1	0	74	5	8	105
Regular	620	8	1	0	111	7	12	140
Fettuccine Alfredo	530	15	4	15	80	3	3	170

GODFATHER'S PIZZA

Menu Item	Cal	Fat	Sat	Chol	Carb	Fib	Sug	Sod
Pasta (cont'd)								
Broccoli Fettuccine Alfredo	560	15	4	15	85	6	5	190
Regular	830	23	6	20	125	8	7	250
Spaghetti w/Meat Sauce	450	8	2	10	74	5	8	370
Regular	670	11	3	10	111	8	11	530
Peppery Chicken Alfredo	610	16	4	50	80	3	3	410
Cheese Ravioli w/Marinara	480	15	7	65	65	4	9	530
PIZZAS								
Cheese Pizza, double slice	460	15	8	40	58	2	6	970
SUBS & PANINIS								
Chicken Pesto Panini	510	20	6	60	51	3	1	1350
Four Cheese and Tomato Panini	720	43	16	75	55	3	3	1450
SALADS *(W/O DRESSING)*								
Garden Salad	30	0	0	0	6	2	4	20
Chicken Finger Salad	190	9	3	45	8	2	4	540
Side Pasta Salad	240	10	3	5	29	2	4	580
SALAD DRESSINGS								
Honey French	150	12	2	0	9	0	9	210
Ranch	150	17	3	5	1	0	1	210
Thousand Island	130	13	2	15	4	0	4	220
Italian, Reduced Calorie	50	5	1	0	3	0	2	390
SOUPS								
Minestrone	120	1	0	0	23	8	8	910
BREADSTICKS								
Dry Breakstick, 1	90	1	0	0	17	1	1	170
DESSERTS								
Lemon Ice	190	0	0	0	45	0	44	95
Choc Chip Cheesecake	300	22	14	85	22	1	19	200
Plain Cheesecake	290	22	14	95	17	0	17	220
Turtle Cheesecake	420	34	17	100	24	2	21	220

(GODFATHER'S PIZZA)

Contact Godfather or their website (www.godfathers.com) for nutritional info.

PIZZAS
500MG SODIUM OR LESS
Cheese, Original Crust, Large, 1/10 slice

(HÄAGEN-DAZS)

Häagen-Dazs products are low sodium, the following have the least in each category.

SORBET *(1/2 CUP UNLESS NOTED)*

	Cal	Fat	Sat	Chol	Carb	Fib	Sug	Sod
Orange, Tropical, or Zesty Lemon (avg)	120	0	0	0	31	1	28	0

Menu Item	Cal	Fat	Sat	Chol	Carb	Fib	Sug	Sod
Sorbet (cont'd)								
Strawberry or Raspberry	120	0	0	0	31	1	28	0
Mango or Orchard Peach (avg)	120	0	0	0	32	1	29	0
FROZEN YOGURT (*1/2 CUP UNLESS NOTED*)								
Vanilla Raspberry Swirl	170	3	2	30	31	1	24	30
Strawberry, Nonfat................................	140	0	0	5	31	0	20	40
Peach Melba.......................................	210	4	2	50	37	0	29	45
Coffee	200	5	3	65	31	0	20	50
Vanilla	200	5	3	65	31	0	21	55
Choc Choc Chip	230	7	4	60	32	2	26	55
ICE CREAM (*1/2 CUP UNLESS NOTED*)								
Belgian Choc	330	21	12	85	29	3	26	50
Mango	250	14	8	85	28	1	27	50
Choc Choc Chip or Tres Leches (avg)	295	20	12	105	26	1	24	55
Pineapple Coconut...............................	230	13	8	90	25	0	24	55
Cherry Vanilla	240	15	9	100	23	0	22	60
Choc or Rum Raisin	270	18	10	110	22	0	21	60
Choc Raspberry Torte	270	15	9	95	29	1	26	65
Strawberry	250	16	10	95	23	1	22	65
GELATO (*1/2 CUP UNLESS NOTED*)								
Hazelnut	260	12	4	75	33	1	23	55
Choc	240	8	5	80	37	2	26	70
Raspberry or Cappuccino (avg)	240	7	4	77	40	1	24	75

(HARDEE'S)

Contact Hardee's or their website (www.hardees.com) for nutritional info.

BREAKFAST

SANDWICHES
EXCEED 1000MG SODIUM
Sunrise Croissant w/Sausage • Sunrise Croissant w/Ham

BREAKFAST SIDES
500MG SODIUM OR LESS
Apple, Cinnamon 'N' Raisin Biscuit

BURGERS & SANDWICHES
500MG SODIUM OR LESS
Slammer
750MG SODIUM OR LESS
Slammer w/Cheese • Chicken Slammer • Grilled Chicken Sandwich
1000MG SODIUM OR LESS
Regular Roast Beef • Fish Supreme Sandwich

HUNGRY HOWIES PIZZA

Menu Item	Cal	Fat	Sat	Chol	Carb	Fib	Sug	Sod

CHICKEN
750MG SODIUM OR LESS
   Leg • Wing

SIDE ITEMS
500MG SODIUM OR LESS
   Cole Slaw • Mashed Potatoes w/o Gravy, small • French Fries, small

DESSERTS
250MG SODIUM OR LESS
   Apple Turnover

HUNGRY HOWIES PIZZA

Contact Hungry Howies or their website (www.hungryhowies.com) for nutritional info.

PIZZAS
500MG SODIUM OR LESS
   Cheese Pizza:
      Small, 1/8 slice • Medium, 1/10 slice • Large, 1/12 slice
   TOPPINGS *(PER MEDIUM PIZZA SLICE)*
      150MG SODIUM OR LESS
      Mushrooms, Pineapple, Onions, Green Peppers, or Bacon • Olives • Pepperoni • Ham

CHICKEN
1000MG SODIUM OR LESS
   Howie Wings, approx 6 wings

IN-N-OUT BURGER

BURGERS

Menu Item	Cal	Fat	Sat	Chol	Carb	Fib	Sug	Sod
Hamburger	390	19	5	40	39	3	10	650
Protein Style *(lettuce leaves are substituted for the bun)*	240	17	4	40	11	3	7	370

SIDES

Menu Item	Cal	Fat	Sat	Chol	Carb	Fib	Sug	Sod
French Fries	400	18	5	0	54	2	0	245

SHAKES *(15 OZ UNLESS NOTED)*

Menu Item	Cal	Fat	Sat	Chol	Carb	Fib	Sug	Sod
Strawberry	690	33	22	85	91	0	75	280
Chocolate	690	36	24	95	83	0	62	350
Vanilla	680	37	25	90	78	0	57	390

JACK IN THE BOX

BREAKFAST

Menu Item	Cal	Fat	Sat	Chol	Carb	Fib	Sug	Sod
Hashbrowns	150	10	3	0	13	2	0	230
French Toast Sticks, 4 pc	430	18	4	10	57	2	11	460

Menu Item	Cal	Fat	Sat	Chol	Carb	Fib	Sug	Sod
BREAKFAST SANDWICHES								
Breakfast Jack	310	14	5	205	3	1	4	720
Sausage Biscuit	380	27	8	35	25	2	2	730
Sausage Croissant	680	50	15	250	41	2	5	760
BURGERS								
Hamburger	310	14	6	45	30	1	6	600
w/Cheese	360	18	8	60	31	1	6	740
To reduce sodium, omit pickles, ketchup, and/or mustard.								
CHICKEN & MORE								
Chicken Sandwich	410	21	5	35	39	2	4	740
Grilled Chicken Fillet	430	22	6	60	34	2	6	910
Chicken Fajita Pita	330	11	5	55	35	3	4	910
To reduce sodium and fat, omit cheese.								
TACOS								
Taco	170	9	3	20	15	2	2	210
Monster Taco	260	15	5	30	21	3	4	340
Tacquitos, 3	320	17	7	40	28	3	1	440
SALADS (W/O DRESSING)								
Side Salad	50	3	2	10	5	2	3	65
SALAD DRESSINGS (2 OZ UNLESS NOTED)								
Buttermilk House Dressing	310	33	5	20	3	0	2	470
Thousand Island	160	12	2	15	12	0	10	490
Low Calorie Italian	15	0	0	0	4	0	2	510
SIDE ITEMS								
Egg Roll, 1	130	6	2	5	15	2	1	310
Onion Rings, 6.8 oz	500	30	5	0	51	3	3	420
Cheese Sticks, 3	240	12	5	25	21	1	1	420
CONDIMENTS (1 OZ UNLESS NOTED)								
Grape Jelly, 0.5 oz	35	0	0	0	9	0	9	10
Sour Cream	60	5	3	15	2	0	0	20
Syrup, 1.5 oz	130	0	0	0	32	0	27	30
Country Crock Spread	25	3	1	0	0	0	0	45
Mustard, 0.2 oz	0	0	0	0	1	0	0	50
Taco Sauce, 0.3 oz	0	0	0	0	0	0	0	80
Ketchup, 0.3 oz	10	0	0	0	2	0	2	105
DESSERTS & SHAKES								
Cheesecake	310	16	9	55	34	0	23	220
Vanilla Shake, 16 oz	570	29	18	115	65	0	54	220
Strawberry Shake, 16 oz	640	28	18	110	84	0	71	220
Cappuccino Shake, 16 oz	640	28	18	110	85	0	75	220
Strawberry Banana Shake, 16 oz	700	28	18	110	100	0	67	230

KFC

Menu Item	Cal	Fat	Sat	Chol	Carb	Fib	Sug	Sod

(KFC)

Contact KFC or their website (www.kfc.com) for nutritional info.

CHICKEN *(1 PIECE)*
500MG SODIUM OR LESS
Whole Wing, Original Recipe • Drumstick, Hot and Spicy •
Whole Wing, Extra Crispy

SANDWICHES
750MG SODIUM OR LESS
Honey BBQ Flavored Sandwich • Triple Crunch w/o Sauce •
Triple Crunch Zinger w/o Sauce • Tender Roast w/o Sauce

SIDE ITEMS
150MG SODIUM OR LESS
Corn on the Cob
250MG SODIUM OR LESS
Mashed Potatoes w/o Gravy
500MG SODIUM OR LESS
Cole Slaw

DESSERTS
150MG SODIUM OR LESS
Strawberry Creme Pie
250MG SODIUM OR LESS
Fudge Brownie Parfait • Strawberry Shortcake Parfait • Double Choc Chip Cake

(KOO-KOO-ROO)

Contact Koo-Koo-Roo or their website (www.kookooroo.com) for nutritional info.

ENTREES
150MG SODIUM OR LESS
Fresh Roasted Turkey, Sliced Breast
500MG SODIUM OR LESS
Original Chicken, Breast
750MG SODIUM OR LESS
Rotisserie Chicken, Leg and Thigh

SANDWICHES
1000MG SODIUM OR LESS
Hand Carved Turkey Breast

WRAPS
EXCEED 1750MG SODIUM
Caesar Chicken

CHICKEN BOWLS
1000MG SODIUM OR LESS
Spicy Ginger Garlic

180

Menu Item	Cal	Fat	Sat	Chol	Carb	Fib	Sug	Sod

SOUPS
500MG SODIUM OR LESS
Chicken Noodle • Ten Vegetable

SALADS *(W/O DRESSING)*
250MG SODIUM OR LESS
House Salad
1000MG SODIUM OR LESS
Chinese Chicken Salad

SALAD DRESSINGS
250MG SODIUM OR LESS
Ranch • Caesar

KID'S MEAL
500MG SODIUM OR LESS
Turkey w/Fruit by the Foot and Baked French Fries

SIDE ITEMS
150MG SODIUM OR LESS
Sticky Rice • Butternut Squash • Tossed Salad w/o Dressing •
Baked Yams • Cantaloupe and Honeydew • Celery Sticks, 6 •
Steamed Vegetables • Lahvash, 1 pc
250MG SODIUM OR LESS
Kernel Corn • Tangy Tomato Salad • Green Beans
Cucumber Salad • Garlic Potatoes

SAUCES & CONDIMENTS *(1 OZ UNLESS NOTED)*
150MG SODIUM OR LESS
Cranberry Sauce • Sour Cream • Pico De Gallo • Salsa • Chipotle Sauce

KRISPY KREME DOUGHNUTS

YEAST DOUGHNUTS

Menu Item	Cal	Fat	Sat	Chol	Carb	Fib	Sug	Sod
Glazed Twist	210	9	3	5	28	1	16	80
Cinnamon Twist	230	9	3	5	33	1	19	85
Sugar	200	12	3	5	21	0	10	95
Glazed Ring	200	12	3	5	22	1	10	95
Choc Iced Glazed Ring	250	12	3	5	33	1	21	100
Choc Iced Glazed Ring w/Sprinkles	260	12	3	5	36	1	23	100
Glazed Cinnamon	210	12	3	5	24	1	12	100
Maple Iced Glazed Ring	250	12	3	5	34	1	22	100
Cinnamon Bun	260	16	4	5	28	1	13	125
Cranapple Crunch Filled	330	18	5	5	38	1	20	140
Dulce De Leche Filled	290	18	5	5	30	1	12	160

CAKE DOUGHNUTS

Menu Item	Cal	Fat	Sat	Chol	Carb	Fib	Sug	Sod
Glazed Blueberry Old Fashioned	300	15	3	5	37	1	29	200
Honey and Oat Old Fashioned	270	13	3	5	36	1	25	200

KRYSTAL

Menu Item	Cal	Fat	Sat	Chol	Carb	Fib	Sug	Sod
Cake Doughnuts (cont'd)								
Sour Creme Old Fashioned	280	11	3	20	41	0	22	210
Powdered Sugar Mini Cake	210	10	3	5	26	1	16	230
Glazed Cruller	240	14	4	15	26	1	14	240
Choc Iced Glazed Cruller	280	15	4	15	35	1	23	240
Choc (Enrobed) Mini Cake	270	17	9	10	26	3	16	240
FILLED DOUGHNUTS								
Yeast, Powdered Raspberry Filled	300	16	4	5	36	1	17	125
Glazed Creme Filled	350	20	5	5	39	1	24	135
Yeast, Glazed Lemon Filled	290	16	4	5	34	1	18	135
Yeast, Vanilla Iced Custard Filled	290	16	4	5	33	1	16	150
Choc Iced Creme Filled	340	18	5	5	39	14	22	160
Yeast, Glazed Cherry Filled	290	14	4	5	36	5	18	160
Yeast, Vanilla Iced Creme Filled	360	19	5	5	41	5	22	160
Yeast, Glazed Custard Filled	290	16	4	5	34	1	17	160
Yeast, Blueberry Filled Powdered Sugar	270	13	4	5	33	1	12	170
Choc Iced Custard Filled	310	16	4	5	39	5	21	170
Apple Filled Cinnamon Sugar Coated	280	13	3	5	35	3	13	180
Glazed Raspberry Filled	350	21	5	10	36	2	19	180
OTHER DOUGHNUTS & PIES								
Powdered Sugar Holes, 3	220	13	4	10	23	2	12	170
Glazed Holes, 3	220	13	3	10	25	1	16	170
Honey Bun, 1	410	24	6	10	44	1	22	170
Glazed Mini Crullers, 3	230	10	3	10	32	1	24	190
Cherry Pie, 1	410	19	6	0	56	1	34	200
Choc (Enrobed) Holes, 3	270	17	8	15	27	2	16	210
Peach Pie, 1	370	17	5	0	51	0	29	220
FROZEN BEVERAGES *(16 OZ UNLESS NOTED)*								
Raspberry	349	8	5	30	65	-	-	66
Latte	248	12	8	45	32	-	-	86
Orig Kreme	268	12	8	45	37	-	-	86
w/Coffee	244	12	8	45	32	-	-	86

(KRYSTAL)

	Cal	Fat	Sat	Chol	Carb	Fib	Sug	Sod
BREAKFAST								
Sunriser Sandwich	240	14	5	255	14	2	1	460
BREAKFAST SIDES								
Hash Browns	190	13	5	10	17	2	0	340
Plain Biscuit, 1	260	15	4	0	27	2	2	570
SANDWICHES								
Krystal Sandwich	160	7	3	20	17	1	1	260
Cheese Krystal	180	9	4	25	16	2	1	430

182

Menu Item	Cal	Fat	Sat	Chol	Carb	Fib	Sug	Sod
Sandwiches (cont'd)								
Bacon Cheese Krystal	190	10	5	25	16	2	2	430
Corn Pup	260	19	8	50	19	1	5	480
Plain Pup	170	9	4	25	15	1	-	500
Chili Cheese Pup	210	12	5	40	17	2	2	510
SIDE ITEMS								
Fries, regular	370	18	7	15	49	6	0	85
DESSERTS								
Lemon Meringue Pie, 1 slice	360	10	4	55	60	1	48	190

(LA SALSA FRESH MEXICAN GRILL)

Contact LaSalsa or their website (www.lasalsa.com) for nutritional info.

EGG DISHES
1000MG SODIUM OR LESS
   Huevos Mex (Pinto or Black Bean)

TACOS *(1 TACO)*
250MG SODIUM OR LESS
   Mexico City, Chicken
500MG SODIUM OR LESS
   Mexico City, Steak • La Salsa, Chicken • La Salsa, Steak •
   Baja Style Shrimp • Vegetarian • Baja Mahi Mahi
   NOTE: Values do not include chips served with tacos.

BASKETS
500MG SODIUM OR LESS
   Mexico City, Chicken
750MG SODIUM OR LESS
   Mexico City, Steak
   NOTE: Values do not include chips served with baskets.

BURRITOS
EXCEED 1000MG SODIUM
   Bean and Cheese, w/Pinto or Black Beans

QUESADILLAS
EXCEED 1250MG SODIUM
   Classic

SALADS
EXCEED 1250MG SODIUM
   Chile-Lime w/Chili-Lime Dressing • Caesar Salad

KIDS PLATES
500MG SODIUM OR LESS
   Taco, Chicken w/Pinto or Black Beans

SIDES & APPETIZERS
150MG SODIUM OR LESS
   Chips served w/1 Taco

183

LITTLE CAESAR'S

Menu Item	Cal	Fat	Sat	Chol	Carb	Fib	Sug	Sod

Sides & Appetizers (cont'd)
  250MG SODIUM OR LESS
  Chips served w/Baskets and Burritos

LITTLE CAESAR'S

Contact Little Caesar's or their website (www.littlecaesars.com) for nutritional info.

PIZZA *(1 SLICE)*
500MG SODIUM OR LESS
  Cheese:
    12" or 14" Thin Crust • 12" Round • 16" Round • 12" Deep Dish, Sq •
    18" Round • 14" Deep Dish, Square
  Pepperoni:
    12" Thin Crust • 14" Thin Crust • 14" Round • 16" Round •
    12" Deep Dish, Sq
  Veggie, 14" Round

CHICKEN
750MG SODIUM OR LESS
  Chicken Wings, 1

SANDWICHES
EXCEED 1000MG SODIUM
  Deli Veggie

SALADS
150MG SODIUM OR LESS
  Tossed Salad
750MG SODIUM OR LESS
  Antipasto

  SALAD DRESSINGS
  500MG SODIUM OR LESS
    Ranch • FF Italian

LONG JOHN SILVER'S

Contact Long John Silver's or their website (www.longjohnsilver.com) for nutritional info.

ENTREES *(1 PIECE)*
150MG SODIUM OR LESS
  Battered Shrimp
500MG SODIUM OR LESS
  Battered Chicken
750MG SODIUM OR LESS
  Battered Fish

Menu Item	Cal	Fat	Sat	Chol	Carb	Fib	Sug	Sod

SANDWICHES

1000MG SODIUM OR LESS
Chicken Sandwich
EXCEED 1000MG SODIUM
Fish Sandwich

SOUPS

1000MG SODIUM OR LESS
Clam Chowder, bowl

SIDE ITEMS

150MG SODIUM OR LESS
Corn Cobbette
250MG SODIUM OR LESS
Hushpuppie
500MG SODIUM OR LESS
Cheesestick • Cole Slaw • Fries, regular

DESSERTS

250MG SODIUM OR LESS
Choc Cream Pie • Pecan Pie • Pineapple Creme Cheesecake Pie

MANHATTAN BAGEL

Contact Manhattan Bagel or their website (www.manhattanbagel.com) for nutritional info.

BAGELS

500MG SODIUM OR LESS
Jalapeño Cheddar • Sun-Dried Tomato • Oat Bran Raisin and Walnut • Whole Wheat • Oat Bran

MCDONALD'S

Contact McDonald's or their website (www.mcdonalds.com) for nutritional info.

BREAKFAST

250MG SODIUM OR LESS
Scrambled Eggs, 2
750MG SODIUM OR LESS
Sausage Breakfast Burrito

BREAKFAST SIDES

250MG SODIUM OR LESS
Cinnamon Roll • English Muffin w/o Margarine
500MG SODIUM OR LESS
English Muffin w/Margarine

SANDWICHES

500MG SODIUM OR LESS
Hamburger w/o Ketchup and/or Pickles

185

MCDONALD'S

Menu Item	Cal	Fat	Sat	Chol	Carb	Fib	Sug	Sod

Sandwiches (cont'd)

750MG SODIUM OR LESS

Hamburger

CHICKEN AND FISH SANDWICHES

750MG SODIUM OR LESS

Filet-O-Fish

1000MG SODIUM OR LESS

Hot 'n Spicy McChicken • McChicken

CHICKEN

500MG SODIUM OR LESS

Chicken McNuggets, 4 pc

SALADS *(W/O DRESSING)*

150MG SODIUM OR LESS

Side Salad

250MG SODIUM OR LESS

Caesar Salad w/o Chicken

500MG SODIUM OR LESS

Bacon Ranch w/o Chicken • California Cobb w/o Chicken

750MG SODIUM OR LESS

Caesar Salad w/Grilled Chicken

SALAD DRESSINGS AND TOPPINGS

150MG SODIUM OR LESS

Butter Garlic Croutons

500MG SODIUM OR LESS

Newman's Own Cobb • *Newman's Own* Creamy Caesar

SIDE ITEMS

150MG SODIUM OR LESS

French Fries, small

CONDIMENTS & DIPPING SAUCES

150MG SODIUM OR LESS

Honey • Honey Mustard • Light Mayonnaise • Sweet 'N Sour

DESSERTS & SHAKES

150MG SODIUM OR LESS

Vanilla Ice Cream Cone, Reduced Fat • Fruit 'n Yogurt Parfait, 5 oz •
Fruit 'n Yogurt Parfait w/o Granola, 5 oz • Strawberry Sundae •
Fruit 'n Yogurt Parfait w/o Granola, 11 oz • Strawberry Triple Thick Shake, 12 oz

250MG SODIUM OR LESS

McDonaldland Choc Chip Cookies • Hot Fudge Sundae w/ or w/o Nuts •
Hot Caramel Sundae w/o Nuts • Baked Apple Pie

Menu Item	Cal	Fat	Sat	Chol	Carb	Fib	Sug	Sod

(MRS. FIELDS COOKIES)

Contact Mrs. Fields or their website (www.mrsfields.com) for nutritional info.

BITE-SIZED NIBBLERS (2 COOKIES)

150MG SODIUM OR LESS
White Chunk Macadamia • Semi-Sweet Choc • Milk Choc w/Walnuts •
Triple Choc • Milk Choc • Debra's Special • Butter • Cinnamon Sugar

BROWNIES

250MG SODIUM OR LESS
Pecan Pie • Pecan Fudge • Double Fudge

COOKIES (1 COOKIE)

150MG SODIUM OR LESS
Oatmeal Choc Chip

250MG SODIUM OR LESS
Peanut Butter w/Milk Choc Chips • Semi-sweet Choc and Walnuts •
Semi-Sweet Choc • Oatmeal, Raisins and Walnuts • Milk Choc w/o Nuts •
Milk Choc and Walnuts

BUNDT CAKE

250MG SODIUM OR LESS
Banana Walnut w/Choc Chips

(MY FAVORITE MUFFIN)

Contact My Favorite Muffin or their website (www.bigapplebagels.com) for nutritional info.

MUFFINS

250MG SODIUM OR LESS
Plain • Chocolate • FF Plain

500MG SODIUM OR LESS
FF Chocolate

BAGELS

500MG SODIUM OR LESS
Honey Grain • Whole Wheat

(PANDA EXPRESS)

APPETIZERS

Menu Item	Cal	Fat	Sat	Chol	Carb	Fib	Sug	Sod
Veggie Spring Rolls, 1.7 oz roll	80	3	0	0	14	1	0	270
ENTREES								
Sweet and Sour Chicken, 4 oz	310	14	3	50	28	2	0	330
Sweet and Sour Pork, 4 oz	410	30	7	55	17	3	0	350
Mixed Vegetables, 5.5 oz	70	3	1	0	8	1	1	420
RICE								
Steamed Rice, 8 oz	330	1	0	0	74	2	0	20

187

PAPA JOHN'S PIZZA

Menu Item	Cal	Fat	Sat	Chol	Carb	Fib	Sug	Sod
SAUCES								
Hot Mustard, 2 tsp	18	0	0	0	1	0	0	90
Sweet and Sour Sauce, 1.5 oz	60	0	0	0	15	0	13	120
Hot Sauce, 2 tsp	10	1	0	0	2	0	1	130

PAPA JOHN'S PIZZA

Menu Item	Cal	Fat	Sat	Chol	Carb	Fib	Sug	Sod
PIZZAS (1/8 SLICE UNLESS NOTED)								
Spinach Alfredo, 14" thin crust	227	13	5	24	20	1	1	429
Garden, 14" thin crust	224	12	4	16	23	2	1	489
Cheese, 14" thin crust	231	13	4	19	22	1	2	490
SIDE ITEMS								
Papa's Chickenstrips, 1.3 oz	83	4	1	13	5	1	1	178
Breaksticks, 1	140	2	0	0	26	1	-	260
SAUCES								
Pizza Sauce, 2 tbsp	25	2	0	0	3	2	1	125
Honey Mustard, 2 tbsp	190	19	3	10	6	0	6	150

PAPA MURPHY'S

Menu Item	Cal	Fat	Sat	Chol	Carb	Fib	Sug	Sod
PIZZAS (FAMILY-SIZE, 1/12 SLICE)								
Papa's Pizza, Cheese	270	10	5	20	29	2	1	470
Papa's Pizza, Veggie Combo	300	13	5	20	32	2	2	570
Gourmet Pizza, Gourmet Veggie	300	14	6	25	31	2	1	570
Papa's Pizza, Hawaiian	290	11	5	25	34	2	4	580
Gourmet Pizza, Chicken Garlic	320	15	6	35	30	1	1	600

Pizzas are topped with 1 lb of cheese, to reduce sodium, omit half the cheese.

Menu Item	Cal	Fat	Sat	Chol	Carb	Fib	Sug	Sod
STUFFED PIZZAS (FAMILY-SIZE, 1/12 SLICE)								
Chicken and Bacon	370	16	6	35	38	2	1	750
Chicago-Style	370	16	7	30	39	2	2	770
Big Murphy	380	17	7	30	39	2	1	800
CALZONES (FAMILY-SIZE, 1/8 SLICE)								
Veggie Calzone	410	17	7	30	46	3	1	720
SALADS (W/O DRESSING)								
Veggie Salad	140	8	5	30	7	4	3	170

PIZZA HUT

Contact Pizza Hut or their website (www.pizzahut.com) for nutritional info.

PIZZAS (1 SLICE)

500MG SODIUM OR LESS

The Chicago Dish:

Veggie Lover's • Supreme • Pepperoni or Pepperoni, Sausage & Mushroom Stuffed Crust Gold, Super Supreme

Menu Item	Cal	Fat	Sat	Chol	Carb	Fib	Sug	Sod

Pizzas (cont'd)
  750MG SODIUM OR LESS
  Pan Pizza:
    Veggie Lover's • Chicken Supreme • Cheese
  Thin n'Crispy:
    Veggie Lover's • Cheese
  Hand Tossed, Veggie Lover's

PASTA
  750MG SODIUM OR LESS
  Spaghetti w/Marinara Sauce
    To reduce sodium request half the sauce.

SANDWICHES
  EXCEED 2000MG SODIUM
  Ham & Cheese or Supreme

SALADS - *nutritional info unavailable*

  SALAD DRESSINGS
    250MG SODIUM OR LESS
    Buttermilk • Garlic Parmesan Mayonnaise • Thousand Island •
    French • Ranch, refrg

SIDE ITEMS
  150MG SODIUM OR LESS
  White Pizza Sauce
  250MG SODIUM OR LESS
  Breakstick w/Dipping Sauce • Garlic Bread, 1 slice

DESSERTS
  250MG SODIUM OR LESS
  Cinnamon Sticks, 2 pcs • Cherry Dessert Pizza, 1 slice •
  Apple Dessert Pizza, 1 slice

(**RAX**)

Contact Rax or their website (www.rax-online.com) for nutritional info.

SANDWICHES
  500MG SODIUM OR LESS
  Jr. Deluxe w/o Mayo and Oil
  750MG SODIUM OR LESS
  Jr. Deluxe • Cheddar Melt

SALADS *(W/O DRESSING)*
  150MG SODIUM OR LESS
  Side Salad
  1000MG SODIUM OR LESS
  Garden Salad

ROUND TABLE PIZZA

Menu Item	Cal	Fat	Sat	Chol	Carb	Fib	Sug	Sod

Salads (cont'd)

SALAD DRESSINGS

150MG SODIUM OR LESS
Vinaigrette

250MG SODIUM OR LESS
Honey French • 1000 Island • FF Catalina • Buttermilk Ranch

BAKED POTATOES

150MG SODIUM OR LESS
Plain Potato • Potato w/Butter and/or Sour Topping

750MG SODIUM OR LESS
Baked Potato w/Cheese • Baked Potato w/Cheese and Broccoli

SOUPS

500MG SODIUM OR LESS
Chicken Noodle • Chili

750MG SODIUM OR LESS
Cream of Broccoli

ROUND TABLE PIZZA

Contact Round Table or their website (www.roundtablepizza.com) for nutritional info.

PIZZAS *(1/12 SLICE)*

500MG SODIUM OR LESS
Thin Crust, 14" Large, Gourmet Veggie

750MG SODIUM OR LESS
Thin Crust, 14":
Cheese • Guinevere's Garden Delight • Chicken & Garlic Gourmet

CHICKEN *(3 PIECES)*

500MG SODIUM OR LESS
Honey BBQ Wings

750MG SODIUM OR LESS
Spicy Buffalo Wings • Honey BBQ Buffalo Wings

SANDWICHES

EXCEED 1500MG SODIUM
RT Veggie Sandwich

SALADS *(W/O DRESSING)*

250MG SODIUM OR LESS
Garden Salad

500MG SODIUM OR LESS
Caesar Salad

SALAD DRESSING *- nutritional info unavailable*

Menu Item	Cal	Fat	Sat	Chol	Carb	Fib	Sug	Sod

RUBIOS FRESH MEXICAN GRILL

Contact Rubios or their website (www.rubios.com) for nutritional info.

TACOS
150MG SODIUM OR LESS
HealthMex Taco w/Grilled Fish
250MG SODIUM OR LESS
Grilled Fish Taco
500MG SODIUM OR LESS
HealthMex Taco w/Chicken • Fish Taco • Grilled Chicken Taco •
Fish Taco Especial

PESKY MEALS
150MG SODIUM OR LESS
Fish Taco
500MG SODIUM OR LESS
Fish Taco w/Mini Churro and Chips

BURRITOS
EXCEED 1000MG SODIUM
HealthMex Veggiee • HealthMex Grilled Fish
NOTE: Values do not include rice served with burritos.

QUESADILLAS
EXCEED 1500MG SODIUM
Cheese Quesadilla

BOWLS & SALADS
EXCEED 1250MG SODIUM
Grilled Chicken Chopped Salad

LOS OSTROS
250MG SODIUM OR LESS
Guacamole, small
500MG SODIUM OR LESS
Chips

SALSA
250MG SODIUM OR LESS
Roasted Chipotle • Salsa Verde

DESSERTS
150MG SODIUM OR LESS
Churro, 1

SCHLOTZSKY'S DELI

Menu Item	Cal	Fat	Sat	Chol	Carb	Fib	Sug	Sod

(SCHLOTZSKY'S DELI)

Contact Schlotzsky's or their website (www.schlotzskys.com) for nutritional info.

SANDWICHES
1000MG SODIUM OR LESS

Western Vegetarian, small • The Vegetarian, small • BLT, small
Nutritional analysis based on sourdough bread.

BREADS
750MG SODIUM OR LESS

Dark Rye Bun, small • Sourdough Bun, small • Wheat Bun, small

WRAPS
EXCEED 1000MG SODIUM

Zesty Albacore Tuna

PIZZAS *(8" SOURDOUGH)*
EXCEED 1500MG SODIUM

Fresh Tomato and Pesto

SOUPS
750MG SODIUM OR LESS

Santa Fe Vegetable

SALADS *(W/O DRESSING)*
150MG SODIUM OR LESS

Small Garden w/o Croutons • Caesar w/o Croutons • Garden w/o Croutons
500MG SODIUM OR LESS

Chinese Chicken w/o Noodles • Chicken Caesar w/o Croutons

SALAD DRESSINGS AND TOPPINGS
150MG SODIUM OR LESS

Chow Mein Noodles • Garlic Cheese Croutons
250MG SODIUM OR LESS

Olde World Caesar

SIDE ITEMS
150MG SODIUM OR LESS

Fresh Fruit Salad
250MG SODIUM OR LESS

Regular Potato Chips • Sour Cream & Onion Potato Chips •
Jalapeño Potato Chips • California Pasta Salad

DESSERTS
150MG SODIUM OR LESS

Fudge Brownie Cake • Golden Raisin Oatmeal Cookie •
Oatmeal Raisin Cookie • White Choc Macadamia Cookie • Choc Chip Cookie •
M&M's Cookie • Cranberry Walnut Crunch Cookie
250MG SODIUM OR LESS

Fudge Choc Chip or Triple Choc Chip Cookie • Peanut Butter Cookie •
Sugar Cookie • NY Creamstyle Cheesecake • Strawberry Swirl Cheesecake

SONIC DRIVE-IN

Menu Item	Cal	Fat	Sat	Chol	Carb	Fib	Sug	Sod

SKIPPER'S

Contact Skipper's or their website (www.skippers.net) for nutritional info.

ENTREES
500MG SODIUM OR LESS
Grilled Cod Fillet • Grilled Salmon Fillet • Grilled Chicken Breast
Grilled Halibut Fillet • Battered Halibut
750MG SODIUM OR LESS
Battered Salmon

SIDES
150MG SODIUM OR LESS
Plain Baked Potato
250MG SODIUM OR LESS
Texas Toast, 1 slice

SONIC DRIVE-IN

Contact Sonic Drive-in or their website (www.sonicdrivein.com) for nutritional info.

BREAKFAST
EXCEED 1000MG SODIUM
Sonic Sausage Egg and Cheese Toaster

BREAKFAST SIDES
150MG SODIUM OR LESS
Sonic Sunrise, regular or large

BURGERS & SANDWICHES
500MG SODIUM OR LESS
Breaded Chicken Sandwich
1000MG SODIUM OR LESS
#1 Sonic Burger • #2 Sonic Burger • Grilled Cheese Toaster Sandwich

CONEYS
750MG SODIUM OR LESS
Regular Coney Plain

CHICKEN
1000MG SODIUM OR LESS
Chicken Strip Snack, 3

WRAPS
1000MG SODIUM OR LESS
Grilled Chickenw/o Ranch Dressing • Chicken Strip w/o Ranch Dressing

WACKY PACK KID'S MEAL
500MG SODIUM OR LESS
Corn Dog
750MG SODIUM OR LESS
Chicken Strips, 2

SOUPLANTATION / SWEET TOMATOES

ADD-ONS
150MG SODIUM OR LESS
Sonic Green Chiles • Slaw • Sonic Chili
250MG SODIUM OR LESS
1000 Island Dressing • Ranch Dressing

SIDE ITEMS
500MG SODIUM OR LESS
Onion Rings, regular

DESSERTS
250MG SODIUM OR LESS
Dish of Vanilla • Strawberry Sundae • Ice Cream Cone • Banana Split • Pineapple Sundae • Slush Floats, reg • CreamSlush, reg

TOPPINGS
150MG SODIUM OR LESS
Vanilla Syrup • Cherry Syrup • Maraschino Cherry • Strawberry Topping • Pineapple Topping • Hot Fudge Topping • Full Flavor Choc Syrup

---

(SOUPLANTATION / SWEET TOMATOES)

Menu Item	Cal	Fat	Sat	Chol	Carb	Fib	Sug	Sod
PASTAS *(1 CUP UNLESS NOTED)*								
Carbonara	280	8	4	20	43	2	3	250
Creamy Pepper Jack	290	15	6	50	35	2	6	360
Creamy Herb Chicken	310	17	8	80	32	2	7	360
Italian Sausage w/Red Pepper Puree	250	10	4	45	35	2	7	380
Smoked Salmon and Dill	380	16	8	45	41	2	2	390
Nutty Mushroom	390	20	9	45	42	2	4	410
Southwestern Alfredo	350	16	9	50	42	1	3	420
Bruschetta	260	4	2	10	41	3	3	450
Garden Veg w/Meatballs	270	7	3	10	42	3	2	460
Italian Veg Beef	270	6	2	10	43	4	3	470
Lemon Cream and Asparagus	230	9	2	0	34	1	4	470
Vegetable Ragu	250	5	2	10	41	3	4	480
SALADS								
TOSSED SALADS *(1 CUP UNLESS NOTED)*								
Strawberry Fields w/Walnuts	130	8	1	0	15	3	12	75
Watercress and Orange	90	4	1	0	12	2	6	90
Mandarin Spinach w/Walnuts	170	11	1	0	14	3	11	150
Roma Tomato, Mozzarella and Basil	120	9	2	10	7	1	2	180
California Cobb	180	8	2	25	4	2	1	190
Barlett Pear and Walnut	160	12	2	5	13	2	10	220
Won Ton Chicken Happiness	150	8	1	10	12	2	4	220
Ensalada Azteca	130	9	3	15	7	4	3	230
Summer Lemon w/Spiced Pecans	220	15	3	10	18	2	13	250

Menu Item	Cal	Fat	Sat	Chol	Carb	Fib	Sug	Sod
SIGNATURE SALADS *(1/2 CUP UNLESS NOTED)*								
Carrot Ginger w/Herb Vinaigrette	150	12	1	0	9	3	8	40
Dijon Potato Salad w/Garlic Dill	150	12	1	0	9	3	6	40
Carrot Raisin, LF	90	3	0	5	17	2	15	80
Oriental Ginger Slaw w/Krab, LF	70	3	0	2	8	4	3	80
Poppyseed Coleslaw	120	9	1	10	9	3	5	130
Baja Bean and Cilantro, LF	180	3	0	0	29	5	2	190
Pineapple Coconut Slaw	150	10	3	15	14	2	10	190
Marinated Summer Vegetables, FF	80	0	0	0	19	4	14	210
Tomato Cucumber Marinade	80	5	0	0	8	1	2	220
Moroccan Marinated Vegetables, LF	90	3	0	0	9	2	2	230
Citrus Noodles w/Snow Peas	140	6	1	0	19	2	5	240
Italian Garden Vegetable	110	8	1	0	9	2	2	240
Roasted Potato w/Chipotle Chile	140	6	1	0	18	4	3	250
Joan's Broccoli Madness	180	14	3	10	11	3	9	250
SALAD DRESSINGS AND TOPPINGS *(2 TBSP UNLESS NOTED)*								
Tomato Basil Croutons, 5 pcs	45	4	1	0	3	0	0	90
Garlic Parmesan Croutons, 5 pcs	40	3	1	2	2	0	2	160
FF Honey Mustard	45	0	0	10	10	0	9	160
Basil Vinaigrette	160	17	1	0	1	0	0	160
FF Ranch	50	0	0	0	2	0	1	180
Ranch	130	13	2	10	1	0	1	180
Balsamic Vinaigrette	180	19	2	0	1	0	1	190
SOUPS *(1 CUP UNLESS NOTED)*								
Garlic Kickin Roasted Chicken	140	6	3	30	10	3	4	310
Country Corn and Red Potato Chowder	160	6	3	15	24	4	6	330
Cream of Chicken	250	15	6	40	21	2	3	350
Living on the Veg	90	1	0	0	15	3	3	380
Sweet Tomato Onion, LF	110	3	1	0	12	1	5	450
Tomato Parmesan and Veg, LF	120	3	1	5	18	3	3	460
Big Chunk Chicken Noodle, LF	160	3	2	20	17	2	3	480
Chunky Potato Cheese w/Thyme	210	10	6	30	19	2	3	480
MUFFINS & BREADS								
MUFFINS								
French Quarter Praline	290	15	2	20	38	2	21	100
Bran Muffins, Apple Cinnamon, Fruit Medley, or Cranberry Orange (avg)	80	1	0	0	17	1	14	110
Cappuccino Chip	160	4	2	25	28	1	15	160
Big Blue Blueberry	140	5	1	10	22	1	9	180
Pauline's Apple Walnut Cake	180	7	3	25	28	1	21	180
Apple Raisin or Banana Nut	150	7	1	10	22	1	9	190
Cherry Nut or Zucchini Nut	150	7	1	10	22	1	9	190
Lemon	140	4	1	10	24	1	13	190

STEAK ESCAPE

Menu Item	Cal	Fat	Sat	Chol	Carb	Fib	Sug	Sod
Muffins & Breads (cont'd)								
Choc Brownie or Choc Chip	170	8	2	10	22	1	10	190
Country Blackberry	170	6	2	15	27	1	13	190
Taffy Apple	160	6	1	10	25	1	18	190
Black Forest	230	9	2	10	36	1	19	190
BREADS								
Garlic Parmesan Focaccia, LF	100	3	0	0	15	1	1	170
DESSERTS *(1/2 CUP UNLESS NOTED)*								
Apple Medley or Banana Royale	75	0	0	0	19	1	12	5
Jello, Sugar Free	10	0	0	0	0	0	0	10
Regular	80	0	0	0	20	0	19	40
Rice Pudding	110	2	1	10	20	1	12	50
Vanilla Soft Serve, Reduced Fat	140	4	3	20	22	0	19	70
Choc Frozen Yogurt, FF	95	0	0	0	21	0	16	80
Nutty Waldorf Salad, LF	80	3	0	0	12	3	5	80
Choc Chip Cookie, 1 small	70	3	1	5	10	0	6	90
Butterscotch Praline Cake	220	12	5	90	24	1	17	140
Butterscotch or Tapioca Pudding, LF	140	3	0	10	24	0	24	160
Vanilla Pudding	140	4	0	10	24	0	24	160
Apple Cobbler	350	10	2	0	64	1	10	160
Cherry Cobbler	340	10	2	0	61	2	10	180

(STEAK ESCAPE)

7" SANDWICHES

Menu Item	Cal	Fat	Sat	Chol	Carb	Fib	Sug	Sod
Vegetarian	500	13	-	41	67	-	-	868
Great Escape	508	12	-	40	63	-	-	1080
Grand Escape	513	12	-	40	65	-	-	1080
To reduce sodium, omit peppers, cheese, olives and/or BBQ sauce.								
KIDS SANDWICHES								
Steak and Cheese	260	9	-	22	33	-	-	667
Chicken and Cheese	255	7	-	32	32	-	-	687
Turkey and Cheese or Ham and Cheese	233	5	-	17	64	-	-	982
SALADS *(W/O DRESSING)*								
Side Salad	192	14	-	45	6	-	-	288
Grilled Salad w/Steak	339	20	-	70	7	-	-	657
Grilled Salad w/Chicken	330	19	-	100	8	-	-	697
SALAD DRESSINGS								
Ranch, 0.5 oz	83	9	-	5	0	-	-	137
Italian, 0.5 oz	51	5	-	0	1	-	-	248
SMASHED POTATOES								
Smashed Potato, Plain	369	0	0	0	86	-	-	18

Menu Item	Cal	Fat	Sat	Chol	Carb	Fib	Sug	Sod
Smashed Potato, Loaded								
Ranch and Bacon	692	34	-	29	87	-	-	501
w/Steak	540	20	-	70	54	-	-	705
w/Chicken	530	21	-	100	53	-	-	744
SIDE ITEMS								
Kids Meal Fries	249	13	-	0	34	-	-	205
French Fries, 12 oz cup	498	26	-	0	67	-	-	409
CONDIMENTS & TOPPINGS								
Lettuce and tomato	2-24	0	0	0	2	-	-	7
Sour Cream, 1 oz	61	6	-	13	1	-	-	15
Swiss Cheese, 1 oz	100	8	-	26	1	-	-	60
Mayonnaise, 1 oz	101	11	-	5	0	-	-	76
Cheddar Cheese, 1 oz	116	9	-	30	1	-	-	179
Black Olives, 1 oz	32	3	-	0	2	-	-	248
BBQ Sauce, 1 oz	40	0	0	0	9	-	-	252

(**SUBWAY**)

BREAKFAST

OMELETS AND FRENCH TOAST

Menu Item	Cal	Fat	Sat	Chol	Carb	Fib	Sug	Sod
Veg Egg Omelet	210	14	4	560	4	1	1	250
Bacon and Egg Omelet	240	17	6	570	2	0	0	350
French Toast w/Syrup	350	8	3	280	57	2	33	350
Western and Egg Omelet	220	14	5	565	4	1	0	360
Cheese and Egg Omelet	240	17	6	570	2	0	0	370

SANDWICHES

On Deli Round:

Menu Item	Cal	Fat	Sat	Chol	Carb	Fib	Sug	Sod
Veg and Egg	290	12	3	175	36	3	4	430
Bacon and Egg	320	15	5	185	34	3	3	520
Western and Egg	300	12	4	180	36	3	4	530
Cheese and Egg	320	15	5	185	34	3	3	550
On 6" Italian or Whole Wheat:								
Veg and Egg	410	16	5	560	44	4	5	610

SUBS & SANDWICHES

SUBS (ON ITALIAN OR WHEAT BREAD)

Menu Item	Cal	Fat	Sat	Chol	Carb	Fib	Sug	Sod
6" Vegie Delite	230	3	1	0	44	4	6	510
6" Roast Beef	290	5	2	20	45	4	7	910
6" Roasted Chicken Breast	320	5	2	45	47	5	8	1000
6" Turkey Breast	280	5	2	20	46	4	6	1010

NOTE: To reduce sodium by more than 120mg, substitute sourdough bread.

SANDWICHES (ON DELI ROUND)

Menu Item	Cal	Fat	Sat	Chol	Carb	Fib	Sug	Sod
Roast Beef	220	5	2	15	35	3	4	660
Turkey Breast	220	4	2	15	36	3	4	730

SUBWAY

Menu Item	Cal	Fat	Sat	Chol	Carb	Fib	Sug	Sod
Sandwiches (cont'd)								
Ham	210	4	2	10	35	3	4	770
Tuna	330	16	5	25	36	3	3	830
NOTE: Sub and sandwich values include lettuce, tomato, onion, green pepper, olives and pickles.								
SOUPS								
Tomato Bisque	90	3	1	0	15	3	7	750
SALADS *(W/O DRESSING)*								
Veggie Delite Salad	50	1	0	0	9	3	2	310
Roast Beef	120	3	2	20	10	3	3	720
Roasted Chicken Breast	140	3	1	45	12	3	4	800
Turkey Breast	100	2	0	20	11	3	3	820
To reduce sodium, omit cheese, pickles, hot peppers and/or olives.								
SALAD DRESSINGS								
FF French, 2 oz	70	0	0	0	17	0	12	390
FF Ranch, 2 oz	60	0	0	0	14	0	6	530
BREADS								
6" Sourdough	210	3	1	0	41	3	2	210
Deli Style Roll	170	3	1	0	32	3	2	280
6" Italian (White)	210	3	2	0	38	3	5	340
6" Hearty Italian	210	3	2	0	41	3	5	340
TOPPINGS & CONDIMENTS								
Lettuce, Tomato, Onions, Green Peppers, or Cucumbers (avg)	5	0	0	0	1	0	0	0
Vinegar, 1 tsp	0	0	0	0	0	0	0	0
Olive Oil Blend, 1 tsp	45	5	1	0	0	0	0	0
Banana Peppers, 3 rings	0	0	0	0	0	0	0	20
Olives, 3 rings	5	0	0	0	0	0	0	25
Swiss Cheese, 2 triangles	53	4	3	13	0	0	0	30
NOTE: Other cheeses have 3 times or more sodium.								
Jalapeño Peppers, 3 rings	0	0	0	0	0	0	0	70
Mayonnaise, 1 tbsp	110	12	3	10	0	0	0	80
Light, 1 tbsp	45	5	1	10	1	0	0	100
Mustard, Yellow or Deli Brown, 2 tsp	5	0	0	0	1	0	0	115
Pickles, 3 chips	0	0	0	0	0	0	0	125
SAUCES *(0.8 OZ UNLESS NOTED)*								
FF Sweet Onion	40	0	0	0	9	0	8	100
FF Mustard	30	0	0	0	7	0	6	140
Dijon Horseradish	90	10	2	10	1	0	0	160
COOKIES								
Choc Chunk or MandM (avg)	220	10	4	12	30	1	17	105
Sugar	230	12	4	15	38	0	14	135
White Macadamia Nut or Choc Chip	220	10	4	15	29	1	17	160

Menu Item	Cal	Fat	Sat	Chol	Carb	Fib	Sug	Sod

(TACO BELL)

Contact Taco Bell or their website (www.tacobell.com) for nutritional info.

BREAKFAST

750MG SODIUM OR LESS
Breakfast Gordita

TACOS

500MG SODIUM OR LESS
Taco, Regular • Taco Supreme

750MG SODIUM OR LESS
Chicken Soft Taco • Chicken Soft Taco Supreme

CHALUPAS & GORDITAS

750MG SODIUM OR LESS
Chalupa Supreme, Steak or Chicken • Gordita Supreme, Steak or Chicken

BURRITOS

EXCEED 1000MG SODIUM
Chili Cheese Burrito • Fiesta Burrito, Steak or Chicken

SPECIALTIES

750MG SODIUM OR LESS
Tostada

1000MG SODIUM OR LESS
MexiMelt

BORDER BOWLS

EXCEED 1250MG SODIUM
Zesty Chicken w/o Dressing

SIDE ITEMS

750MG SODIUM OR LESS
Nachos

CONDIMENTS & SAUCES

150MG SODIUM OR LESS
Sour Cream • Cheddar Cheese • Three Cheese Blend • Guacamole

SAUCES

150MG SODIUM OR LESS
Fiesta Salsa • Creamy Lime Sauce • Creamy Jalapeño Sauce •
Pepper Jack Cheese Sauce • Green Sauce

250MG SODIUM OR LESS
Border Sauce, Mild

DESSERTS

150MG SODIUM OR LESS
Cinnamon Twists

TACO DEL MAR

Menu Item	Cal	Fat	Sat	Chol	Carb	Fib	Sug	Sod

(TACO DEL MAR)

TACOS

Menu Item	Cal	Fat	Sat	Chol	Carb	Fib	Sug	Sod
Soft Taco, Beef	252	9	-	-	-	-	-	308
Hard Taco, Fish	260	19	-	-	-	-	-	378
Soft Taco, Chicken	250	7	-	-	-	-	-	407
Hard Taco, Chicken	265	18	-	-	-	-	-	408
Hard Taco, Pork	256	17	-	-	-	-	-	436
Soft Taco, Pork	237	6	-	-	-	-	-	450

BURRITOS *(FLOUR TORTILLA WITH WHOLE BEANS)*

Menu Item	Cal	Fat	Sat	Chol	Carb	Fib	Sug	Sod
Jumbo, Vegetarian, flour tortilla	731	17	-	-	-	-	-	1531
Jumbo, Beef, flour tortilla	847	20	-	-	-	-	-	1620
Jumbo, Fish, flour tortilla	856	42	-	-	-	-	-	1649

OTHER STUFF

Menu Item	Cal	Fat	Sat	Chol	Carb	Fib	Sug	Sod
Taco Salad, Veggie w/whole beans	773	37	-	-	-	-	-	1292
Taco Salad, Beef w/whole beans	847	42	-	-	-	-	-	1295
Taco Salad, Fish w/whole beans	782	42	-	-	-	-	-	1439

(TACO JOHN'S)

Contact Taco John or their website (www.tacojohns.com) for nutritional info.

TACOS

250MG SODIUM OR LESS
Crispy Taco
500MG SODIUM OR LESS
Softshell Taco
750MG SODIUM OR LESS
Sierra Taco, Beef

BURRITOS

1000MG SODIUM OR LESS
Bean Burrito • Combination Burrito • Beefy Burrito

SPECIALTIES

1000MG SODIUM OR LESS
Cheese Quesadilla

PLATTERS & LOCAL FAVORITES - *not available at all locations*

250MG SODIUM OR LESS
Bean Tostada • Tostada • Cheese Crisp

PLATTERS

EXCEED 1500MG SODIUM
Beef & Bean Chimi Platter

Menu Item	Cal	Fat	Sat	Chol	Carb	Fib	Sug	Sod

SALADS
750MG SODIUM OR LESS
Side Salad
1000MG SODIUM OR LESS
Chicken Festiva w/o Dressing

SIDE ITEMS
750MG SODIUM OR LESS
Nachos

DESSERTS
150MG SODIUM OR LESS
Cinnamon Mint Swirl • Choco Taco • Churro
250MG SODIUM OR LESS
Apple Grande

(TACO TIME)

NOTE: Taco Time is updating their nutritional guides. Check with individual restaurants or their website (www.tacotime.com) for nutritional info. The following is the most current info.

TACOS
750MG SODIUM OR LESS
Super Soft Taco, Beef • Soft Taco, Beef • Crisp Taco

BURRITOS
500MG SODIUM OR LESS
Crsip Bean Burrito
750MG SODIUM OR LESS
Chicken and Black Bean Burrito • Veggie Burrito • Soft Bean Burrito

SALADS *(w/o DRESSING)*
1000MG SODIUM OR LESS
Chicken Fiesta Salad • Chicken Taco Salad

  SALAD DRESSINGS - *nutritional info unavailable*

SIDE ITEMS
750MG SODIUM OR LESS
Refritos (Cheese, Sauce, Chips) • Mexi-Rice

SAUCES
150MG SODIUM OR LESS
Green Sauce • Hot Sauce

DESSERTS
150MG SODIUM OR LESS
Fruit-Filled Empanada • Cinnamon Crustos

TCBY

Menu Item	Cal	Fat	Sat	Chol	Carb	Fib	Sug	Sod
(TCBY)								
FROZEN YOGURT & SORBET (1/2 CUP UNLESS NOTED)								
NF Frozen Yogurt	110	0	0	5	23	0	20	60
No Sugar Added	80	0	0	5	20	0	7	35
NF and Nondairy Sorbet	100	0	0	0	24	0	19	30
99% FF Frozen Yogurt	130	3	2	15	23	0	20	60
HAND-DIPPED ICE CREAM (1/2 CUP UNLESS NOTED)								
No Sugar LF Ice Cream	100	3	2	10	20	0	6	20
LF Ice Cream	120	3	1	5	22	0	18	75
(WENDY'S)								
SANDWICHES (W/LETTUCE, ONION AND TOMATO ONLY)								
Jr. Hamburger	270	9	3	30	34	2	6	590
Chicken Breast Fillet	430	16	6	65	34	2	6	690
Grilled Chicken	300	7	2	55	36	2	8	700
CONDIMENTS								
Mustard, 1/2 tsp	0	0	0	0	0	0	0	50
Mayonnaise, 1 1/2 tsp	30	3	0	5	1	0	0	60
Ketchup, 1 tsp	10	0	0	0	2	0	1	80
Dill Pickles, 4	0	0	0	0	0	0	0	105
CRISPY CHICKEN NUGGETS								
4 Piece Kids' Meal	180	11	3	25	10	0	0	380
5 Piece Kids' Meal	220	14	3	35	13	0	0	480
DIPPINGS SAUCES (1 PKT UNLESS NOTED)								
Sweet and Sour Sauce	45	0	0	0	12	0	10	115
Barbecue Sauce	40	0	0	0	10	0	7	160
SALADS (W/O DRESSING)								
Side Salad	35	0	0	0	7	3	4	20
Spring Mix Salad w/o Pecans	180	11	6	30	12	5	5	230
w/Pecans	310	24	7	30	17	7	8	295
Caesar Side Salad w/o Croutons	70	4	2	15	2	1	1	250
SALAD DRESSINGS AND TOPPINGS (1 PKT UNLESS NOTED)								
Homestyle Garlic Croutons	70	3	0	0	9	0	0	120
FF French Dressing	80	0	0	0	19	0	16	210
Caesar Dressing	150	16	3	20	1	0	0	240
LF Honey Mustard Dressing	110	3	0	0	21	0	16	340
BAKED POTATOES								
Potato, Plain	310	0	0	0	72	7	5	25
w/Sour Cream and Chives	370	6	4	15	73	7	5	40
w/Whipped Margarine, 1 pkt	370	7	2	0	72	6	5	140
Broccoli and Cheese Potato	480	14	3	5	80	9	6	510

Menu Item	Cal	Fat	Sat	Chol	Carb	Fib	Sug	Sod
SIDE ITEMS								
French Fries, Kids' Meal	250	11	2	0	36	4	0	220
French Fries, medium	390	17	3	0	56	6	0	340
DESSERTS								
Frosty, Junior, 6 oz	170	4	3	20	28	0	21	100
Frosty, Small, 12 oz	330	8	5	35	56	0	43	200

WHATABURGER

Contact Whataburger or their website (www.whataburger.com) for nutritional info.

BREAKFAST
500MG SODIUM OR LESS
Egg Sandwich w/o Cheese
750MG SODIUM OR LESS
Egg Sandwich w/Cheese • Taquito w/Sausage and Egg •
Taquito w/Potato and Egg

BREAKFAST SIDES
500MG SODIUM OR LESS
Cinnamon Roll

SANDWICHES
500MG SODIUM OR LESS
Whataburger, Jr. w/o Mustard and/or Pickles
750MG SODIUM OR LESS
Whataburger, Jr. w/o Pickles • Whataburger, Jr.

FISH SANDWICHES
1000MG SODIUM OR LESS
Whatacatch

CHICKEN SANDWICHES
1000MG SODIUM OR LESS
Grilled Chicken on Sm White Bun w/Salad Dressing, Lettuce and Tomato
EXCEED 1000MG SODIUM
Grilled Chicken Sandwich

CHICKEN
750MG SODIUM OR LESS
Chicken Strips, 2 strips

SALADS *(W/O DRESSING)*
150MG SODIUM OR LESS
Garden Salad w/o Cheese
250MG SODIUM OR LESS
Garden Salad w/Cheese
750MG SODIUM OR LESS
Grilled Chicken w/o Cheese

WHITE CASTLE

Menu Item	Cal	Fat	Sat	Chol	Carb	Fib	Sug	Sod

Salads (cont'd)

SALAD DRESSINGS
500MG SODIUM OR LESS
Ranch • 1000 Island Dressing

SIDE ITEMS
250MG SODIUM OR LESS
French Fries, small
500MG SODIUM OR LESS
Onion Rings, medium

CONDIMENTS
150MG SODIUM OR LESS
Salad Dressing (on Small Sandwiches) • Mustard (on Small Sandwiches) •
Ketchup (on Small Sandwiches)
500MG SODIUM OR LESS
Ketchup, 1 pkt

DESSERTS & SHAKES
150MG SODIUM OR LESS
Cookies, all
250MG SODIUM OR LESS
Strawberry, Vanilla, or Choc Shake, 16 oz

(WHITE CASTLE®)

Menu Item	Cal	Fat	Sat	Chol	Carb	Fib	Sug	Sod
SANDWICHES								
Hamburger, 1	135	7	3	10	11	2	0	135
Double Hamburger, 1	235	14	6	20	16	4	0	200
Fish Sandwich, 1	160	6	1	15	18	0	1	220
Cheeseburger, 1	160	9	4	15	11	2	0	250
Chicken Sandwich, 1	190	8	2	20	21	-	1	360
Bacon Cheeseburger, 1	200	13	6	25	12	3	0	400
Double Cheeseburger, 1	285	18	8	30	16	5	0	430
SIDE ITEMS								
French Fries, small	115	6	1	-	15	2	2	15
SHAKES								
Chocolate Shake, 14 oz	220	7	1	25	32	-	27	140
Vanilla Shake, 14 oz	230	7	1	25	35	-	28	150

Menu Item	Cal	Fat	Sat	Chol	Carb	Fib	Sug	Sod

RESTAURANT QUICK REFERENCE

Use this guide to find the fast food restaurants offering the lowest sodium items in each of the following categories.

BURGERS & FRIES

WHITE CASTLE

Menu Item	Cal	Fat	Sat	Chol	Carb	Fib	Sug	Sod
Hamburger, 1	135	7	3	10	11	2	0	135
Double Hamburger, 1	235	14	6	20	16	4	0	200
Fish Sandwich, 1	160	6	1	15	18	0	1	220
Cheeseburger, 1	160	9	4	15	11	2	0	250
French Fries, small	115	6	1	-	15	2	2	15

KRYSTAL

Menu Item	Cal	Fat	Sat	Chol	Carb	Fib	Sug	Sod
Krystal Sandwich	160	7	3	20	17	1	1	260
Cheese Krystal	180	9	4	25	16	2	1	430
Bacon Cheese Krystal	190	10	5	25	16	2	1	430
Fries, regular	370	18	7	15	49	6	0	85

IN-N-OUT BURGER

Menu Item	Cal	Fat	Sat	Chol	Carb	Fib	Sug	Sod
Hamburger Protein Style *(lettuce leaves are substituted for the bun)*	240	17	4	40	11	3	7	370
French Fries	400	18	5	0	54	2	0	245

CARL'S JR.

Menu Item	Cal	Fat	Sat	Chol	Carb	Fib	Sug	Sod
Hamburger w/o Mustard and Pickles	-	-	-	-	-	-	-	<500
French Fries, kids	-	-	-	-	-	-	-	<150

MCDONALD'S

Menu Item	Cal	Fat	Sat	Chol	Carb	Fib	Sug	Sod
Hamburger w/o Ketchup and Pickles	-	-	-	-	-	-	-	<500
French Fries, small	-	-	-	-	-	-	-	<250

WHATABURGER

Menu Item	Cal	Fat	Sat	Chol	Carb	Fib	Sug	Sod
Whataburger, Jr. w/o Mustard and/or Pickles	-	-	-	-	-	-	-	<500
French Fries, small	-	-	-	-	-	-	-	<250

DAIRY QUEEN / BRAZIER

Menu Item	Cal	Fat	Sat	Chol	Carb	Fib	Sug	Sod
DQ Homestyle Hamburger w/o Ketchup and Pickles	-	-	-	-	-	-	-	<500
Onion Rings	-	-	-	-	-	-	-	<250

SANDWICHES

BOJANGLES

Menu Item	Cal	Fat	Sat	Chol	Carb	Fib	Sug	Sod
Cajun Filet w/o Mayo	337	11	5	45	41	3	-	401
Cajun Filet w/Mayo	437	22	7	55	41	3	-	506
Grilled Filet w/o Mayo	235	5	3	51	25	2	-	540

205

QUICK REFERENCE

Subs

Menu Item	Cal	Fat	Sat	Chol	Carb	Fib	Sug	Sod
Sandwiches (cont'd)								
D'ANGELO								
Pokket Sandwiches *(SMALL HONEY WHEAT POKKET)*								
Steak	-	-	-	-	-	-	-	<500
Classic Veggie No Cheese	-	-	-	-	-	-	-	<500
Hamburger	-	-	-	-	-	-	-	<500
Salad	-	-	-	-	-	-	-	<500
Turkey	-	-	-	-	-	-	-	<500
SONIC DRIVE-IN								
Breaded Chicken Sandwich	-	-	-	-	-	-	-	<500
RAX								
Jr. Deluxe w/o Mayo and Oil	-	-	-	-	-	-	-	<500
Jr. Deluxe	-	-	-	-	-	-	-	<750
Cheddar Melt	-	-	-	-	-	-	-	<750
KFC								
Honey BBQ Flavored Sandwich	-	-	-	-	-	-	-	<750
BRUEGGER'S BAGELS								
Garden Veggie Bagel Sandwich	-	-	-	-	-	-	-	<750
Atlantic Smoked Salmon Bagel Sandwich	-	-	-	-	-	-	-	<750

(SUBS)

Menu Item	Cal	Fat	Sat	Chol	Carb	Fib	Sug	Sod
D'ANGELO *(SMALL ON HONEY WHEAT)*								
Steak	-	-	-	-	-	-	-	<500
Hamburger	-	-	-	-	-	-	-	<500
Salad	-	-	-	-	-	-	-	<500
Turkey	-	-	-	-	-	-	-	<500
SUBWAY								
6" Vegie Delite	230	3	1	0	44	4	6	510
COUSINS SUBS								
Seafood w/Crab, mini 4"	-	-	-	-	-	-	-	<750
Tuna, mini 4"	-	-	-	-	-	-	-	<750
Cold Veggie, 7 1/2"	-	-	-	-	-	-	-	<750

(WRAPS)

Menu Item	Cal	Fat	Sat	Chol	Carb	Fib	Sug	Sod
D'ANGELO *(WHITE WRAP)*								
Steak	-	-	-	-	-	-	-	<500
Salad	-	-	-	-	-	-	-	<500
Hamburger	-	-	-	-	-	-	-	<500
Turkey	-	-	-	-	-	-	-	<500
Roast Beef	-	-	-	-	-	-	-	<750

Menu Item	Cal	Fat	Sat	Chol	Carb	Fib	Sug	Sod
Wraps (cont'd)								
AU BON PAIN								
Fields and Feta	570	17	4	10	91	13	6	850
Chicken Caesar	600	25	8	80	63	5	3	930
Mediterranean	560	23	3	5	77	8	5	960
SONIC DRIVE-IN								
Grilled Chicken w/o Ranch Dressing	-	-	-	-	-	-	-	<1000
Chicken Strip w/o Ranch Dressing	-	-	-	-	-	-	-	<1000

CHICKEN NUGGETS

Menu Item	Cal	Fat	Sat	Chol	Carb	Fib	Sug	Sod
WENDY'S								
4 Piece Kids' Meal	180	11	3	25	10	0	0	380
BURGER KING								
Chicken Tenders, 4 pc	-	-	-	-	-	-	-	<500
MCDONALD'S								
Chicken McNuggets, 4 pc	-	-	-	-	-	-	-	<500

POULTRY OR FISH W/SIDE DISHES

Menu Item	Cal	Fat	Sat	Chol	Carb	Fib	Sug	Sod
EL POLLO LOCO								
Leg, Flame-Broiled	-	-	-	-	-	-	-	<150
Wing, Flame-Broiled	-	-	-	-	-	-	-	<250
Thigh, Flame-Broiled	-	-	-	-	-	-	-	<250
Breast, Flame-Broiled	-	-	-	-	-	-	-	<500
Add a side:								
3" Corn Cobbette, 1	-	-	-	-	-	-	-	<150
Tortilla Chips, unsalted, 2.8 oz	-	-	-	-	-	-	-	<150
Tortilla, corn, 4 1/2", 1	-	-	-	-	-	-	-	<150
Corn, 6", 1	-	-	-	-	-	-	-	<150
Fresh Vegetables, 4 oz	-	-	-	-	-	-	-	<150
CHURCH'S CHICKEN								
Leg	-	-	-	-	-	-	-	<250
w/o Batter, Skin Removed	-	-	-	-	-	-	-	<150
Add a side:								
Corn on the Cob, 1 cob	-	-	-	-	-	-	-	<150
French Fries, regular	-	-	-	-	-	-	-	<150
Collard Greens, regular	-	-	-	-	-	-	-	<250
Cole Slaw, regular	-	-	-	-	-	-	-	<250
BOSTON MARKET								
Marinated Grilled Chicken, 1 breast	-	-	-	-	-	-	-	<250
Add a side:								
Cranberry Walnut Relish	-	-	-	-	-	-	-	<150
Fruit Salad	-	-	-	-	-	-	-	<150
Hot Cinnamon Apples	-	-	-	-	-	-	-	<150

Menu Item	Cal	Fat	Sat	Chol	Carb	Fib	Sug	Sod
Poultry or Fish w/Side Dishes (cont'd)								
Steamed Vegetables, 1 cup	-	-	-	-	-	-	-	<150
Jumpin Juice Squares, 1 serv	-	-	-	-	-	-	-	<150
New Potatoes	-	-	-	-	-	-	-	<150
Whole Kernel Corn	-	-	-	-	-	-	-	<250
Sweet Potato Casserole	-	-	-	-	-	-	-	<250
LONG JOHN SILVER'S								
Battered Shrimp	-	-	-	-	-	-	-	<150
Battered Chicken	-	-	-	-	-	-	-	<500
Add a side:								
Corn Cobbette, 1	-	-	-	-	-	-	-	<150
Hushpuppie, 1	-	-	-	-	-	-	-	<250
KFC								
Whole Wing, Original Recipe	-	-	-	-	-	-	-	<500
Drumstick, Hot and Spicy	-	-	-	-	-	-	-	<500
Whole Wing, Extra Crispy	-	-	-	-	-	-	-	<500
Add a side:								
Corn on the Cob,	-	-	-	-	-	-	-	<150
Mashed Potatoes w/o Gravy	-	-	-	-	-	-	-	<250
Cole Slaw, 5 oz	-	-	-	-	-	-	-	<500
SKIPPER'S								
Cod Fillet, Grilled, 5.1 oz	-	-	-	-	-	-	-	<500
Salmon Fillet, Grilled, 5.3 oz	-	-	-	-	-	-	-	<500
Chicken Breast, Grilled, 4 oz	-	-	-	-	-	-	-	<500
Halibut Fillet, Grilled, 5.3 oz	-	-	-	-	-	-	-	<500
Add a side:								
Baked Potato, 10 oz	-	-	-	-	-	-	-	<150
Texas Toast, 1.3 oz slice	-	-	-	-	-	-	-	<250

TACOS, BURRITOS & OTHER MEXICAN

Menu Item	Cal	Fat	Sat	Chol	Carb	Fib	Sug	Sod
RUBIOS FRESH MEXICAN GRILL								
HealthMex Taco w/Grilled Fish	-	-	-	-	-	-	-	<150
Grilled Fish Taco	-	-	-	-	-	-	-	<250
HealthMex Taco w/Chicken	-	-	-	-	-	-	-	<500
Fish Taco	-	-	-	-	-	-	-	<500
DEL TACO								
Taco	-	-	-	-	-	-	-	<150
Soft Taco	-	-	-	-	-	-	-	<500
EL POLLO LOCO								
Taco Al Carbon	-	-	-	-	-	-	-	<150
Chicken Tamale	-	-	-	-	-	-	-	<500

Menu Item	Cal	Fat	Sat	Chol	Carb	Fib	Sug	Sod
Tacos, Burritos & Other Mexican (cont'd)								
JACK IN THE BOX								
Taco	170	9	3	20	15	2	2	210
Monster Taco	260	15	5	30	21	3	4	340
Taquitos, 3 pc	320	17	7	40	28	3	1	440
TACO JOHN'S								
Bean Tostada	-	-	-	-	-	-	-	<250
Crispy Taco	-	-	-	-	-	-	-	<250
Tostada	-	-	-	-	-	-	-	<250
Cheese Crisp	-	-	-	-	-	-	-	<250
LA SALSA FRESH MEXICAN GRILL								
Mexico City, Chicken Taco	-	-	-	-	-	-	-	<250
Mexico City, Steak Taco	-	-	-	-	-	-	-	<500
La Salsa, Chicken Taco	-	-	-	-	-	-	-	<500
La Salsa, Steak Taco	-	-	-	-	-	-	-	<500
NOTE: Values do not include chips served with tacos.								
TACO DEL MAR								
Soft Taco, Beef	252	9	-	-	-	-	-	308
Hard Taco, Fish	260	19	-	-	-	-	-	378
Soft Taco, Chicken	250	7	-	-	-	-	-	407
Hard Taco, Chicken	265	18	-	-	-	-	-	408
Hard Taco, Pork	256	17	-	-	-	-	-	436
Soft Taco, Pork	237	6	-	-	-	-	-	450
BAJA FRESH MEXICAN GRILL								
Baja Style, Charbroiled Steak	-	-	-	-	-	-	-	<500
Baja Style, Charbroiled Chicken	-	-	-	-	-	-	-	<500
Baja Style, Wild Gulf Shrimp	-	-	-	-	-	-	-	<500
TACO BELL								
Taco, Regular	-	-	-	-	-	-	-	<500
Taco Supreme	-	-	-	-	-	-	-	<500
Soft Taco, Chicken	-	-	-	-	-	-	-	<750
Soft Taco Supreme, Chicken	-	-	-	-	-	-	-	<750
TACO TIME								
Crisp Bean Burrito	-	-	-	-	-	-	-	<500

(**PIZZA**)

DOMINO'S PIZZA								
Cheese, hand tossed, 12" medium, 1/8 slice	176	6	5	12	28	2	3	388
LITTLE CAESAR'S *(1 slice)*								
Cheese:								
12" or 14" Thin Crust	-	-	-	-	-	-	-	<500
12" Round	-	-	-	-	-	-	-	<500

Menu Item	Cal	Fat	Sat	Chol	Carb	Fib	Sug	Sod
Pizza (cont'd)								
Cheese (cont'd):								
16" Round	-	-	-	-	-	-	-	<500
12" Deep Dish, Square	-	-	-	-	-	-	-	<500
18" Round	-	-	-	-	-	-	-	<500
14" Deep Dish, Square	-	-	-	-	-	-	-	<500
Pepperoni:								
12" Thin Crust	-	-	-	-	-	-	-	<500
14" Thin Crust	-	-	-	-	-	-	-	<500
14" Round	-	-	-	-	-	-	-	<500
16" Round or 12" Deep Dish, Sq	-	-	-	-	-	-	-	<500
Veggie, 14" Round	-	-	-	-	-	-	-	<500
HUNGRY HOWIES PIZZA								
Cheese:								
Small, 1/8 slice	-	-	-	-	-	-	-	<500
Medium, 1/10 slice	-	-	-	-	-	-	-	<500
Large, 1/12 slice	-	-	-	-	-	-	-	<500
PIZZA HUT								
The Chicago Dish:								
Veggie Lover's	-	-	-	-	-	-	-	<500
Pepperoni	-	-	-	-	-	-	-	<500
Pepperoni, Sausage and Mushroom	-	-	-	-	-	-	-	<500
Supreme	-	-	-	-	-	-	-	<500
Stuffed Crust Gold, Super Supreme	-	-	-	-	-	-	-	<500

POTATOES

Menu Item	Cal	Fat	Sat	Chol	Carb	Fib	Sug	Sod
RAX								
Potato, Plain	-	-	-	-	-	-	-	<150
w/Sour Topping	-	-	-	-	-	-	-	<150
w/Butter	-	-	-	-	-	-	-	<150
STEAK ESCAPE								
Smashed Potatoes, Plain	369	0	0	0	786	-	-	18
CARL'S JR.								
Baked Potato, Plain	-	-	-	-	-	-	-	<150
w/Margarine	-	-	-	-	-	-	-	<150
w/Sour Cream and Chives	-	-	-	-	-	-	-	<250
WENDY'S								
Potato, Plain	310	0	0	0	72	7	5	25
w/Sour Cream and Chives	370	6	4	15	73	7	5	40
w/Whipped Margarine, 1 pkt	370	7	2	0	72	6	5	140
ARBY'S								
Baked Potato, Plain	-	-	-	-	-	-	-	<150
Baked Potato w/Butter and Sour Cream	-	-	-	-	-	-	-	<250

Menu Item	Cal	Fat	Sat	Chol	Carb	Fib	Sug	Sod

SALADS

AU BON PAIN *(W/O DRESSING)*

Menu Item	Cal	Fat	Sat	Chol	Carb	Fib	Sug	Sod
Charbroiled Salmon Fillet	210	7	1	50	9	2	5	135
Tomato, Mozzarella w/Basil Pesto	280	19	11	60	11	3	7	180
Mozzarella and Red Pepper	360	25	16	90	10	2	6	380
Garden	160	4	1	0	26	5	6	400
Add salad dressing:								
FF Raspberry	35	0	0	0	8	0	7	80
Caesar	160	16	3	15	3	0	2	220
Lite Olive Oil Vinaigrette	60	6	1	0	3	0	2	230
Lite Honey Mustard	100	6	1	15	11	0	8	240

D'ANGELO *(W/O DRESSING)*

Menu Item	Cal	Fat	Sat	Chol	Carb	Fib	Sug	Sod
Tossed	-	-	-	-	-	-	-	<150
Turkey	-	-	-	-	-	-	-	<150
Roast Beef	-	-	-	-	-	-	-	<250
Add salad dressing:								
Honey Mustard	-	-	-	-	-	-	-	<250

SCHLOTZSKY'S DELI *(W/O DRESSING)*

Menu Item	Cal	Fat	Sat	Chol	Carb	Fib	Sug	Sod
Caesar w/o Croutons	-	-	-	-	-	-	-	<150
Garden w/o Croutons	-	-	-	-	-	-	-	<150
Chinese Chicken w/o Noodles	-	-	-	-	-	-	-	<500
Chicken Caesar w/o Croutons	-	-	-	-	-	-	-	<500
Add salad dressing:								
Olde World Caesar	-	-	-	-	-	-	-	<250
Spicy Rancy	-	-	-	-	-	-	-	<500
Light Spicy Ranch	-	-	-	-	-	-	-	<500

CARL'S JR. *(W/O DRESSING)*

Menu Item	Cal	Fat	Sat	Chol	Carb	Fib	Sug	Sod
Garden Salad-to-Go	-	-	-	-	-	-	-	<150
Add salad dressing:								
Blue Cheese	-	-	-	-	-	-	-	<500

EL POLLO LOCO *(W/O DRESSING)*

Menu Item	Cal	Fat	Sat	Chol	Carb	Fib	Sug	Sod
Garden Salad	-	-	-	-	-	-	-	<150
Add salad dressing:								
Hidden Valley Ranch	-	-	-	-	-	-	-	<250

WENDY'S *(W/O DRESSING)*

Menu Item	Cal	Fat	Sat	Chol	Carb	Fib	Sug	Sod
Spring Mix Salad w/o Pecans	180	11	6	30	12	5	5	230
w/Pecans	310	24	7	30	17	7	8	295
Caesar Side Salad w/o Croutons	70	4	2	15	2	1	1	250
Add salad dressing:								
Homestyle Garlic Croutons	70	3	0	0	9	0	0	120
FF French Dressing	80	0	0	0	19	0	16	210
Caesar Dressing	150	16	3	20	1	0	0	240

211

Menu Item	Cal	Fat	Sat	Chol	Carb	Fib	Sug	Sod
Salads (cont'd)								
KOO-KOO-ROO (w/o DRESSING)								
House Salad	-	-	-	-	-	-	-	<250
Add salad dressing:								
Ranch	-	-	-	-	-	-	-	<250
Caesar	-	-	-	-	-	-	-	<250
ARBY'S (w/o DRESSING)								
Caesar Salad	-	-	-	-	-	-	-	250
Add salad dressing:								
Honey French	-	-	-	-	-	-	-	<500
Light Buttermilk Ranch	-	-	-	-	-	-	-	<500
SUBWAY (w/o DRESSING)								
Veggie Delite Salad	50	1	0	0	9	3	2	310
Add salad dressing:								
FF French, 2 oz	70	0	0	0	17	0	12	390
MCDONALD'S (w/o DRESSING)								
Caesar Salad w/o Chicken	-	-	-	-	-	-	-	<250
Bacon Ranch w/o Chicken	-	-	-	-	-	-	-	<500
California Cobb w/o Chicken	-	-	-	-	-	-	-	<500
Add salad dressing:								
Newman's Own Cobb	-	-	-	-	-	-	-	<500
Newman's Own Creamy Caesar	-	-	-	-	-	-	-	<500

SOUPS & CHILI

Menu Item	Cal	Fat	Sat	Chol	Carb	Fib	Sug	Sod
AU BON PAIN								
Southwest Vegetable	150	3	1	0	23	4	3	250
Southern Black-Eyed Pea	190	1	0	5	34	12	2	400
Mediterranean Pepper	190	4	0	0	30	7	3	450
SOUPLANTATION / SWEET TOMATOES								
Garlic Kickin Roasted Chicken	140	6	3	30	10	3	4	310
Country Corn and Red Potato Chowder	160	6	3	15	24	4	6	330
Cream of Chicken	250	15	6	40	21	2	3	350
Living on the Veg	90	1	0	0	15	3	3	380
RAX								
Chicken Noodle	-	-	-	-	-	-	-	<500
Chili	-	-	-	-	-	-	-	<500
KOO-KOO-ROO								
Chicken Noodle, 5 oz	-	-	-	-	-	-	-	<500
Ten Vegetable, 5 oz	-	-	-	-	-	-	-	<500

Menu Item	Cal	Fat	Sat	Chol	Carb	Fib	Sug	Sod

(BREAKFAST - EGGS, FRENCH TOAST & SANDWICHES)

CARL'S JR.

Menu Item	Cal	Fat	Sat	Chol	Carb	Fib	Sug	Sod
Scrambled Eggs	-	-	-	-	-	-	-	<150
Sourdough Breakfast Sandwich w/o Ham and/or American Cheese	-	-	-	-	-	-	-	<500
Sunrise Sandwich w/o Meat and/or Cheese	-	-	-	-	-	-	-	<500
French Toast Dips w/o Syrup	-	-	-	-	-	-	-	<500
w/Table Syrup, 1 oz	-	-	-	-	-	-	-	<500
w/Grape or Strawberry Jam, 1 serv	-	-	-	-	-	-	-	<500

MCDONALD'S

Menu Item	Cal	Fat	Sat	Chol	Carb	Fib	Sug	Sod
Scrambled Eggs, 2	-	-	-	-	-	-	-	<250
English Muffin w/o margarine	-	-	-	-	-	-	-	<250

KRYSTAL

Menu Item	Cal	Fat	Sat	Chol	Carb	Fib	Sug	Sod
Sunriser Sandwich	240	14	5	255	14	2	1	460

JACK IN THE BOX

Menu Item	Cal	Fat	Sat	Chol	Carb	Fib	Sug	Sod
French Toast Sticks, 4 pc	430	18	4	10	57	2	11	460
w/Grape Jelly, 0.5 oz	465	18	4	10	66	2	20	470
w/Syrup, 1.5 oz	560	18	4	10	89	2	38	490

BURGER KING

Menu Item	Cal	Fat	Sat	Chol	Carb	Fib	Sug	Sod
French Toast Sticks, 5 sticks	-	-	-	-	-	-	-	<500

ARBY'S

Menu Item	Cal	Fat	Sat	Chol	Carb	Fib	Sug	Sod
French Toastix w/Syrup	-	-	-	-	-	-	-	<500

(BAGELS)

BIG APPLE BAGELS

Menu Item	Cal	Fat	Sat	Chol	Carb	Fib	Sug	Sod
Cinnamon Raisin or Vegetable	-	-	-	-	-	-	-	<500
Plain or Eight Grain	-	-	-	-	-	-	-	<500
Whole Wheat	-	-	-	-	-	-	-	<500

MANHATTAN BAGEL

Menu Item	Cal	Fat	Sat	Chol	Carb	Fib	Sug	Sod
Jalapeño Cheddar	-	-	-	-	-	-	-	<500
Sun-Dried Tomato	-	-	-	-	-	-	-	<500

(DOUGHNUTS)

KRISPY KREME DOUGHNUTS

Yeast Doughnuts:

Menu Item	Cal	Fat	Sat	Chol	Carb	Fib	Sug	Sod
Glazed Twist	210	9	3	5	28	1	16	80
Cinnamon Twist	230	9	3	5	33	1	19	85
Sugar	200	12	3	5	21	0	10	95
Glazed Ring	200	12	3	5	22	1	10	95
Choc Iced Glazed Ring	250	12	3	5	33	1	21	100
Choc Iced Glazed Ring w/Sprinkles	260	12	3	5	36	1	23	100

Menu Item	Cal	Fat	Sat	Chol	Carb	Fib	Sug	Sod
Doughnuts (cont'd)								
Glazed Cinnamon	210	12	3	5	24	1	12	100
Maple Iced Glazed Ring	250	12	3	5	34	1	22	100
Cinnamon Bun	260	16	4	5	28	1	13	125
Cranapple Crunch Filled	330	18	5	5	38	1	20	140
Filled Doughnuts:								
Yeast, Powdered Raspberry Filled	300	16	4	5	36	1	17	125
Glazed Creme Filled	350	20	5	5	39	1	24	135
Yeast, Glazed Lemon Filled	290	16	4	5	34	1	18	135
Yeast, Vanilla Iced Custard Filled	290	16	4	5	33	1	16	150
DUNKIN' DONUTS								
Lemon Glazed Cake	-	-	-	-	-	-	-	<150
Sugar Raised	-	-	-	-	-	-	-	<250
Glazed	-	-	-	-	-	-	-	<250
Vanilla Kreme Filled	-	-	-	-	-	-	-	<250

MUFFINS, ROLLS & DANISHES

CHICK-FIL-A								
Danish	430	17	5	25	63	2	16	160
MY FAVORITE MUFFIN								
Plain	-	-	-	-	-	-	-	<250
FF	-	-	-	-	-	-	-	<250
Chocolate	-	-	-	-	-	-	-	<250

RESOURCES

DASH DIET

NHLBI Health Information Center (Publication #01-4082)
P.O. Box 30105
Bethesda, MD 20824-0105
301.592.8573 or 240.629.3255 (TTY)
www.nhlbi.nih.gov

ONLINE PRODUCTS FROM MANUFACTURERS

Alvarado Street Bakery
500 Martin Ave.
Rohnert Park, CA 94928
707.585.3293
www.alvaradostreetbakery.com

Annie's Naturals
792 Foster Hill Rd.
North Calais, VT 05650
800.434.1234 or 802.456.8866
www.anniesnaturals.com

Authentic Foods
1850 W. 169th St., Suite B
Gardena, CA 90247
800.806.4737 or 310.366.7612
www.glutenfree-supermarket.com

Barbara's Bakery
707.765.2273
www.barbarasbakery.com

'Cause You're Special
P.O. Box 316
Phillips, WI 54555
866.669.4328 or 715.339.6959
www.causeyourespecial.com

Drew's Salad Dressings
926 Vermont Route 103
Chester, Vermont 05143
800-228-2980
www.chefdrew.com

Eden Foods, Inc.
701 Tecumseh Rd.
Clinton, MI 49236
888.424.EDEN
www.edenfoods.com

Ener-G Foods
5960 First Ave. So.
Seattle, WA 98001
800.331.5222 or 206.870.4740
www.ener-g.com

French Meadow Bakery
2610 Lyndale Ave. So.
Minneapolis, MN 55408
877.NO.YEAST or 612.870.4740
www.frenchmeadow.com

Garden of Eatin'
800.434.4246
www.gardenofeatin.com

Ginny's Vegan Foods
102 Chipman Park
Middlebury, VT 05753
888.59.EARTH
www.ginnysveganfoods.com

Gloria's Gourmet Foods
425 2nd St. Alley
Lake Oswego, OR 97034
800.782.5881 or 802.388.6581
www.gloriasgourmet.com

215

RESOURCES

Grey Owl Foods
www.greyowlfoods.com

HolGrain c/o Conrad Rice Mill Inc.
P.O. Box 10640
New Iberia, LA 70562
800.551.3245 or 337.364.7242
www.holgrain.com

The Lollipop Tree, Inc.
www.lollipoptree.com

Med-Diet Labs, Inc.
800.MED.DIET
www.med-diet.com

Melissa's
P.O. 21127
Los Angeles, CA 90021
800.588.0151
www.melissas.com

Montana Mills Bread Co.
2171 Monroe Ave., #205A
Rochester, NY 14618
877.MMBREAD
www.montanamills.com

Mozzarella Company
800.798.2954 or 214.741.4072
www.mozzco.com

Mr. Spice c/o Lang Naturals
850 Aquidneck Ave.
Newport, RI 02842
800.SAUCE.IT or 401.848.7700
www.mrspice.com

Natural Ovens Bakery
P.O. Box 730
Manitowoc, WI 54221-0730
800.772.0730
www.naturalovens.com

Nu-World Foods
P.O. Box 2202
Naperville, IL 60567
630.369.6851
www.nuworldfoods.com

Pacific Bakery
P.O. Box 950
Oceanside, CA 92049
www.pacificbakery.com

Papa Cheese Country Store
715.669.7620
www.papacheese.com

Rising Sun Farms
5126 So. Pacific Hwy.
Phoenix, OR 97535-6606
800.888.0795 X-211
www.risingsunfarms.com

Roberts American Gourmet
P.O. Box 326
Sea Cliff, NY 11579
800.626.7557 or 516.656.4545
www.robscape.com

Seneca Foods
3736 S. Main St.
Marion, NY 14505
315.926.8100
www.senecafoods.com

Tasty Baking Co. (Tastykake)
2801 Hunting Park Ave.
Philadelphia, PA 19129
800.33-TASTY
www.tastykake.com

Uncle Dave's Kitchen
www.vermontfinest.com

Wax Orchards Inc.
22744 Wax Orchards Rd. SW
Vashon Island, WA 98070
800. 634.6132
www.waxorchards.com

Wolferman's
PO Box 15913
Shawnee Mission, KS 66285-5913
800.999.0169
www.wolfermans.com

(ONLINE GROCERY STORES WITH LOW-SODIUM PRODUCTS)

Atkins Nutritionals
www.atkins.com
Carries Atkins, Carbolite, Fran Gare's, Genisoy, Keto and Steel's

The Better Health Store
305 N. Clippert
Lansing, MI 48912
877.876.8247
www.thebetterhealthstore.com
Carries Amy's Kitchen, Annie's Homegrown, Arrowhead Mills, Atkins, Barbara's Bakery, Bearitos, Bob's Red Mill, Breadshop, Carbolite, Carbsense, Cascadian Farm, Clif, Eden Foods, Ener-G, Enrico's, Erewhon, Garden of Eatin, Guiltless Gourmet, Hain, Health Valley, Keto, Low Carb Success, Muir Glen, Nature's Path, Terra Chips, Tree of Life, Westbrae Natural and more

eDiet Shop
P.O. Box 1037
Evanston, IL 60204-1397
800.325.5409 or 847.679.5409
www.edietshop.com
Carries Bagel Buddy, Baja Bob, Bernard, Calorie Control, Joseph's, Longhorn Grill, San Sucre, Spice Up Your Life, Steel's, Sweet N' Low, To Market To Market

eFood Pantry
2520 S. Grand Ave. East
Springfield, IL 62703
800.238.8090
www.efoodpantry.com
Carries Aunt Patsy's, Erewhon, Featherweight, Fifty/50, Just Delicious, Kavli, Magic Seasonings, Pritikin, Robbie's, Rustler's, Sans Sucre, Steel's, Sweet'N Low and more

F3 Fat Free Foods
770 Second Ave. (41st)
New York, NY 10017
212.972.0191
www.fatfreefoods.com
Carries Alvarado St Bakery, American Spoon, Aunt Gussie's, Bake Boy, Barbara's Bakery, Bobby Flay, Bon Appetito, BP Gourmet, Brad's, Busha Browne, Cary Randall, Casa Visco, Cathy's, Chef Allen, Dimitria Delights, Fischer & Wieser, Floribbean, Food for Life, Fox's Fine Foods, Frieda's Kitchen, Golden Star, Heavenly Desserts, Irene's, Miss Meringue, Muffin Delight, Nantucket Offshore, Natural Exotic, Nature's Path, No Pudge, Nutritious Creations, Olde Cape Cod, The Original, Our Daily Muffin, Pantry Shelf, Peanut Wonder, Prairie Thyme, Private Harvest, Royal, Scotto's, Toufayan, Tree of Life, Wholesome Classics, Wild Thyme and more

www.glutenfreemall.com
Carries Authentic Foods, 'Cause You're Special, Creme De La Creme, Glutano, Mr. Spice, Nu-World Foods, Tartex and more

The Gluten-Free Pantry
P.O. Box 840
Glastonbury, CT 06033
800.291.8386
www.glutenfree.com
Carries Bumble Bar, Ener-G, Glenny's, Glutano, Gluten-Free Pantry, Omega Smart, Orgran

Healthy Heart Market
800.753.0310
www.healthyheartmarket.com
4C, Bearitos, Bernard, Breadshop, Consorzio, Eden, Ener-G, Enrico's, Featherweight, Frog Ranch, Frontier, Garden of Eatin, Gloria's, Hain, Minnesota Wild, Mr. Spice, Muir Glen, New Traditions, Sheila's Select, Sweet 'N Low, Vonn's and more

RESOURCES

www.kosherkingdomonline.com
Carries Empire, Frankel, J&J, Kemach, Kineret, Manischewitz, Oronoque, Osem, Rokeach, Season, Tabachnick, Tuv Taam and more

Low Carb Living, Inc.
1465 Encinitas Blvd., Suite H
Encinitas, CA 92024
888.569.2272 or 760.634.5316
www.lowcarbliving.com
Carries Atkins, Baja Bob, Bran-a-Crisp, Carbolite, Carbsense, Cheeters, Heavenly Desserts, Keto, Low Carbolicious, LowCarb Success, Steel's, Walden Farms and more

www.lowcarboutfitters.com
Carries Atkins, Carbolite, Carbsense, Heavenly Desserts, Jok 'N Al, Keto, Steel's, Walden Farms

www.mykoshermarket.com
Carries A&M, Billy Bee, Empire Kosher, Gefen, Goodman's, Hain, J&J, Kineret, Mikee, Miko, Osem, Ratner's, Rokeach, Season, Streit, Tabatchnick and more

www.mothernature.com
Carries Atkins, Eden, Ener-G, Genisoy, Golden Temple, Nature's Path, Spice Hunter and more

www.netgrocer.com
Online grocer carrying many low-sodium products

www.peapod.com
Online market carrying many low-sodium foods

www.shopnatural.com
Carries Amy's, Annie's Homegrown, Arrowhead Mills, Atkins, Barbara's Bakery, Breadshop, Cascadian Farm, Deb-El, Drew's, Eden, Enrico's, Garden of Eatin, Genisoy, Glenny's, Golden Temple, Hain, Heaven Sent, Lundberg, Melissa's, Nature's Path, Pamela's, Westbrae and more

Strictly Natural, Inc.
31 Seabreeze Ave.
Thornhill, ON L4J 8R6 Canada
877.771.1230 or 905.771.0095
www.strictlynatural.com
Carries Annie's Homegrown, Cascadian Farm, Eden, Erewhon, Lifestream, Mr. Spice, Nature's Path, Tree of Life, Westbrae and more

www.sugarfreemarket.com
6710 N. University Dr.
Tamarac, FL 33321
800.726.6191 or 954.726.9747
www.sugarfreemarket.com
Carries Arrowhead Mills, Atkins, Cheeters, Drews, Estee, Fifty/50, Grainfields, Health Valley, Joseph's, Koslowski Farms, Murray, Millina's Finest, Sans Sucre, Sorbee, Steel's, Sweet'N Low, Walden Farms and more

www.sugarlessshop.com
Carries Bernard, Calorie Control, Estee, Joseph's, Steel's, Sweet'N Low, Wax Orchards, Westbrae Naturals and more

www.synergydiet.com
Carries Adios Carbs, Atkins, Baja Bob's, Better Bakery, Carbolite, Carbsense, Cheeters, Fran Gare's, Grainfield's, Keto, LowCarb Success, Jok 'n'Al, Murray, Sans Sucre, Steel's, Walden Farms and more

www.truefoodsonline.com
Carries Annie's Naturals, Barbara's Bakery, Bearitos, Breadshop, Eden, Food for Life, French Meadow, Garden of Eatin, Pamela's and more

WorldPantry.com, Inc.
1024 Illinois St.
San Francisco, CA 94107
866.972.6879 or 415.581.0067
www.worldpantry.com
Carries Annie Chun's, Bette's Diner, Heaven & Earth, Neera's, Prairie Thyme, Upper Crust and more

INDEX

A

Albacore, 117
Alcoholic Beverages, 12
Alfredo sauce, 51
Almond paste, 3
Anchovy Paste, 115
Anchovies, 115
Appetizers & Snacks, 92
Asian foods, 107
Asian meals, 94
Aspartame, 11

B

Bacon, 123
Bacon bits, 47
Bagels, 21
Baking Chocolate & Chips, 3
Baking Mixes, 3
Baking powder, 7
Baking soda, 7
Bamboo shoots, 110
Barbecue sauce, 37
Batter, Seasoning & Coating Mixes, 3
BBQ sauce, 37
Bean sauce, 108
Bean sprouts, 110
Beans & Legumes, 147-150
Bearnaise sauce, 39
Beef, Lamb & Veal, 124
Beer, 12
Biscotti, 74
Biscuits, 21
Blintzes & Crepes, 92
Bouillon, Broths & Bases, 143
Bran, 132
Bread, 22
Bread Dough & Mixes, 25
Breadcrumbs, Cracker & Sweet Crumbs, 4

Breadsticks, 26
Breakfast bars, 31
Breakfast Drinks, 31
Breakfast Meals, 93
Breakfast meat alternatives, 123
Breakfast Meals, 123
Broths, 143
Brownies & Dessert Bars, 64
Browning & seasoning sauce, 49
Buffalo (Bison), 126
Buns, Rolls & Croissants, 27
Burgers & patties, 119, 125, 128
Butter, Margarine & Spreads, 55
Butter substitutes, 55
Buttermilk, 7, 61

C

Cake mixes, 65
Cake decorations, 7
Cake frosting, 6
Cakes, 65
Canadian bacon, 123
Candy, 67
Capers, 38
Caramel corn, 141
Carob powder, 16
Catsup (ketchup), 38
Caviar, 115
Cereal, 33
Cereal, Granola & Breakfast Bars, 31
Cheese, 55
Cheese - Cottage, 58
Cheese - Ricotta, 59
Cheese alternatives, 58
Cheesecakes, 66
Cheese sauce, 50, 113
Chewing gum, 68
Chicken & Turkey, 125
Chili, 144

219

Chili/garlic sauce, 108
Chili peppers, 111
Chili sauce, 113
Chips & Nibblers, 134
Chinese food products, 107
Chocolate, 3
Chocolate chips, 3
Chocolate drinks, 15
Chocolate milk, 61
Chocolate syrup, 16
Chow mein noodles, 107
Chutneys & Fruit Relishes, 43
Clam Juice, 115
Clam sauce, 50
Clams, 115, 118
Coating mixes, 3
Cocktail Mixers, 12
Cocktail sauce, 48
Cocoa - Hot Chocolate, 3, 15
Coconut, 4
Coffee, 13
Coffee Flavored Drinks, 13
Coffeecakes, 81
Coffee Creamers & Flavorings, 13
Coffee Substitutes, 14
Condensed milk, 7
Cookie mixes, 69
Cookies, 68
Cooking wine, 12
Corn chips, 134
Corn syrup, 11
Cornbread, 25, 29
Cornmeal, 5
Cornstarch, 5
Cottage cheese, 59
Crab, 115, 118
Crackermeal, 4
Crackers, 136
Cranberry sauce/relish, 43
Cream, 59
Cream - Sour, 60
*Cream Cheese & Alternative
   Spreads*, 60

Cream cheese alternatives, 60
Cream Cheese Spreads, 60
Cream of tartar, 7
Creamers, 13
Crepes, 92
Crispbread, 137
Croissants, 27
Croutons, 46
Crumbs & breading, 4
Curry sauce, 48

D
Deer, 126
Deli salads, 105
Dessert bars, 65
Dessert breads, 26
Diet & Nutritional Drinks, 88
Diet, Energy & Nutritional Bars, 89
Dinner Mixes & Helpers, 99
Dinners & Entrees, 94-98
Dips, 139
Doughnuts, 74
Dressing, 46, 105
Dried fruit, 120
Dried vegetables, 154
Drink mixes, 13, 15
Duck, 126

E
Egg rolls, 92
Egg roll wrappers, 110
Eggs & Egg Substitutes, 61
Eggs - Dried/Powder, 5
Eggnog, 61
Elk, 126
Enchilada sauce, 113
Energy bars, 89
Energy drinks, 18
English Muffins, 28
Entree substitutes, 129
Entrees, 94, 125, 128
Evaporated milk, 7
Extracts, 5

F

Fats, Oils & Cooking Sprays, 5
Fat Substitutes, 5
Fillo (phyllo) dough, 8
Fish & Seafood, 115
Fish & seafood meals, 94, 118
Fish & Seafood Substitutes, 119
Fish burgers & patties, 119
Flavored drinks, 61
Flavored milk, 15
Flavorings & Extracts, 5
Flour, 6
Fortune cookies, 107
Frankfurters, 127, 130
French Toast, 35, 93
Fried Rice, 107
Frosting, Icing & Decorations, 6
Frozen dough, 8
Frozen Desserts, 75
Frozen dinners, 94
Frozen yogurt, 76
Fructose, 11
Fruit, 120-122
Fruit Fillings, 9
*Fruit Juice & Fruit-Flavored
  Drinks*, 15
Fruit relishes, 43
Fruit spreads, 38
Fruit sweetener, 11

G

Game Meat, 126
Garlic sauce, 108
Gefilte fish, 116
Gelatin, 83
Gelato, 76
Goat milk, 7, 61
Goose, 126
Gourmet sauce, 50
Granola bars, 31
Graham crackers, 137
Grain side dishes, 104
Grains, 132
Gravy, 50

Green chilis, 111
Grilling sauce, 47
Guacamole, 139
Gum, 68

H

Ham & Pork, 126
Hamburger mix, 83
Hard sauce, 50
Hawaiian foods, 110
Herbs & spices, 10
Herring & kipper snacks, 116
Hispanic foods, 111
Hispanic meals, 95
Hoisin sauce, 108
Hollandaise sauce, 50
Honey, 11
Horseradish, 38
Hot sauce, 51, 113
*Hot Dogs, Frankfurters &
  Sausages*, 127, 130

I

Ice cream alternatives, 80
Ice cream bars, pops &
  sandwiches, 79
Ice Cream, Ices & Frozen Yogurt, 75
Ice Cream Cones & Toppings, 80
Icing & decorations, 7
Instant breakfast, 31
International meals, 96

J

Jams, Jellies & Fruit Spreads, 38
Japanese noodles, 107
Jellies & preserves, 38
Jerky & Meat Snacks, 140
Juices & juice concentrate, 15

K

Ketchup, 38
Kim chee, 107
Kipper snacks, 116
Knishes, 104

L

Lamb, 124
Leavening Agents, 7
Liquor & spirits, 12
Lunch Packs, 99
Luncheon, Deli & Sandwich Meats, 127
Luncheon & sandwich meat substitutes, 130

M

MSG, 10
Macaroni & cheese, 94, 97, 98, 99
Malted milk, 16
Maraschino Cherries, 39
Margarine & spreads, 55
Marinades, 47
Marshmallows, 7
Matzos & tam tams, 138
Mayonnaise & Sandwich Spreads, 39
Meat & poultry meals, 96, 125
Meat & poultry substitutes, 123, 129
Meat snacks, 140
Meat tenderizer, 10
Melba toast, 138
Mexican foods, 111
Milk-Based Drinks & Additives, 15
Milk - Canned/Powdered, 7
Milk Products & Non-Dairy Alternatives, 61
Milk shake, 15
Milk substitutes, 7, 62
Mineral water, 20
Mint sauce, 51
Molasses, 11
Mole, 113
Muffins & Scones, 29
Mussels, 116, 118
Mustard, 40

N

Neufchatel, 60
Nibblers, 135

Non-dairy alternatives, 62, 63, 80
Non-Meat Substitutes, 129
Noodles, Asian, 107
Noodles, 132
Nut Butters, 40
Nutritional bars, 89
Nutritional drinks, 88
Nuts & Seeds, 140
Nuts - Baking, 8

O

Oils & shortenings, 5
Olives, 41
Oyster crackers, 138
Oyster sauce, 108
Oysters, 116, 118

P

Packaged meats, 127
Pancake & Waffle Syrup, 36
Pancakes & Waffles, 35, 98
Pasta & Noodles, 132
Pasta meals & entrees, 97, 100
Pasta sauce, 51
Pastries & Coffeecakes, 81
Pastry Fillings, 8
Pastry Dough, 8
Patés & Spreads, 41
Peanut bars, 141
Peanut butter, 40
Peanut sauce, 108
Peppers, 42, 111
Pesto sauce, 53
Phyllo dough, 8
Pickle relish, 43
Pickled Vegetables, 42
Pickles, 42
Pie Fillings, 9
Pie Crusts, 9
Pierogies, 103
Pies & Cobblers, 82
Pies - snack, 86
Pimiento, 43
Pita & Pocket Breads, 30

Pizza, 101
Pizza Crust & Dough, 102
Pizza sauce, 53
Plum pudding, 84
Plum sauce, 109
Pocket bread, 30
Pockets, Sandwiches, & Wraps, 103
Polenta, 104
Popcorn, 141
Popcorn and rice cakes, 142
Pork, 126
Pork sausage, 123
Potato chips, 136
Potato dishes, 104
Potato salad, 105
Potatoes, 104, 152, 156
Poultry, 125
Poultry meals, 96
Powdered drink mix, 15
Powdered milk, 7
Preserves, 38
Pretzels, 141
Puddings & Gelatins, 83
Puff pastry, 8
Pumpkin pie filling, 10

Q
Quiches, pies & souffles, 98

R
Refried beans, 111
Relishes, 43
Rice & grains, 132
Rice beverages, 61
Rice cakes, 142
Rice crackers, 138
Rice & Rice Dishes, 107, 132
Rice milk, 62
Rice pudding, 85
Rice syrup, 11
Ricotta cheese, 59
Rolls, 27

S
Saccharin, 11
Salad dressing (mayo-type), 39
Salad Dressings & Toppings, 46
Salads, 105
Salmon, 116
Salsas, 112
Salt, 9
Salt Substitutes, 9
Saltines, 138
Sandwich buns, 27
Sandwich crackers, 139
Sandwich meats, 127
Sandwich spreads, 39, 41, 131
Sandwiches, 103
Sardines, 116
Sauces, 47-54
Sauces & Toppings (Desserts), 85
Sausage, 123, 127
Scones, 30
Seasoning & Coating Mixes, 3
Seasoning mixes, 3, 113, 144
Seasonings, 10
Seaweed, 91
Seeds, 140
Seltzer, 20
Sherbet & sorbet, 79
Side Dishes, 104
Sloppy Joe sauce, 53
Snack Cakes, Pies & Sweet Snacks, 86
Snacks, 134
Sodas/soft drinks, 16
Sorbet, 79
Souffles, 98
Soup bases & mixes, 143
Soups & Stews, 145
Sour cream, 60
Sour cream alternatives, 60
Soy beverages, 19, 61
Soy milk, 61
Soy sauce, 109
Spaghetti & pasta, 96, 98, 99

Spaghetti sauce, 51
Spices & seasonings, 10
Sports & Energy Drinks, 18
Spreads, 39, 41, 131
Sprinkles, 7
Steak sauce, 53
Stews, 145
Stir-fry sauce, 109
Stir-fry vegetables, 110,
Stuffing & dressing, 105
Sucralose, 11
Sugar, 11
Sugar substitutes, 11
Sweet & sour sauce, 109
Sweet crumbs, 4
Sweet rolls, 81
Sweeteners, 11
Syrup, chocolate, 16
Syrup, pancake/waffle, 36

T

Taco sauce, 112
Taco shells, 114
Tahini, 40
Tam Tams, 138
Tapioca, 85
Tartar sauce, 53
Tea, 19
Tempeh, 130
Tempura batter, 3
Teriyaki sauce, 110
Toaster Foods & Pastries, 37
Tofu, 131
Tofu ice cream, 80
Tofu mixes, 99
Tofu yogurt, 63
Tomatillos, 113
Tomato, 153, 155
Tomato juice, 19
Tomato sauce/puree, 153
Tonic, 20
Toppings - salad, 46

Toppings - ice cream, 81, 85
Tortilla chips, 134
Tortillas & taco shells, 114
Trail mix, 140
Tuna, 117
Tuna mix, 98
Turkey, 125

V

Veal, 124
Vegetable chips, 134
Vegetable dishes, 106
Vegetable Juices, 19
Vegetable relishes, 44
Vegetables, 150-156
Vegetarian meat dishes, 97
Vinegar, 54

W

Waffles, 35, 98
Water, 20
Wheat Germ, 91
Whipped Toppings, 62
Whipping cream, 59
Whiskey, 12
White sauce, 54
Wine, 12
Wonton wrappers, 110
Worcestershire sauce, 54

Y

Yeast, 7
Yogurt, 62
Yogurt, tofu, 63
Yogurt (frozen), 76

InData Group, Inc.
P.O. Box 11908
Olympia, WA 98508-1908
360.432.7844 (tel)
800.897.8440 (toll free)
360.432.7838 (fax)

Pocket Guide to Low Sodium Foods is available from your local bookstore and online book retailers. To order books directly from the publisher:

Internet orders: www.lowsaltfoods.com

Fax orders: 360.432.7838 (send this form)

Telephone orders: 800.897.8440 (credit card orders)

Mail orders: InData Group, Inc.
P.O. Box 11908
Olympia, WA 98508-1908, USA
(send this form)

Please send me:

____autographed copies of *Pocket Guide to Low Sodium Foods* at $7.95 each.   _____

Sales tax: Washington residents, please add 8.3%   _____

Shipping: U.S.(Priority) - $4.00 for first book and $2.00 for each additional book. International - $9.00 for first book and $5.00 for each additional book.   _____

TOTAL   _____

Credit Card ___VISA ___MasterCard   Exp. Date _____

Credit Card # _____

Name _____

Address_____

City _____State_____ Zip_____